Clinical Examination of Farm Animals

BY

Peter G.G. Jackson
BVM&S, MA, DVM&S, FRCVS
University of Cambridge UK

&

Peter D. Cockcroft
MA, VetMB, MSc, DCHP, DVM&S, MRCVS,
University of Cambridge UK

Illustrations by
Samantha Elmhurst, BA Hons & Mike Pearson

T0312196

Blackwell
Science

© 2002 by Blackwell Science Ltd,
a Blackwell Publishing Company
Editorial Offices:
Osney Mead, Oxford OX2 0EL, UK
    Tel: +44 (0)1865 206206
Blackwell Science, Inc., 350 Main Street,
Malden, MA 02148-5018, USA
    Tel: +1 781 388 8250
Iowa State Press, a Blackwell Publishing
Company, 2121 State Avenue, Ames, Iowa
50014-8300, USA
    Tel: +1 515 292 0140
Blackwell Science Asia Pty, 54 University
Street, Carlton, Victoria 3053, Australia
    Tel: +61 (0)3 9347 0300
Blackwell Wissenschafts Verlag,
Kurfürstendamm 57, 10707 Berlin, Germany
    Tel: +49 (0)30 32 79 060

The right of the Author to be identified as the
Author of this Work has been asserted in
accordance with the Copyright, Designs and
Patents Act 1988.

First published 2002 by Blackwell Science Ltd

Library of Congress
Cataloging-in-Publication Data
Jackson, Peter G. G.
    Clinical examination of farm animals / by Peter G.G. Jackson
    & Peter D. Cockcroft.
        p.   cm.
    Includes bibliographical references (p.   ).
    ISBN 0-632-05706-8
    1. Veterinary medicine—Diagnosis.   I. Cockcroft,
    Peter D.   II. Title.
SF771 .J23 2002
636.089'6075—dc21
                                                2002023213

ISBN 0-632-05706-8

A catalogue record for this title is available
from the British Library

Set in 9/12 Palatino
by SNP Best-set Typesetter Ltd., Hong Kong

For further information on
Blackwell Science, visit our website:
www.blackwell-science.com

Contents

This book is dedicated to our families

Preface

More mistakes are made by not looking than by not knowing.

Anon.

Clinical examination is a fundamental part of the process of veterinary diagnosis. It provides the veterinarian with the information required to determine the disease or diseases producing the clinical abnormalities. In addition, the information derived from the clinical examination should assist the veterinarian in determining the severity of the pathophysiological processes present. Without a proficient clinical examination and an accurate diagnosis it is unlikely that the treatment, control, prognosis and welfare of animals will be optimised.

The purpose of this book is to assist clinicians in performing a detailed clinical examination of the individual animal and to increase the awareness of more advanced techniques used in further investigations. The structure and content of the book should assist veterinary students in their understanding of farm animal clinical examination, act as a quick reference for clinicians who are called upon to examine an unfamiliar species and provide a more detailed account for experienced clinicians in their continuing professional development.

In this book the authors have attempted to describe and illustrate the ways in which clinical examination of farm animal species can be performed. Throughout the book conditions are used to illustrate the predisposing risk factors and the clinical abnormalities that may be present. In doing so the authors have tried to provide information that may assist the reader in formulating differential diagnoses. Numerous illustrations are provided to complement the text.

In the first part of the book the principles of clinical examination are described. The second and largest part of the book is devoted to the clinical examination of cattle. Following a chapter on the general examination of cattle, each body system or region has a chapter in which the applied anatomy is briefly reviewed and the clinical examination is described in detail. Within each of these chapters there are checklists on how to perform the examination and what abnormalities may be present. Further parts of the book are devoted to the clinical examination of sheep, goats and pigs. Where the examination of the ovine, caprine or porcine body system is similar to the bovine, the reader is referred back to the appropriate cattle chapter.

The book is largely based on the experience of the authors as practitioners, as consultants in referral clinics and as teachers of clinical veterinary students. The authors hope that the reader will find this book both interesting and useful.

Acknowledgements

The authors would like to thank the graphic artists for the illustrations in this book. The pictures in Chapters 5 and 6 were drawn by Mike Pearson. The front cover and the other pictures in the book were drawn by Samantha Elmhurst. The authors would also like to acknowledge Antonia Seymour of Blackwell Publishing for her support and guidance during the writing of this book.

Part I

Introduction

Principles of Clinical Examination

Introduction

The purpose of the clinical examination is to identify the clinical abnormalities that are present and the risk factors that determine the occurrence of the disease in the individual or population. From this information the most likely cause can be determined. In addition, the organs or systems involved, the location, type of lesion present, the pathophysiological processes occurring and the severity of the disease can be deduced from the information gained during the clinical examination. Without a proficient clinical examination and an accurate diagnosis it is unlikely that the control, prognosis and welfare of animals will be optimised.

There are several different approaches to the clinical examination. The *complete clinical examination* consists of checking for the presence or absence of all the clinical abnormalities and predisposing disease risk factors. From this information a ranked list of differential diagnoses is deduced. This is a fail-safe method and ensures no abnormality or risk factor is missed.

The problem orientated method (hypothetico-deductive method) combines clinical examination and differential diagnosis. The sequence of the clinical investigation is dictated by the differential diagnoses generated from the previous findings. This results in a limited but very focused examination. The success of the method relies heavily on the knowledge of the clinician and usually assumes a single condition is responsible for the abnormalities.

Many clinicians begin their examination by performing a *general examination* which includes a broad search for abnormalities. The *system or region* involved is identified and is then examined in greater detail using either a complete or a problem orientated examination.

The clinical examination

The clinical examination ideally proceeds through a number of steps (Table 1.1). The owner's complaint, the history of the patient, the history of the farm and the signalment of the patient are usually established at the same time by interview with the owner or keeper of the animal. Observations of the patient and environment are performed next. Finally a clinical examination of the patient occurs, followed by additional investigations if required.

Owner's complaint

This information usually indentifies which individuals and groups of animals are affected. It may also indicate the urgency of the problem. The owner may include the history of the patient and the signalment in the complaint. Stockpersons usually know their animals in detail, and reported subtle changes in behaviour should not be dismissed. However, opinions expressed regarding the aetiology should be viewed with caution as these can be misleading. The extent of the problem or the exact nature of the problem may not be appreciated by the owner, and the clinician should attempt to maintain an objective view.

Signalment of the patient

Signalment includes the identification number, breed, age, sex, colour and production class of animal. Some diseases are specific to some of these groupings and this knowledge can be useful in reducing the diseases that need to be considered.

Table 1.1 The clinical examination

Owner's complaint
Signalment of the patient
History of the patient(s)
History of the farm
Observation of the environment
Observation of the animal at a distance
Detailed observations of the animal
Examination of the animal
Further investigations

History of the patient(s)

Disease information
Disease information should include the group(s) affected, the numbers of animal affected (morbidity) and the identities of the animals affected; the number of animals that have died (mortality) should be established. Information regarding the course of the disease should be obtained including the signs observed.

Risk factors
Possible predisposing risk factors should be identified. These may include the origin of the stock, current disease control programmes (vaccination, anthelmintic programmes, biosecurity) and nutrition.

Response to treatment
Clinical improvement following treatment may support a tentative diagnosis.

History of the farm

The disease history of the farm will indicate diseases that should be considered carefully and may indicate some of the local disease risk factors operating. The sources of information may include farm records, practice records, colleagues and the owner. Husbandry standards, production records, biosecurity protocols, vaccination and anthelmintic programmes may all be relevant.

Observation of the environment

The environment in which the animals were kept at the time of the onset or just before the onset of the illness should be carefully examined. The animals may be housed or outside. Risk factors outdoors may include the presence of toxic material, grazing management, biosecurity and regional mineral deficiencies. Risk factors indoors may include ventilation, humidity, dust, stocking density, temperature, lighting, bedding, water availability, feeding facilities and fitments.

Observation of the animal at a distance

Ideally this procedure should be performed with the patient in its normal environment. This enables its behaviour and activities to be monitored without restraint or excitement. These can be compared with those of other member of the group and relative to accepted normal patterns. However, sick animals have often been separated from their group and assembled in collecting yards or holding pens awaiting examination. Observations are most frequently made in this situation; they may include feeding, eating, urinating, defaecation, interactions between group members and responses to external stimuli. The patient can be made to rise and walk. The posture, contours and gait can be assessed, and gross clinical abnormalities detected.

Useful information is often derived from these observations and this stage in the clinical examination should not be hurried.

Detailed observations of the animal

Detailed observations can be made in docile animals without restraint; however, restraint may be necessary to facilitate this procedure. Closer observation of the patient may detect smaller and more subtle abnormalities.

Examination of the animal

Restraint is usually necessary for the examination and to ensure the safety of the animal and clinician.

Table 1.2 Examination by topographical region

Region	Common sequences used		
	Head to tail	Tail to head	Tail to tail
Head and neck	1	5	3
Left thorax and abdomen	2	4	2
Right thorax and abdomen	3	3	4
Tail end	4	1	1
Vaginal examination	5	6	5
(Rectal examination)	6	7	6
(Udder/Male: external genitalia)	7	2	7

The clinical examination usually proceeds topographically around the animal, with clinicians starting at different points dependent upon personal preference. Each topographical area may encompass several components of the different body systems and these are examined concurrently (Table 1.2). Frequently the topographical approach is used to identify major clinical abnormalities which are then examined in a more detailed manner using a systems approach.

Further investigations

Further investigations may be required before a diagnosis can be made. These may include laboratory tests, post-mortem examination, and a wide range of advanced techniques. Careful consideration should be given to the additional cost and what additional diagnostic or prognostic information will be gained from the additional procedures.

Techniques used during a physical examination

Palpation (touching)

Changes in shape, size, consistency, position, temperature and sensitivity to touch (pain response) can be assessed by palpation.

Auscultation (listening)

Changes in the frequency, rhythm and intensity of normal sounds can be detected. Abnormal sounds can be identified. Stethoscopes are often used to increase the acuity.

Percussion (tapping)

The resonance of an object can be determined by the vibrations produced within it by the application of a sharp force. The sound produced provides information regarding the shape, size and density of the object.

Manipulation (moving)

Manipulation of a structure indicates the resistance and the range of movements possible. Abnormal sounds may be produced, and the pain produced in response to the movement can be assessed.

Ballottement (rebound)

This is performed by pushing the body wall sharply and forcefully so that internal structures are first propelled against the body wall then on recoil rebound against the operator's fingers. This enables the presence or character of an internal structure to be assessed.

Succussion (shaking)

Succussion is performed to determine the fluid content of a viscus. The shaking induces the fluid inside the viscus to produce an audible sloshing sound which can be detected by auscultation.

Visual inspection

This is used to identify abnormalities of conformation, gait, contour and posture. Visual appraisal may help determine the size and character of a lesion.

Olfactory inspection

This is used to identify and characterise abnormal smells which may be associated with disease.

CHAPTER 1

CHECKLIST OF USEFUL EQUIPMENT FOR THE CLINICAL EXAMINATION

Scissors

Forceps

Battery operated hair clippers

Sample bottles

   Heparin

   EDTA

   Plain

   Sterile urine collection bottle

   Faecal sample pot

Rotheras tablets for ketone detection

Nasogastric tube

Stomach tube

Wide range pH papers

Surgical scrub

Thermometer (digital or mercury)

Long stethoscope with a phonoendoscope

Watch with a second hand

Torch

Paddle and Californian milk test reagent

Plastic rectal gloves and lubricant

Hoof knife, hoof testers and clippers

Assorted needles and syringes

Local anaesthetic with and without adrenalin

Spinal needles

Oral gag

Vaginal speculum

Ophthalmoscope

Auriscope

Part II

Cattle – Clinical Examination by Body System and Region

The General Clinical Examination of Cattle

General approach to the clinical examination

The patient should always be treated humanely. A quiet word as the patient is approached will often help to reassure the animal and calm an anxious owner.

A *thorough examination* of the patient should always be carried out. The consequences of not doing so can be embarrassing and potentially dangerous.

Respiratory rate

This should be counted over a period of 1 minute before the animal is caught or restrained for examination. Inspiratory or expiratory movements of the chest wall or flank can be counted. In cold weather exhaled breaths can be counted. If the animal is restless the clinician should count the rate of breathing for a shorter period and use simple multiplication to calculate the respiratory rate in breaths/minute. Mouth breathing is abnormal in cattle and is usually an indication of very poor lung function or a failing circulation.

Normal respiratory rate in cattle

- Adult 25 breaths/minute (range 15 to 30)
- Calf 30 breaths/minute (range 24 to 36)

Restraint for examination

The animal must be restrained so that it can be examined carefully, safely and with confidence. Calves are usually held by an assistant with one arm round their necks and may be backed into to a corner. Adult cattle can be restrained in a crush if available or (less satis-factorily) behind a swing gate. Quiet animals can be held using a halter or head collar. Unhandled cattle may be caught with a lasso if no crush is available. Additional control can be achieved using bulldogs or the nose ring in the case of a bull. An antikick bar may also be useful.

Chemical restraint

The use of a drug such as xylazine is helpful with nervous or difficult animals, but the restrictions of milk or meat withdrawal times must be observed.

Detailed observation

Once the animal has been restrained it should be visually examined more closely to see if any further abnormalities can be detected at close quarters. A small eye lesion that might not be spotted from a distance in an animal with profuse epiphora (excessive production of tears) may now be readily visible. Any swelling or other lesions on the body seen earlier can now be inspected more closely and palpated.

Temperature

The body temperature is taken using a mercury or digital electronic thermometer placed carefully into the rectum. The thermometer should be lubricated before insertion and checked (in the case of a mercury thermometer) to ensure that the mercury column has been shaken down before use. It should be held whilst it is in the rectum. Sudden antiperistaltic movements in the rectum may pull the thermometer out of reach towards the colon. The thermometer is left in position for at least 30 seconds; the clinician should ensure the instrument is in contact with the rectal mucosa, especially if a lower than expected reading is obtained. The thermometer must be cleaned after removal from the patient. It must not be wiped clean on the patient's coat. If the animal's temperature is higher or lower than anticipated it should be checked again.

Normal temperature in cattle

- Adult 38.5°C (range 38.0 to 39.0°C)
- Calf 39.0°C (range 38.5 to 39.5°C)

Pulse

The patient's pulse is taken from the caudal artery palpable along the midline of the ventral surface of the tail approximately 5 to 10 cm from the tail head. Alternative sites are the median artery or the digital arteries of the forelegs. The median artery is palpable as it runs subcutaneously on the medial aspect of the forelimb at the level of the elbow joint. The digital arteries are palpable on the lateral aspect of the forelimb just caudal to the metacarpus. In calves the femoral artery can be used. It is located on the medial aspect of the thigh between the gracilis and sartorius muscles. If a peripheral pulse is not palpable direct measurement of the heart rate can be used – by auscultating the heart and counting the beats per minute. There is a small chance of missing a pulse deficit by this latter method.

The pulse rate can rise rapidly in nervous animals or those which have undergone strenuous exercise. In such cases the pulse should be checked again after a period of rest lasting 5 to 10 minutes.

Normal pulse in cattle

- Adult 60 to 80 beats/minute
- Calf 80 to 120 beats/minute

Examination of the mucous membranes

Those of the eye can be demonstrated using the single or two handed technique. In both methods the eyelids are everted as the eye (protected by the eyelids) is gently pushed into the orbit. The colour of the mucosa of the conjunctiva is revealed. Alternative accessible mucosae are the vulva in the female and the mouth in both sexes. In some cattle black pigmentation makes assessment of the oral mucosal colour in parts of the mouth difficult.

The ocular and other visible mucosae should be salmon pink in colour. *Pallor of the mucous membranes* may indicate anaemia caused by direct blood loss or by haemolysis – in the latter case the pallor may be accompanied by jaundice. A *blue tinge* may indicate cyanosis caused by insufficient oxygen in the blood. A *yellow colour* is a sign of jaundice. The mucosae may be *bright red* (sometimes described as being 'injected mucous membranes') in febrile animals with septicaemia or viraemia. Bright red colouration of the conjunctiva is often seen, for example, in cases of bovine respiratory syncitial virus infection. A *cherry-red* colouration may be a feature of carbon monoxide poisoning. A *greyish tinge* in the mucosae may be seen in some cases of toxaemia – such membranes are sometimes said to be 'dirty'. High levels of methaemoglobin, seen in cases of nitrate and/or nitrite poisoning, may cause the mucosae to be *brown* coloured.

Capillary refill time (CRT)

This is taken by compressing the mucosa of the mouth or vulva to expel capillary blood, leaving a pale area, and recording how long it takes for the normal pink colour to return. In healthy animals the CRT should be less than 2 seconds. A CRT of more than 5 seconds is abnormal, and between 2 and 5 seconds it may indicate a developing problem. An increase in CRT may indicate a poor or failing circulation causing reduced peripheral perfusion of the tissues by the blood.

Further examination

It is essential that every case is examined fully, and for this reason a routine system for examination of the patient should be adopted. The patient's temperature, pulse, respiratory rate, colour of the mucous membranes and CRT are recorded and assessed. The clinician then moves on to examine every body system and region to identify any abnormality of form or function.

As mentioned in Chapter 1, the clinician can start the examination anywhere in the body. Many clinicians start at the head or the tail of the patient and then target their examination systematically over the whole body so that nothing is missed.

CHECKLIST FOR THE GENERAL CLINICAL EXAMINATION

Tail end 1
Record respiratory rate, temperature and pulse
Check colour of the mucous membranes
Examine the skin and coat
Assess condition score

Head and neck
Check symmetry of the head
Check the eyes, ears, muzzle and nostrils
Examine the mouth, palpate the tongue and lymph nodes of the head
Check the jugular vein, brisket and prescapular lymph nodes

Left side
Palpate and auscultate the heart – check for abnormalities
Auscultate and percuss the lung field – check for abnormalities
Check the abdominal shape and contour
Palpate and auscultate the rumen
Percuss and auscultate the body wall
Ballott the lower flank

Right side
Palpate and auscultate the heart – check for abnormalities
Auscultate and percuss the lung field – check for abnormalities
Check the abdominal shape and contour
Check the position and size of the liver
Percuss and auscultate the body wall
Palpate and auscultate the sublumbar fossa
Ballott the lower flank

Tail end 2
Examine the udder, teats and milk or the penis, prepuce, testes and epididymes
Vaginal examination
Rectal examination

Limbs
Observe for signs of lameness
Palpate the limbs
Raise and examine the feet

Samples
Collect samples as required

Dealing with the animal found dead

The clinician may encounter this problem when a patient has died before it has been examined and the cause of death is unknown. In such cases it is important to be sure that it has not died from anthrax. A blood smear should be made using blood collected by incising an ear vein (the lower ear in an animal in lateral recumbency). Pressure should be applied after collection to ensure that blood does not escape from the vein. Smears should be heat-fixed and then stained with polychromatic methylene blue. Anthrax bacilli are often found in chains. The rectangular bacilli have truncated ends and a pink staining capsule.

Clinical Examination of the Lymphatic System

Lymphatic system

The lymphatic system consists of the carcase lymph nodes, the network of lymph vessels which connect them and the lymphatic parts of the spleen. Many of the nodes are readily palpable in the healthy animal. Others can be palpated only when enlarged. Details of the location of the individual nodes and their ease of palpation are given below. The lymph vessels are normally palpable only if they are enlarged. Some vessels may be seen and palpated as they run sub-cutaneously towards the regional lymph nodes.

Clinical examination of the lymphatic system

Grossly enlarged lymph nodes may have been seen during observation of the patient before it is handled. Further observation and palpation is possible when the animal is restrained. The lymph nodes can be examined as a separate system or checked during the examination of the skin when the clinician's hands run over the whole body surface. Each paired node should be compared for size and consistency with the contralateral node.

Lymph node enlargement

This may occur for two main reasons.
(1) *Enlargement of one or more lymph nodes* may occur in cases of *infection of the lymphatic system*. This can occur in a number of diseases including bovine tuberculosis, actinobacillosis and a number of other bacterial infections. It can also occur in both forms of bovine leucosis – *enzootic bovine leucosis* (EBL) and *sporadic bovine leucosis*. EBL is an uncommon but notifiable disease in the UK. Infection is widespread in some other countries.

Any animal over 2 years of age with enlargement of the carcase lymph nodes and in which bovine leucosis is suspected is blood tested for serological evidence of EBL. Positive cases of EBL are slaughtered.

Cases of *sporadic bovine leucosis* may be examined further to determine which carcase and palpable visceral lymph nodes are involved. Gross lymph node enlargement may be seen, for example, in the prescapular lymph nodes. In most cases some enlargement is present in other lymph nodes. Ulceration of affected lymph nodes may occur. Areas of tumour tissue may be seen in the skin and in the thymus. Internal lymphoid tumours may be found in many locations including the heart base, the mediastinum and wherever lymph nodes are present. Affected lymph nodes are usually non-painful to the touch but may interfere with many body functions. Heart base and thymic tumours may obstruct venous return. Mediastinal tumours may compress the oesophagus causing bloat or dysphagia.

(2) *Lymph node enlargement in response to local infection or inflammation* in the region of the body drained by the lymph node involved. In these circumstances the lymph node is acting as a sentinel of local disease. The enlarged node may be warm and inflamed, and sensitive to the touch. On finding an enlarged lymph node the clinician should examine the area draining into the affected node for evidence of any pathological problem. As with tumour infiltration, the enlarged lymph nodes may affect the function of adjacent organs.

Location of the carcase lymph nodes

Many of the nodes are paired and should be compared for size and consistency. Lymph nodes are normally firmer than adjacent muscle and other soft tissues (Fig. 3.1).

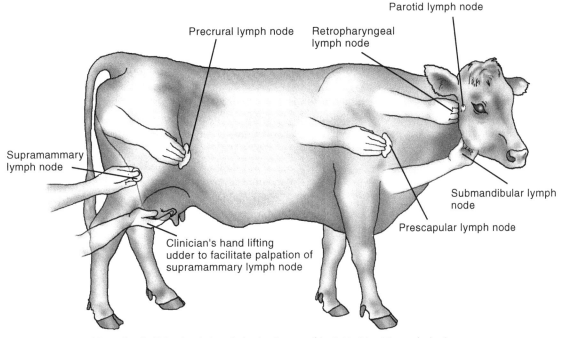

Figure 3.1 Locations of the readily palpable lymph nodes in cattle showing placement of the clinician's hand. See text for details.

Submandibular lymph nodes

These are situated and are palpable on the medial aspect of the 'angle of the jaw' where the horizontal and vertical rami of the mandible meet. Normal size is 1.5 to 2 cm at maximum diameter.

Parotid lymph nodes

Often these are not palpable unless they are enlarged through local infection or tumour formation. These small nodes lie subcutaneously just below the temperomandibular joint. Normal size is 0.5 cm.

Retropharyngeal lymph nodes

These nodes lie in the midline dorsal to the pharynx. If enlarged they can be palpated by placing two fingers of one hand on either side of the larynx. The fingers of the two hands are advanced towards each other just dorsal to the larynx. In normal animals the retropharyngeal nodes are rarely palpable and it is possible to advance the fingers (as described above) towards each other until they are separated only by the compressed pharynx. Dysphagia and dyspnoea with stertorous breathing may be seen in animals in which the retropharyngeal nodes are enlarged. The nodes may be up to 4 cm in diameter when enlarged.

Prescapular lymph nodes

These nodes lie subcutaneously and underneath the cutaneous muscle just anterior to the shoulder joint. It is often possible to palpate them directly in front of the shoulder. They may also be reliably located by extending the fingers and pressing them forward from the shoulder joint onto the neck. The fingers push against the prescapular node even if it is small, thus identifying its position. Further advance causes the fingers to rise over the node and down onto the neck in front of it, thus obtaining an estimate of the size of the node. The prescapular nodes vary in size and may be small and round or elongated in a dorsoventral direction. Normal size in adult is 1 cm × 3.5 cm.

Axillary lymph nodes

Normally only palpable in young calves without heavy muscling, these nodes are found on the medial aspect of the upper limb close to the point where the median artery and brachial plexus leave the thoracic cavity to run down the forelimb. The axillary nodes are located by deep palpation through the pectoral muscles. In adult cattle muscle tension, especially in the standing animal, normally prevents palpation of the axillary lymph nodes. Normal maximum diameter is 1.5 cm.

Precrural lymph nodes

These nodes lie beneath the cutaneous trunci muscles of the caudal flank just anterior to the stifle joint. Their size is very variable and in many cases they are palpable as an elongated chain running in a dorsoventral direction. They are most readily palpated by using the same technique as was described for the prescapular lymph nodes. The precrural nodes are found by advancing the flattened fingers anteriorly from the stifle joint. Normal size is 0.75 cm ×3 cm.

Popliteal lymph nodes

These nodes are found surrounded by dense muscle tissue immediately behind the stifle. They are sometimes palpable in young calves (normal maximum diameter 1 to 1.5 cm). Unless grossly enlarged they are seldom palpable in adult cattle.

Inguinal lymph nodes

These are usually palpable as a small group of fairly mobile and firm structures adjacent to the inguinal canal. In the male they are found just anterior to the scrotum, and in the female just anterior and lateral to the udder. Normal maximum diameter is 0.5 cm.

Supramammary lymph nodes

These two nodes are normally readily palpated on the caudal aspect of the udder just above the upper limit of the mammary glandular tissue. The nodes may seem to be contiguous with the mammary glandular tissue but are denser on palpation than the mammary tissue. Although they may be slightly enlarged in many cases of mastitis, unilateral enlargement may be particularly noticeable in cases of *Streptococcus uberis* infection. Location and palpation of the nodes is facilitated by the clinician supporting some of the weight of the udder with the hand. This will reduce the tension on the skin of the udder. Normal maximum diameter is 2.5 cm.

Internal iliac lymph nodes

These are palpable on rectal examination just anterior to the wing of the ilium on either side. Normal maximum diameter is 3 cm.

Spleen

In cattle the spleen is flat, 40 cm in length, 9 cm in width and 2 to 3 cm thick. It lies on the left side of the body with its visceral surface in contact with the dorsolateral walls of the rumen and reticulum. The parietal surface is in contact with the diaphragm. The upper extremity is level with the dorsal parts of the 12th and 13th ribs, and the lower extremity is level with the costochondral junction of the 7th rib (Fig. 6.1). It is normally not palpable, but if grossly enlarged it may be palpated just caudal to left rib cage. The spleen can be palpated at laparotomy either directly or through the wall of the opened rumen. It is seldom involved in disease, although its lymphoid tissue may be involved as part of the bovine leucosis complex.

PHYSICAL SIGNS OF DISEASE ASSOCIATED WITH THE LYMPHATIC SYSTEM

Carcase lymph node enlargement
  Single
  Regional
  General

Carcase lymph nodes
  Abnormally warm
  Suppuration
  Ulceration

Physical obstruction (N.B. These physical signs may also be associated with diseases of other body systems and regions)

Venous return obstructed
  Jugular (thymus and mediastinal lymph nodes)
  Heart base lymphoma
Physical damage or compression
  Oesophagus (thymus and mediastinal lymph nodes)
  Larynx (retropharyngeal lymph nodes)
  Trachea (retropharyngeal lymph nodes)
  Vagal nerve supply to rumen (mediastinal lymph nodes)
  Spinal cord (vertebral column lymphoma)

Clinical Examination of the Skin

Introduction

The skin has been described as the largest organ in the body. It defends the body it covers and is involved in the maintenance of homeostasis including water conservation. The skin is involved in body temperature conservation through insulation and in heat loss through perspiration. The sensory nerves of the skin recognise pain and temperature extremes. The skin provides protection against minor physical injuries, supports hair growth and offers some defence against microbial invasion.

The condition of the skin is a reflection of the general health of the animal, deteriorating in cases of ill health, ill thrift and debility. In some conditions, such as jaundice, the skin may provide through discolouration direct diagnostic evidence of a specific disease process. In other conditions, such as parasitism or severe mineral deficiency, a non-specific general deterioration of skin health may occur causing a greater number of hairs than normal to enter the telogen or resting phase and a delay in their replacement, leaving the coat in poor condition with little hair. Sebaceous secretions may be reduced, allowing the skin to become abnormally dry and inflexible and less able to perform its normal defence role in an already debilitated animal. In other cases sebaceous secretion increases causing the skin to have either a greasy or a dry seborrhoeic, flaky appearance.

The mutual dependency of the skin and the body it covers must be borne in mind during every clinical examination. Abnormalities of the skin may be caused by specific skin disease or by the poor general health status of the patient. A detailed clinical examination of the patient and of its skin are essential parts of the process of diagnosis and should enable the health status of the patient's body and its skin to be determined.

Applied anatomy

The skin has three main layers: the epidermis, dermis and subcutis. The *epidermis* consists largely of epithelial cells and pigment. The epithelial cells of this layer are produced by the stratum germinativum and as further cells are produced reach the outer surface of the skin in about 3 weeks. Here they become keratinised, die and are lost from the skin as a result of contact with the animal's environment. The *dermis* is a connective tissue layer containing blood vessels, nerves, hair follicles, sebaceous and sweat glands. The *subcutis* contains fibrous and fatty tissues which provide insulation for the body and support for the outer skin layers. The skin has considerable elasticity in the normal animal, allowing body movements to occur. This elasticity may be reduced by ill health, especially in dehydrated animals, and also as a result of inflammation and injury to the skin.

Hair follicles cover much of the bovine body but are not present at the mucocutaneous junctions or the surfaces of the muzzle and teats. Most cattle shed part of their coats in the spring. Considerable hair growth occurs as cold weather approaches in the autumn.

History of the case

The general history of the case will have been considered at an earlier stage in the process of diagnosis. There are specific points of history, however, that may have direct bearing on the consideration of skin disease. The *history of the herd* and a knowledge of the geographical area may provide useful information for the clinician. In areas where copper deficiency occurs, changes in coat colour may be seen. Previous skin disease problems on the farm with details of

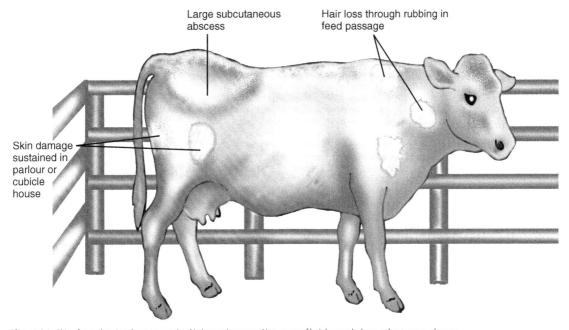

Large subcutaneous abscess

Hair loss through rubbing in feed passage

Skin damage sustained in parlour or cubicle house

Figure 4.1 Skin of cow showing damage sustained in her environment. Note areas of hair loss and a large subcutaneous abscess.

their diagnosis and treatment may provide a useful background of information which will assist in the evaluation of the present case.

The *history of the patient*, including recent contacts with other cattle at shows or markets, may also be important. Recent changes in diet and management should be noted. Poor nutrition can give rise to a dull, dry, thin and brittle coat. Loss of condition may have contributed to poor skin health which can itself then lead to further deterioration in the animal's general health. Specific points in the history of the patient may be useful. The stockperson may report frequent rubbing by the animal, suggesting pruritus. Failure to ensure an adequate supply of minerals and vitamins can contribute to poor skin health. Details of previous treatment given and the response to such treatment may also provide useful information.

The *environment of modern cattle*, especially the dairy cow, contains many features that may damage the skin. The cubicles, the parlour and the floor may have abrasive surfaces or sharp corners that can cause injury to the skin, often repeatedly. Such problems in the environment are especially likely to be important if a number of cattle in the herd are seen with identical superficial injuries. Overcrowding and insufficient feeding facilities may also contribute to poor coat condition including superficial skin damage (Fig. 4.1).

Abnormalities such as a very poor coat, evidence of excessive self-grooming or large areas of alopecia may be seen from a distance, but the areas of the skin must be closely examined too. Opportunities to examine the skin arise as each part of the body is examined, but in order to get a general impression of the skin it can be assessed separately before the more detailed examination of each area begins.

Visual appraisal of the skin

The whole body surface is methodically inspected initially from a distance and then more closely, looking for areas of abnormal skin or hair which will later be subjected to closer scrutiny. Healthy animals have lick marks on their skin, especially over the flank and shoulders. Pruritus, for example that caused by heavy louse infestation, may cause excessive grooming and the presence of more lick marks than normal. Repeated rubbing can lead to hair loss and thickening of the skin. The presence of any obvious abnormalities, including swellings or discharging abscesses, should be noted for further investigation later. Damp areas caused by sweating may be seen in pyrexic animals and in warm weather. Skin loss through injury may be seen. Gangrenous changes in the skin and deeper tissue may have arisen through loss of circulation and may be seen or noted during manual appraisal of the skin.

Manual appraisal of the skin

This should involve as much of the body surface as possible, using caution when touching sensitive areas which might cause the animal to kick. Manual appraisal will enable the clinician to detect lesions which are not immediately visible, for example beneath matted hair. Any abnormalities detected are subjected to further scrutiny which may necessitate removal of hair and examination of the skin in good light with the aid of a hand lens. Enlargement of lymph nodes may be detected at this stage (see below). *The thickness of the skin* and the presence of any subcutaneous oedema or infection should also be noted. The average skin thickness in adult cattle is 6 mm, with decreasing thickness being evident from the dorsal to the ventral body surfaces. The skin over the brisket is quite thick and mobile. This area of skin may have a spongy texture when compressed and may give an impression of subcutaneous oedema although it does not pit on pressure. Genuine *oedema* which *does* pit on pressure may be seen in this area and between the mandibles in cases of right sided cardiac failure. The skin covering the lower limbs is relatively immobile.

Manual examination of the skin will also allow assessment of *skin turgor* – its resilience and flexibility. Picking up a skin fold between finger and thumb and releasing it provides a general assessment of the animal's state of hydration. In a well hydrated animal the pinched skin falls immediately back into place; in a dehydrated animal the return to normal is delayed.

The best site for this test is the skin of the upper eyelid.

Pathological thickening of the skin occurs in a number of skin conditions, including sarcoptic mange. Thickening in the form of *callus formation* can occur in areas of skin, including those covering joints, which are repeatedly subjected to trauma. Examples include the elbows and hocks in animals with poor bedding.

Distribution of skin lesions

This is of diagnostic importance. Lesions caused by photosensitisation are commonly seen in lightly pigmented areas on the dorsal parts of the body which are exposed to sunlight. Such lesions are not normally seen in pigmented areas. Ringworm lesions in calves are particularly common on the head and neck, but also occur elsewhere.

Description of the skin lesions

The clinician should try to determine exactly what abnormalities are present in the skin, which tissues are involved and how deeply the disease process extends into and over the skin. The larger external parasites such as lice may be seen at this stage. Skin temperature, thickness, consistency and colour are observed and compared with adjacent areas. The presence of subcutaneous oedema or increased skin turgor is noted: these abnormalities may be caused by hypoproteinaemia or heart failure and dehydration, respectively, but they can also be the result of local pathology. When numbers of skin lesions are found it is important to determine if they share the same aetiology. They may represent different stages of one disease process. More than one condition can be present at the same time.

There may be abnormalities in the sebaceous and sweat glands or gross proliferation of the superficial layers. *Self-inflicted trauma* can greatly modify and mask the clinical picture. Skin abnormalities may involve some or all of the component structures of the skin: the hair, follicles, epidermal, dermal and subcutaneous tissues.

Lesions may be primary or secondary. *Primary lesions* are the direct result of the skin disease. They are usually most obvious in the early stages of skin disease and are the lesions upon which the definitive diagnosis should be based. *Secondary lesions* are mostly non-specific and result either from further development of the primary lesions or from self-inflicted damage. Examples of the more common lesions in each category are listed below.

Primary lesions

Macule – flattened area of colour change less than 1 cm in diameter; no skin thickening

Papule – flat circumscribed area, mostly rounded and often raised with a necrotic centre; overall size less than 1 cm in diameter; may be associated with the hair follicles

Nodule – a papule more than 1 cm in diameter

Plaque – solid raised flat topped mass more than 1 cm in diameter

Tumour – large nodular structure, often of neoplastic origin

Vesicle – fluid filled blister less than 1 cm in diameter (vesicles larger than 1 cm are called bullae)

Pustule – pus filled vesicle.

Secondary lesions

Scale – accumulation of loose, dry fragments of superficial skin layers

Crust – dried accumulation of debris including blood and pus

Erosion – loss of superficial epidermal layers with intact inner layers

Excoriation – erosion or deep ulcer of traumatic origin

Ulcer – deep erosion penetrating the epidermal basement membrane

Scar – fibrous tissue replacing damaged skin

Fissure – split in the superficial skin layers often caused by drying and thickening

Keratosis – overgrowth of dry horny keratinised epithelium

Pigment changes – hyper- or hypopigmentation

Alopecia – hair loss.

Having identified the extent, distribution and type of skin lesions present, the clinician should try to identify the cause of the problem. Some skin diseases have specific signs which may help to establish a diagnosis. The most important of these are described below.

Clinical signs associated with some of the more common bovine skin diseases

Parasitic skin diseases

Lice

These are one of the most common causes of bovine skin disease. Three species of blue-grey sucking lice, *Haematopinus eurysternus*, *Linognathus vituli* and *Solenopotes capillatus*, and one species of brown chewing lice, *Damalinia bovis*, are found in the UK. All species are capable of rapid multiplication and spread rapidly, especially in housed cattle. Infested cattle show signs of skin irritation, with affected animals rubbing themselves against the walls and fittings in their pen. They may show signs of excessive grooming, and hair loss will occur. Adult lice can be seen with the naked eye, especially along the dorsum of the neck and back. Small white egg cases are visible adhering to hairs (Fig. 4.2). A good light and possibly a hand lens are essential to enable lice to be seen. *Solenopotes capillatus*, the least common species, is found chiefly around the eyes of cattle where it may produce a 'spectacled' appearance similar to that seen in cases of copper poisoning. Heavy infestations by sucking lice may cause anaemia in affected animals.

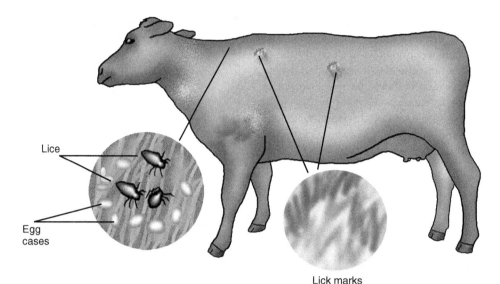

Figure 4.2 Louse infestation.

In *calves* large numbers of lice may be seen all over the body surface and not confined to the dorsum of the neck and back as in adult cattle. Affected calves may show no obvious signs of infestation, but a careful examination of the whole skin surface allows the extent of this serious problem to be determined.

Confirmation of louse infestation is based on the clinical signs and the visible presence of lice moving along the skin surface between the hairs. Microscopic examination of a skin scraping will enable the presence of lice and their egg cases to be confirmed and their species identified.

Flies

During the summer months fly worry can produce tear scalding under the eyes. Superficial skin damage is caused by various biting fly species. Multiple nodules in the skin can be caused by the bites of flies including the species *Haematobia*, *Stomoxys* and *Simulium*. Extensive bites may produce signs of *urticaria* in which prominent oedematous wheals rapidly develop in the epidermis and dermis, especially on the neck and flanks. Open wounds on the lower abdomen, udder and teats can be caused by the bites of flies such as *Haematobia irritans* and *Hippobosca equina* (the 'louse fly'). *Warble flies* are not present in the UK, but occasional cases are seen in imported animals. Caused by flies of the *Hypoderma*

family, the condition is characterised by subcutaneous nodules and cysts along the backs of cattle in the spring and summer; careful opening of these lesions reveals the presence of warble fly larvae.

Diagnosis of fly damage is based on the presence of the various fly species and their associated skin lesions.

Mange mites

Chorioptic, sarcoptic, psoroptic and demodectic mange mites are found in cattle. The first three species produce intense pruritus in infested animals; this can be so severe that milk production and growth are impaired.

Chorioptic mange is the most common (64% of UK mange cases), especially in housed cattle during the winter. Caused by the surface living mite *Chorioptes bovis*, the condition is seen chiefly around the tail head area of cattle where it causes crusty skin lesions (Fig. 4.3). Rubbing by infested cattle produces secondary changes such as alopecia and thickening of the skin.

Sarcoptic mange mites (31% of UK cases) may occasionally infest the tail head of cattle, but are also seen on the head, neck and shoulders. *Sarcoptes scabiei* is a burrowing mite which produces thickening of the skin and secondary damage associated with the intense pruritus seen in this condition.

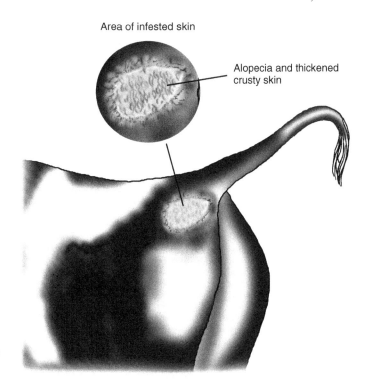

Area of infested skin

Alopecia and thickened crusty skin

Figure 4.3 Chorioptic mange mite infestation of the tail head. Similar lesions occasionally involve sarcoptic mange mites.

Psoroptic mange is rare in the UK (5% of cases), but large numbers of cases occur elsewhere. *Psoroptes natalensis*, the surface living causal mite, is associated with extensive thickening of the skin, pruritus and hair loss over the shoulders, hindquarters and perineum. Thickened crusty skin is seen in chronic cases which may be in very poor condition.

Demodectic mange is often asymptomatic in cattle, but the mite can be found in nodules in the skin covering the thorax. Alopecia involving the skin of the neck but with no pruritus has been found in animals infested with the *cattle itch mite Psorobia bovis*.

Diagnosis of mite infestation is based on the clinical signs associated with each mite and identification of mites in skin scrapings.

Ticks

Ixodes ricinis, Dermacentor reticulatus and *Haemaphysalis punctata* are found in parts of the UK. The ticks may be found on animals imported from these areas and produce particularly severe symptoms in animals which have had no previous exposure to them. The ticks are visible to the naked eye and can be identified under the microscope. Heavy tick infestation can lead to anaemia, and skin lesions on the lower parts of the body are seen; there are small areas of granulation tissue and possibly a hypersensitivity reaction. Ticks carry a number of diseases including babesiosis, tick-borne fever and Lyme disease.

Blow-fly strike

This is initiated by the egg laying of blow flies, including *Lucilia sericata* or *Phormia terraenovae*, whose larvae infest soiled skin especially in warm weather. Blow-fly strike can occur anywhere on the body, including the frontal sinuses exposed by horn removal. The larvae, which are readily seen with the naked eye, penetrate the skin and the deeper body tissues. Adjacent areas of skin may show signs of necrosis. Larvae may also enter the natural orifices of the body, including the anus.

Bacterial skin disease

Superficial trauma, heavy contamination, damp and

dirty conditions, chronic trauma or reduced dermal immunity may predispose to bacterial infection. Local infection is frequently seen on the ears of calves a few days after the insertion of metal tags (less commonly after plastic tags). Pus is seen oozing from around the tag and there may be evidence that infection has invaded the cartilage of the pinna. Staphylococcal infection may be seen as a superficial pustular dermatitis. This is a non-pruritic impetigo-like condition often seen on the udder or perineum. Pustules, from which the organism can be cultured, may be seen on the skin. A staphylococcal folliculitis is sometimes seen on the skin of the hindquarters of young cattle kept in unhygienic conditions. Pustules develop in hair follicles which can be squeezed to reveal their purulent contents.

Dermatophilus infection

This is occasionally seen, especially on the backs of cattle kept in crowded conditions where minor trauma allows the infection to become established. Thick crusty lesions may be seen overlying a granulating skin surface. Hairs from the coat grow through the crusty lesions which are approximately 2 cm across.

Subcutaneous abscesses

These are very frequently seen in cattle and are mostly associated with *Arcanobacterium pyogenes* infection gaining access through superficial injuries. They are often very extensive and are palpable as fluctuating subcutaneous swellings around the tail head and other parts of the body surface (Fig. 4.1). *Infected hygromas* on the knees or hocks are seen as fluctuating, often painful swellings over these and other pressure points. Confirmation of diagnosis and determination of cause can be obtained by ultrasonographic scan and by needle aspiration.

Actinomyces bovis infection is occasionally seen as lumpy jaw when it causes an osteomyelitis in the bovine mandible (Fig. 5.4). Subcutaneous abscesses and fistulae may arise from the underlying pathology. The exudate is thick and honey-like in appearance. *Actinobacillus lignieresii* has been associated with superficial skin lesions on the face and around the muzzle and nostril (Fig. 4.4). Drainage lymph nodes may be enlarged in this and other skin infections.

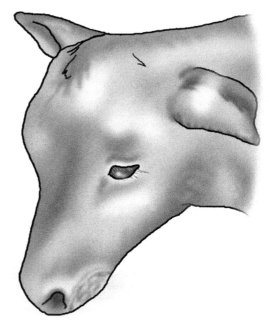

Figure 4.4 Skin lesion on left lip caused by *Actinobacillus lignieresii*.

Fungal skin disease

Ringworm is a very common disease, especially in young cattle. Raised grey crusty lesions often associated with areas of alopecia are seen. The lesions are most often seen on the head or neck (Fig. 4.5). Diagnosis is by demonstration of fungal spores and mycelia in skin scrapings or broken hairs carefully prepared in 10% KOH before microscopic examination. Most cases of bovine ringworm are caused by *Trichophyton verrucosum* which does not fluoresce with Wood's lamp.

Viral skin disease

A large number of viruses can cause specific skin lesions in cattle. In some diseases lesions are confined to the skin, whilst in others skin lesions are just part of spectrum of signs involving a number of body systems.

Bovine viral papillomatosis

Bovine papillomavirus is the cause of warts or angleberries in cattle. At least five strains of the causal

Ringworm lesions

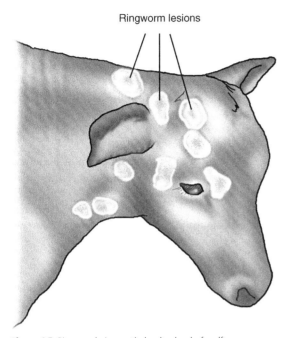

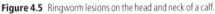

Figure 4.5 Ringworm lesions on the head and neck of a calf.

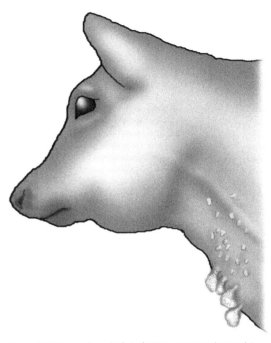

Figure 4.6 Warts on the neck of a heifer. Note variation in shape and size.

agent have been identified, each responsible for a particular type or location of lesion. There is great variation in distribution and size, varying from small individual or multiple warts on the teats or skin 2–3 mm in length to pedunculated angleberries 10 cm or more in diameter (Fig. 4.6). Warts are hard outgrowths from the epidermis, and in the early stages of their development larger warts may be confused with the lesions of ringworm or the cutaneous form of lymphosarcoma. Penile warts may only visible when the bull's penis is extruded at service or are discovered when blood coming from the prepuce is investigated. Penile warts are soft to the touch, bleed easily and arise from peduncles, often near to the external urethral orifice (Fig. 11.6). Diagnosis is based on the appearance, distribution and consistency of the warts confirmed, if necessary, by histology.

Bovine papular stomatitis

This zoonotic disease is seen chiefly on the muzzle, nostrils, dental pad and buccal mucosa of young cattle. The lesions are small red-brown coloured papules approximately 0.5 cm in diameter. The surface of the lesions is roughened and slightly elevated. They are mostly horseshoe shaped (Fig. 4.7). Adjacent lesions sometimes coalesce. Lesions are usually found on several animals in a group. Older lesions may be less distinct (Fig. 5.12). Diagnosis is based on clinical signs and on examination of fresh lesions by electron microscopy for evidence of the characteristic parapoxvirus.

Foot-and-mouth disease

Teat lesions which resemble those of bovine herpes mammillitis may be seen together with characteristic vesicles, bullae and ulcerated areas on the muzzle, tongue and coronary bands (Fig. 5.15). Affected animals are anorexic, pyrexic ($T = 40$–$41°C$), salivate profusely and are lame.

Other viral diseases with possible skin lesions

Infectious bovine rhinotracheitis (IBR)   Areas of erythema, pustule formation, ulceration and localised necrosis may be seen around the muzzle, nos-

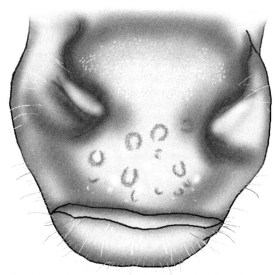

Figure 4.7 Lesions of papular stomatitis on the muzzle of a heifer. See also Fig. 5.12.

trils and less commonly around the perineum and scrotum. Inflammation of the upper respiratory tract and ocular mucosa is often also seen.

Infectious vulvovaginitis/balanoposthitis The related venereal condition of infectious vulvovaginitis/balanoposthitis affects the genitalia of both bull and cow. The mucosa of penis, vulva and vagina are inflamed, painful and ulcerated. Secondary bacterial infection may occur, and in some bulls extrusion of the penis may be difficult.

Mucosal disease Small shallow erosions may be seen on the oral mucosa, muzzle and less commonly around the coronary band. Diagnosis is based on the clinical signs, serology and antigen detection.

Malignant catarrh A superficial necrosis followed by severe ulceration of the oral mucosa is seen. Similar lesions may be found on the muzzle and coronary band. Diagnosis is based on the severe clinical signs and virus detection.

Neoplastic skin disease

The following tumours may found on the skin of cattle.

Squamous cell carcinoma

These tumours are seen in poorly pigmented areas at the mucocutaneous junctions of the body. The mucosa of the third eyelid, the periorbital skin and the vulva are common sites (Fig. 5.9). The tumours are initially small but grow rapidly, invading adjacent tissues.

Cutaneous lymphosarcoma

These tumours may be the precursor of generalised lymphosarcoma or a consequence of it. The tumour masses are mostly multiple and are found chiefly in the skin of the neck or flanks. They are seen as grey elevated plaques in the skin with some hyperkeratosis of surrounding skin.

Fibromas and fibrosarcomas

These are usually seen as large tumours arising from the subcutaneous tissue and covered with normal skin (Fig. 5.2).

Lipomas

Lipomas invading the soft tissues of the head have been described. Diagnosis of tumour type can be confirmed histologically.

Nutritional causes of skin disease

Gross deficiency of the main dietary components or a severe shortage of food can lead to a deterioration in skin condition. A dull, dry non-elastic skin may be seen, with poor growth of scant and brittle hairs. The skin may be more susceptible to bacterial infection. It is important to ensure that no specific condition such as chronic mucosal disease which might predispose to similar lesions is present. *Vitamins A, C and E* deficiencies have all been associated with skin disease. *Copper deficiency* and excess *molybdenum* may produce subtle coat colour changes, especially around the eyes, in addition to other general symptoms of deficiency. Diagnosis is based on the history of the patient, dietary analysis and response to specific therapy.

Toxic causes of skin disease

Excessive intake of some elements may produce

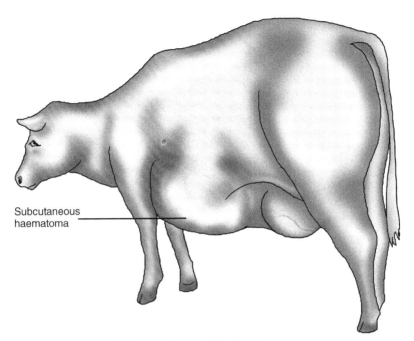

Subcutaneous
haematoma

Figure 4.8 Large subcutaneous haematoma caused by damage to the external abdominal vein.

signs of skin disease along with other symptoms. Chronic *arsenic, selenium* or *molybdenum toxicity* is associated with poor skin quality and in some cases changes in hair colour. Overdosing with potassium iodide may produce signs of *iodism* including widespread dry seborrhoeic dermatitis. Diagnosis is based on a history of exposure to toxic elements and confirmatory analysis.

Snake bites may cause severe swelling and oedema of the skin. Detection of snake venom antitoxins in the blood of bitten animals can be undertaken but is expensive.

Physical causes of skin disease

A poorly designed, uncomfortable environment may produce a number of skin lesions in cattle. Most are the result of chronic injury to the skin. Lack of bedding may predispose to *callus formation* or *decubitus ulcers* over pressure points covered only by skin and connective tissue such as the hock. Subcutaneous *haematomata* are produced by injury, but may be exacerbated by underlying blood clotting defects (Fig. 4.8). Differential diagnosis of a haematoma and an abscess may be aided by aspirating the contents

with a needle and by ultrasonography. *Hair loss* on the necks of cattle through chronic chafing by the bars of the feeding passage is seen on many farms (Fig. 4.1). *Milk scald* is quite frequently seen in calves, especially those fed on high fat or acidified milk. Those parts of the muzzle that are regularly immersed in milk when the animal is feeding suffer complete hair loss (Fig. 4.9). The underlying skin is often normal and hair growth resumes immediately after weaning.

Photosensitisation

This is commonly seen in individual animals on lush pasture. The condition may be primary when photodynamic agents are present in consumed plants such as St John's wort, or secondary when phylocrythrin accumulates as a result of hepatic malfunction. Lesions are seen chiefly in non-pigmented areas. Erythema and pruritus occur and are followed by crusting of the skin and deep fissure formation (Fig. 4.10). Some serum loss occurs through the skin and superficial layers of skin may die and slough.

Chronic diarrhoea

This may lead to the development of sore and cracked areas of skin in the perineal area. Alopecia in

25

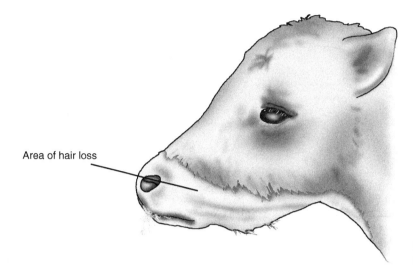

Figure 4.9 Calf with milk scald. See text for details.

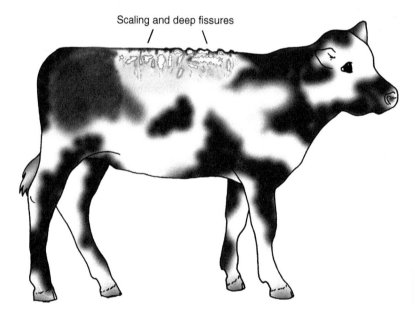

Figure 4.10 Calf with photosensitisation. Note lesions on unpigmented part of the back.

affected areas may also be seen. Local skin necrosis may be caused by faeces adhering to the tail and drying out, compromising the circulation of the skin.

Congenital causes of skin disease

A number of hereditary defects have been recorded in calves. Affected animals are born with partial or complete alopecia, or less commonly the condition develops within the first few weeks of life. There are usually no other abnormalities. The exact nature of the defect may require histological and genetic evaluation.

Telogen effluvium

This is a non-specific skin lesion seen in calves recovering from severe illnesses such as *Escherichia coli* septicaemia. Hair loss may appear to be getting worse as the calf recovers from the primary disease. Lesions, which may be seen on the head, neck and limbs, are non-pruritic. Underlying non-pigmented skin may appear pinker in colour than normal. Visible hair growth resumes after a few weeks.

Special diagnostic procedures

A firm diagnosis may have been made at this point, but if not, further investigation may be required by the use of special diagnostic techniques.

Bacterial culture

The normal bovine skin has a large population of bacteria and fungi. The bacterial population rises in wet weather and also in areas of the body where sebuminous secretion occurs. The bacterial flora normally live symbiotically with their host, but can be opportunist pathogens if the body's defences are lowered in any way. Staphylococci, streptococci, *Arcanobacterium pyogenes* and coliforms are commonly found on the normal bovine skin, but heavy growths of these organisms especially in pure culture may be significant. Swabs from suspicious lesions should be taken with care to avoid contamination and processed quickly. Pustular material from abscess may be aspirated by sterile needle and syringe for culture. Skin biopsies may also be cultured.

Skin scrapings

These are particularly useful in the diagnosis of mange infestation. They should be taken, if possible, in the early stages of the disease. Later on very few mites may be present as they encounter the skin's defence mechanisms. The scraping is best taken with a scalpel blade to a depth at which signs of capillary bleeding just appear. The scraping may be examined microscopically directly or after treatment with potassium hydroxide.

Skin biopsy

This is the most useful of the special diagnostic tests. For good results it should be taken early on in the disease process before secondary and possibly non-specific changes have occurred. Fully developed primary lesions are particularly useful, and multiple biopsies may also be helpful. If the biopsy is to prove useful it must be taken with care. A small piece of skin should be removed either by excision or by punch biopsy. Before removal, hairs should be clipped short and the skin gently cleaned with 70% alcohol, after which local anaesthetic is instilled around and under the proposed biopsy site. The biopsy should be at least 5 mm in size and should be fixed in 10% buffered formalin as soon as it has been taken. The volume of fixative should be at least ten times that of the biopsy.

Other diagnostic tests

Numerous other tests are available, including electron microscopy for virus infections such as bovine papular stomatitis. In other virus diseases with skin lesions, serial serological samples may provide evidence of recent infection.

CLINICIAN'S CHECKLIST

Have signs caused by the following causes of skin disease been seen?

Parasitic causes
Bacterial causes
Fungal causes
Viral causes
Neoplastic causes
Nutritional causes
Toxic causes
Physical causes

PHYSICAL SIGNS OF DISEASE ASSOCIATED WITH THE SKIN

Distribution of hair loss and/or skin lesions
  Generalised
  Periocular
  Head and neck
  Shoulders
  Thorax
  Back
  Body
  Tail head
  Genital system
  Perineum
  Udder
  Teats
  Legs
  Feet
  Pressure points
  Non-pigmented areas
Size, shape and number of lesions
  Diameter
  Circumscribed
  Diffuse
  Single
  Multiple
Skin abnormal
  Dry
  Greasy
  Flaky
  Seborrhoea
  Callus
  Thickened
  Dull
  Inelastic
  Reduced turgor (tent test for
    dehydration)
  Increased/decreased pigmentation
Skin lesion type
  Macule
  Papule
  Nodule
  Plaque
  Mass
  Vesicle
  Pustule
  Scale
  Crust
  Erosion
  Excoriation
  Lacerations
  Ulcer

Scar
Fissure
Sweating
Necrosis
Keratosis
Skin peeling and parchment-like
Skin wheals (urticaria)
Suppurative
Masses
Swellings
Serum oozing
Presence of ticks
Blow-fly strike
Gangrene
Loss of skin
Skin temperature
  Hot
  Cold
Skin colour change
  Jaundice
  Pale
  Cyanotic
Pruritus
  Excessive grooming
  Lick marks
  Repeated rubbing
  Hair loss
Hair
  Change in hair colour
  Hair hypopigmented
  Hair loss
  Symmetrical hair loss
  Hair broken
  Hair easily plucked
  Presence of lice
  Presence of eggs adherent to hairs
  Glossy coat
  Staring coat
Subcutis
  Oedema
  Emphysema
  Swellings over pressure points
  Fistulae
  Masses
  Cellulitis
Lymph nodes
  Regional lymph nodes enlarged
Mucous membranes
  Pale

Clinical Examination of the Head and Neck

Inspection and observation

Before handling the head a further *visual inspection and observation* of the head and neck is advisable (Fig. 5.1). Observation of the head and the animal's behaviour enables an evaluation to be made of parts of the nervous system including the brain and cranial nerves. Initial confirmation may be made that the animal has vision – by its ability to follow movements of the clinician's hand. Also whether it can hear – by its response to clapping the hands outwith its visual field. The presence of abnormal ocular or nasal discharges is noted, as are changes or abnormalities in the outline and contours of the region. Cattle normally produce large quantities of saliva, but drooling of saliva from the mouth is abnormal and should be investigated; it may be associated with painful oral lesions or an inability to swallow, for example as a result of choke.

The head is normally held vertically upright in the undisturbed animal. Persistent head tilting is abnormal and may indicate vestibular disease or unilateral pain in part of the head, e.g. the ear. Abnormal head carriage is seen as part of the posture of opisthotonos and other neurological abnormalities. If the animal is eating it should be closely observed to check that prehension, mastication and swallowing of its food are normal.

The *neck of cattle is normally very mobile* and it should be possible for the animal to turn the head back towards the flanks on either side of the body. Lick marks on both sides of the withers suggest good natural neck mobility.

CLINICIAN'S CHECKLIST – OBSERVATION OF THE HEAD AND NECK

Movements of head and neck – normal or abnormal
Carriage of head – normal or tilted
Can the animal see?
Can the animal hear?
Ocular or nasal discharge
Salivation – normal or excessive
Ability to prehend, masticate and swallow food
Mobility of the neck

Closer examination of the head and neck is aided by restraint of the head, either by applying a halter or manually holding it. In nervous or difficult animals the patient may be further restrained by holding the nose either by hand or using bulldogs.

The head, face and neck should be symmetrical. Abnormalities of outline should be noted and investigated. Unilateral swellings of the head in the adult may be caused by abscess formation or less commonly by tumours such as fibrosarcomas (Fig. 5.2). Gross distortion of the cranial area of the head is seen in cases of hydrocephalus. The maxilla is severely truncated in the so called bulldog calf, caused by a recessive gene in Dexter cattle. Unilateral *facial swelling* over the cheek area in calves is often an external sign of calf diphtheria (necrotic stomatitis) (Fig. 5.2). *Muscular tone* on both sides of the face should be equal. Unilateral *facial paralysis* with local loss of muscle tone may be seen in conditions such as listeriosis.

Sinusitis is uncommon in cattle but the health of the *sinuses* – frontal and maxillary – can be assessed by percussion over their location (Fig. 5.3). In normal animals such percussion is painless, but in the presence of sinus infection discomfort on percussion is evident. The frontal sinuses extend into the horns of adult cattle. Removal of the horns results in exposure of the mucosal surfaces of the frontal sinuses.

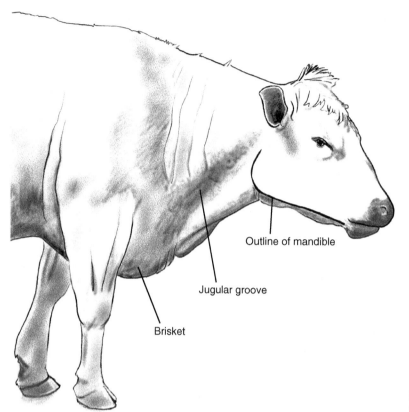

Figure 5.1 Lateral (side) view of the outline of the bovine head and neck.

Outline of mandible

Jugular groove

Brisket

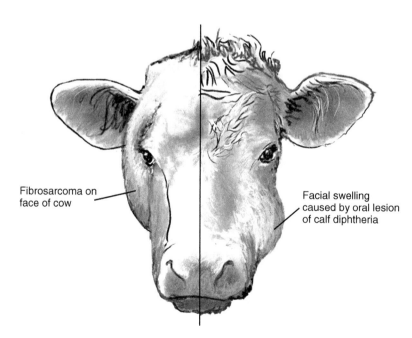

Fibrosarcoma on face of cow

Facial swelling caused by oral lesion of calf diphtheria

Figure 5.2 Abnormal facial swellings on cow and calf.

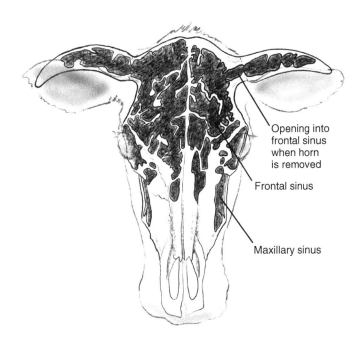

Opening into
frontal sinus
when horn
is removed

Frontal sinus

Maxillary sinus

Figure 5.3 Anterior (front) view of the bovine head and neck.

Infection of the sinuses in recently dehorned cattle may be indicated by the presence of pus or an unpleasant odour in the sinuses. In warm weather there is a risk of blow-fly strike in the exposed sinuses.

The *mandibles* should be inspected and palpated for signs of injury or infection. Some irregularity of the ventral mandibular outline is normal, especially in animals changing their teeth. Discharging sinuses originating from the mandible are seen in cases of *Actinomycosis bovis* (lumpy jaw) (Fig. 5.4). The mandibles may be injured through collision with farm machinery. A fracture may be present in the mandibular symphysis or in the rami if the animal is unable to prehend food, close its mouth and eat. Very occasionally the teeth of neonatal calves may be damaged or displaced during birth. The cheek teeth can be palpated externally through the cheeks. Missing teeth, sharp edges and painful teeth can be detected. The *salivary glands* are rarely involved in disease in cattle. Blockage of gland ducts may result in the formation of a *mucocoele* in the animal's mouth. The *parotid salivary gland* can be palpated as a firm structure just behind and medial to the caudal border of the vertical ramus of the mandible.

CLINICIAN'S CHECKLIST – INSPECTION OF THE HEAD AND NECK

Outline and profile of the head and neck
Cranial or other enlargement
Facial symmetry
Muscular tone of the face
Percussion of the sinuses
Mandible – symphysis and profile
Palpation of the cheek teeth
Palpation of the salivary glands

Ears

The ears are normally held horizontally to the head and *drooping* is abnormal. Animals in poor health may show bilateral drooping of the ears (Fig. 5.5). Unilateral ear drooping may indicate infection of the ear itself, for example caused by an infected ear tag, or compromise of the 7th cranial (facial) nerve supply, for example in listeriosis (Fig. 5.6). Ears may also droop if weighed down by heavy ear tags. Ear tremor

31

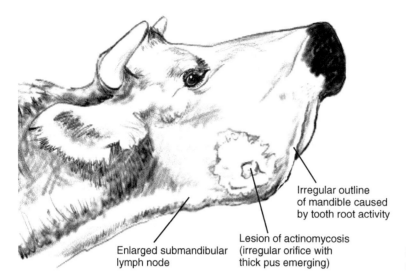

Irregular outline
of mandible caused
by tooth root activity

Enlarged submandibular
lymph node

Lesion of actinomycosis
(irregular orifice with
thick pus emerging)

Figure 5.4 Ventrolateral view of mandibles and proximal throat of cow.

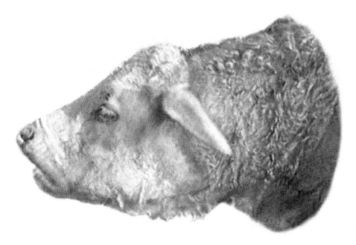

Figure 5.5 Drooping of ears in depressed calf.

has been seen in some cases of bovine spongioform encephalopathy (BSE). Increased muscle tone with stiffness of the ears is seen in tetanus. Despite their dirty and dusty environment, otitis externa and foreign bodies in the ears of cattle are extremely uncommon. If aural discharge is present, the ear canal can be inspected using an auriscope or a small fibreoptic endoscope. *Deafness* may be caused by damage to the auditory part of the 8th cranial (vestibulocochlear) nerve. *Lacerations in the ear* are frequently seen and are often caused by metal tags catching on hooks and other objects. They are then pulled out, tearing the ear. Local infection may be seen around recently inserted ear tags, especially in calves. Aural haematomata are extremely rare in cattle.

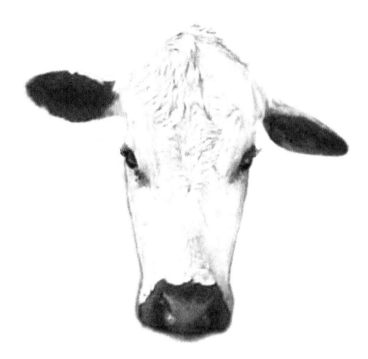

Figure 5.6 Cow with listeriosis showing unilateral drooping of left ear.

Eyes

The eyes must always be examined with great care. *Anophthalmia* or *microphthalmia* are seen occasionally as congenital defects in calves. Anophthalmia is sometimes accompanied by the absence of a tail.

Eye movements

Repeated and spontaneous lateral movements of the eye (nystagmus) may be seen in some neurological conditions. The various presentations of nystagmus are discussed fully under examination of the nervous system in Chapter 14. Some ocular movements are seen in normal animals. The eye moves to a limited extent within the orbit if the animal is visually following a moving object. If the head is tilted upwards the eyes move downwards within the orbit, a movement involving the vestibular system and known as *vestibular eye drop*.

Position of eyeball in orbit

The normal phenomenon of vestibular eye drop has been described above. Abnormal eye positions can occur in cases of damage to the nerves controlling ocular movements and are discussed in Chapter 14.

Intraocular pressure and prominence of eyes

Gentle pressure on the eyeball through the upper eyelid should be exerted to assess intraocular pressure. The pressure should be the same in both eyes. Increased pressure is termed *glaucoma* and may affect one or both eyes. One eye may also be more prominent if it is displaced by a tumour mass or infection within the orbit. The eyes may be sunken in dehydrated cattle, and in severe cases a space is apparent between the eyelids and the eyeball. The eyes may also be sunken in severely emaciated animals which have lost all fat deposits within the orbit. The eye may appear sunken and have a reduced intraocular pressure if it has been accidentally penetrated or ruptured through overwhelming internal pressure.

Examination of ocular reflexes

Fixation, palpebral, corneal, menace and light response reflexes are checked on both sides. Full details of these and the neurological pathways involved are discussed in Chapter 14. Inequality of pupil size may indicate general or specific neurological damage if there is no sign of glaucoma or intraocular infection. When assessing the pupillary light response reflex care must be taken to ensure that no physical damage, such as anterior synechia (see below), interferes with the reflex.

CLINICIAN'S CHECKLIST – OBSERVATION OF THE EYES

Anophthalmia/microphthalmia
Eye movement – normal or abnormal
Position of eyeballs in orbits
Intraocular pressure
Assessment of ocular/cranial nerve reflexes
  Fixation reflex
  Palpebral reflex
  Corneal reflex
  Menace reflex
  Pupillary light reflex

Close examination of the eye

Good access can be difficult if the animal has ocular pain and is very sensitive to further discomfort.

Visual access to the eye is often aided by tilting the head slightly downwards on the side which is being examined. This will cause the animal to rotate the eyeball upwards with wide open eyelids allowing both direct visual access and facilitate the use of the ophthalmoscope.

All parts of the eye and eyelids should be carefully and methodically inspected. Topical anaesthetic instilled into the eye will also facilitate a pain-free examination (Fig. 5.7). Ocular injury, infection and foreign bodies are quite common in cattle.

Sclera

The sclera is occasionally damaged by injury. Its vascularity is also increased in some cases of meningitis. Petechial haemorrhages in the sclera may be seen in cases of septicaemia and yellow discolouration may be present in jaundice.

Cornea

Corneal lesions in cattle are common, being chiefly the result of either New Forest disease or injury. Mild damage or early cases of New Forest disease may appear as a small *corneal ulcer* (Fig. 5.8a) or area of *corneal opacity* caused by local oedema and neutrophil invasion. Growth of blood vessels (neovascularisation) from adjacent sclera leads to repair and in some cases an inert residual scar or *pannus*. Generalised corneal opacity (Fig. 5.8b) in both eyes is seen in keratitis and in some cases of malignant catarrh fever. More severe injuries or untreated corneal infection may cause deeper corneal damage and exposure of Descemet's membrane. If the membrane ruptures a *staphyloma* may form through which some of the interior components of the eye may prolapse (Fig. 5.8c). The exact extent of *corneal injury* or *ulceration* can be highlighted by the use of fluorescein dye strips which stain damaged tissue a luminous green (Fig. 5.7). Fluorescein in the eye passes eventually with the tears into the *nasolachrymal duct*. Patency of the ducts is demonstrated by the presence of the dye placed in the conjunctiva appearing in the ipsilateral nostril. Patency can also be checked by retrograde flushing. A fine catheter is introduced into the small opening of the nasolachrymal duct on the lateral wall of the nostril. Sterile saline or a weak dye solution is introduced into the catheter using a syringe.

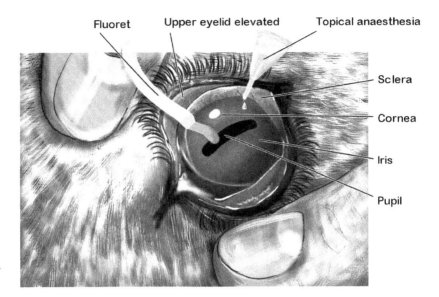

Figure 5.7 Examination of the outer surface of the eye.

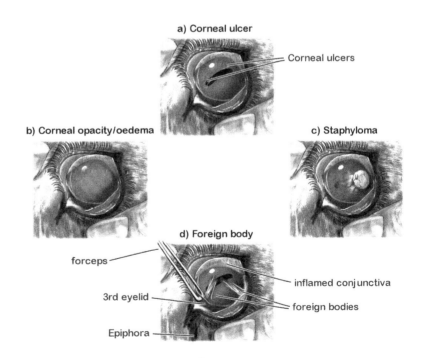

Figure 5.8 Conditions of the eye – 1.

If the duct is patent, fluid appears at the ocular conjunctiva.

Conjunctiva

The *conjunctiva* which lines the eyelids and is reflected onto the eyeballs should be salmon pink in colour and slightly moist. Dark pigment may occasionally prevent recognition of true conjunctival colour. The causes of abnormal colouration of the conjunctiva are discussed in Chapter 2. Tear production is often increased when the conjunctiva is inflamed, and excessive tears may spill down the animal's face (epiphora). *Chemosis* (oedema of the conjunctiva) may be seen in cases of damage and severe inflammation.

Foreign bodies, chiefly chaff and hay seeds, frequently become trapped in the conjunctiva where they cause irritation and corneal damage (Fig. 5.8d). They should always be suspected and searched for when *excessive lachrymation* is seen. The incidence of ocular foreign bodies may reach near epidemic proportions when cattle are eating hay from overhead racks. The presence of sharp foreign bodies often provokes *blepharospasm* and anaesthesia of the cornea and conjunctiva with topical anaesthetic eye drops aids examination and treatment. Foreign bodies may be hidden in folds of conjunctiva and also *behind the third eyelid* which should be carefully lifted with forceps after topical anaesthesia (Fig. 5.8d). Even with care, some foreign bodies may be hard to find and a second search should always be implemented if the first is unsuccessful.

Eyelids – upper and lower

Partial or complete closure of the eyelids may be present in the absence of ocular abnormalities. *Ptosis* (local paralysis) of an upper eyelid may cause it to droop. Unilateral ptosis is seen in cases of Horner's syndrome. In this condition, caused by damage to the cervical sympathetic trunk, miosis (see below) and retraction of the eyeball may also be present. Tight closure of both lids – *blepharospasm* – may occur if a foreign body, corneal ulcer or other painful condition is present.

Third eyelid

The mucous membrane covering the *third eyelid* may be the origin of a *squamous cell carcinoma* which is highly invasive and may rapidly spread to the surrounding tissues including the eyeball (Fig. 5.9c). The third eyelid may flick across the eye in cases of tetanus if the hyperaesthetic animal is stimulated. The third eyelid may also appear more prominent if the eye is sunken or reduced in size.

> ### CLINICIAN'S CHECKLIST – INSPECTION OF THE EYES
>
> Sclera
> Cornea
> Conjunctiva
> Foreign bodies
> Eyelids – upper and lower
> Third eyelid

Internal structures of the eye

These are inspected first visually and then through an ophthalmoscope.

The *anterior chamber of the eye* should be carefully examined. *Hypopyon* – pus and debris in the anterior chamber – is seen occasionally in calves accompanying or following septicaemia (Fig. 5.9a). Infection gaining access to the anterior chamber may result in *damage to and inflammation (iritis) of the iris* as seen in some cases of 'silage eye' caused by listeria or chlamydia (Fig. 5.9d). In *anterior synechia* the inflamed iris may become adherent to the posterior surface of the cornea. In *posterior synechia* the iris is adherent to the anterior surface of the lens. *Cataract* formation (Fig. 5.9b) is seen in some cases of intrauterine infection with bovine virus diarrhoea (BVD). The lens, which is normally supported between the anterior chamber and the vitreous by the ciliary bodies, is sometimes displaced into the anterior chamber. This is usually the result of injury or intraocular infection. The pupil varies greatly in size. In bright light it is constricted and extends as a rectangle laterally across the eye surrounded by the iris. In poor light the dilated pupil assumes a more circular shape. It is also dilated in cases of milk fever. Response to the pupillary light reflex may be com-

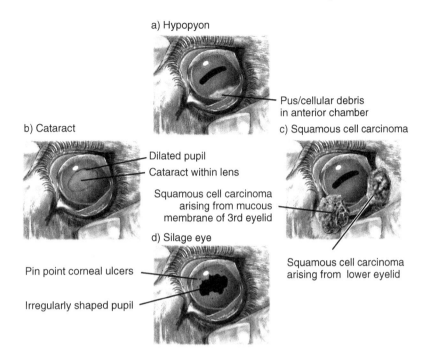

a) Hypopyon

Pus/cellular debris
in anterior chamber

b) Cataract

Dilated pupil
Cataract within lens

c) Squamous cell carcinoma

Squamous cell carcinoma
arising from mucous
membrane of 3rd eyelid

d) Silage eye

Pin point corneal ulcers

Irregularly shaped pupil

Squamous cell carcinoma
arising from lower eyelid

Figure 5.9 Conditions of the eye – 2.

promised in cases of anterior synechia in which the iris is adherent to the lens.

Abnormal pupillary size may be seen in a number of conditions and may involve one or both eyes. *Abnormal dilation* of the pupil (mydriasis) is usually accompanied by absence of the pupillary light reflex. If the animal can see there may be a lesion in the 3rd (oculomotor) cranial nerve. If the animal is blind there may be a problem in the retina or the optic nerve. Retinal damage may be visible through the ophthalmoscope, e.g. in cases of ophthalmitis. Optic nerve damage is seen as papilloedema in some cases of vitamin A deficiency. *Abnormal constriction* of the pupil (miosis) may be seen in cases of organophosphorus poisoning and also in some cases of polioencephalomalacia.

Use of the ophthalmoscope is not normally practised during every routine clinical examination unless there is evidence of eye pathology. Best results are obtained in a well restrained or sedated animal in a darkened area. The ophthalmoscope is held close to the operator's eye with the light source pointing into the ocular fundus of the patient. The instrument is adjusted to the 'O' position and further adjusted as necessary in positive and negative directions to allow visualisation of the entire internal structure of the eye. The *retina* is examined revealing the dorsal bright tapetal fundus and the darker ventral non-tapetal area. The bovine retina (Fig. 5.10) is quite vascular with vessels running in four directions (N, S, E and W) from the optic disc area. The *optic disc* lies slightly medially to the midline at the junction of these retinal areas. *Papilloedema* (oedema of the optic disc) may occur in meningitis and vitamin A deficiency. Absence of normal retinal tissue in some parts of the retina is seen in cases of *coloboma*. In many calves the beautiful, gossamer thin, tubular remnants of the embryological *hyaloid artery* can be seen sweeping up from the optic disc to the cornea (Fig. 5.11).

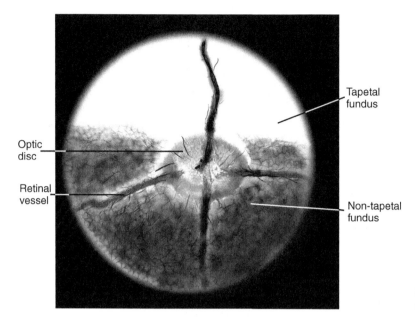

Tapetal
fundus

Optic
disc

Retinal
vessel

Non-tapetal
fundus

Figure 5.10 Fundus of bovine eye as viewed through an ophthalmoscope.

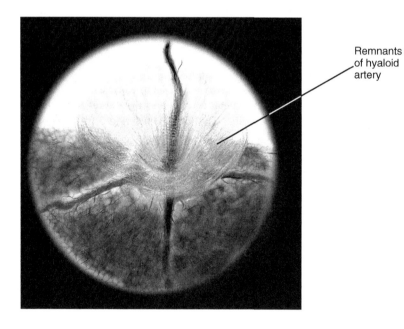

Remnants
of hyaloid
artery

Figure 5.11 Fundus of calf's eye showing remnants of the hyaloid artery.

CLINICIAN'S CHECKLIST – CLOSE INSPECTION OF THE EYE

Anterior chamber
Iris
Lens
Pupil

CLINICIAN'S CHECKLIST – OPHTHALMOSCOPIC EXAMINATION

Retina
Tapetal and non-tapetal fundus
Optic disc
Hyaloid artery remnants

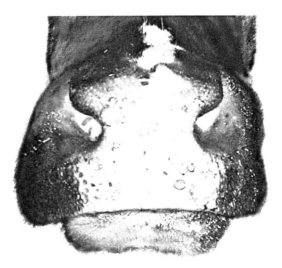

Figure 5.12 Muzzle of heifer showing fading lesions of bovine papular stomatitis. See also Fig. 4.7.

Muzzle and nostrils

The *muzzle or nose* is normally moist with numerous small droplets of fluid being present. A dry nose may be indicative of ill health, especially in pyrexic animals. It may also be found in normal animals which have been resting. The nose may also be very dry in cases of milk fever. A clear mucoidal *nasal discharge* is often seen in normal animals, but a mucopurulent discharge can accompany infection in most parts of the respiratory system. The nose is often dirty in very sick animals. A blood-stained nasal discharge may indicate damage to the nasal mucosa. *Profuse nasal haemorrhage* may be seen as a terminal event in cases of thrombosis of the caudal vena cava. Bovine papular stomatitis is frequently accompanied by the development of small papules, which are often horseshoe shaped, on the muzzle and in the mouth (Fig. 5.12; see also Fig. 4.7).

Air flow through both nostrils should be assessed by holding the hand close to the nose where the pressure of air flow can be appreciated. Air flow should be approximately the same through each nostril and may be reduced by inflammation of the nasal mucosa or by tumour formation within the nasal passages. Further investigation by endoscopy may be necessary to determine where the lesion is and allow a biopsy to

be taken (see below). A foetid odour on the *patient's breath* may be detected in cases of nasal infection and necrosis, pharyngeal infection or pneumonia. The smell of ketones may be detected in cases of ketosis. Chemical detection of ketones in the milk, blood, urine or saliva, may provide a more accurate diagnosis.

CLINICIAN'S CHECKLIST – INSPECTION OF THE MUZZLE AND NOSTRILS

Moist or dry muzzle surface
Nasal discharge – quality and quantity
Air flow through both nostrils
Smell of the breath

Mouth

The *mouth* must be carefully inspected in good light or with the aid of a pen torch. In young animals the mouth can be readily held open by the clinician exerting upward pressure on the hard palate and downward pressure on the diastema. In older animals a gag such as the Drinkwater gag or Young's gag can be used (Fig. 5.13). *Difficulty in opening* the mouth may

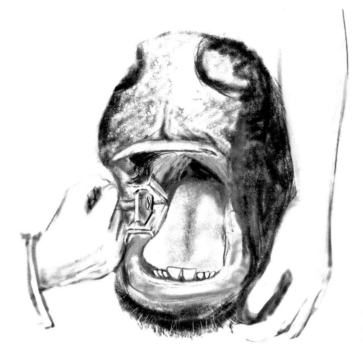

Figure 5.13 Use of Young's gag to open a bullock's mouth. Note the central pair of permanent incisor teeth in this animal aged 1 year 9 months.

be caused by excessive muscular activity such as is seen in *trismus* which may occur in tetanus and sometimes in hypomagnesaemia. Damage to the temperomandibular joint or degenerative changes affecting its articular surfaces may also result in an inability to open the mouth. *Malocclusion* of the upper and lower jaws is seen occasionally as a result of developmental abnormality.

Neurological lesions affecting prehension, mastication and swallowing of food may occur and should be evaluated if difficulty in completing these functions is detected.

Inability to co-ordinate lip movements may occur through damage to the 7th cranial (facial) nerve. This may be unilateral or less commonly bilateral. *Accumulation of food boluses* in the cheeks may also be seen. Facial nerve damage may occur through injury to the nerve and surrounding tissues. It is also seen in some cases of listeriosis (Fig. 5.6).

Inability to move the tongue may arise through damage to the 12th cranial (hypoglossal) nerve. This may be the result of alkaloid toxicity, botulism or in listeriosis.

Inability to swallow may arise through dysfunction of the 9th cranial (glossopharyngeal) nerve and also the 10th cranial (vagus) nerve. Such problems may arise through local damage to nerves by abscess or tumour formation adjacent to the nerves or in the medulla. Damage may also be seen in listeriosis.

All visible areas of the mucosa including the dental pad should be inspected for signs of ulceration or damage. The buccal mucosa which lines the cheeks should be carefully checked – especially in calves – for the presence of *diphtheritic membranes* which are visible adjacent to the cheek teeth in some cases of calf diphtheria (necrotic stomatitis) (Fig. 5.14). A good light is essential for this examination. The buccal mucosa can also be a site for vesicles of foot-and-mouth disease.

The dental pad replaces the incisor teeth in the upper jaw of cattle. It is covered with mucosa but is quite firm and fibrous. In adult cattle it may show small scars sustained when the animal was grazing. It can also be the site for lesions of a number of diseases including bovine papular stomatitis, bovine virus diarrhoea, and foot-and-mouth disease.

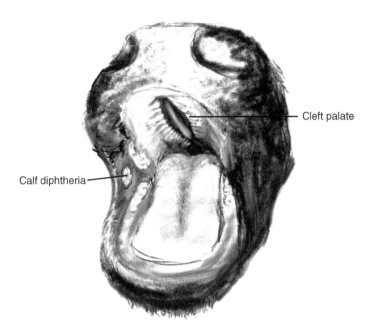

Cleft palate

Calf diphtheria

Figure 5.14 Mouth of calf showing (a) lesions of calf diphtheria (necrotic stomatitis) and also (b) a cleft palate.

The hard palate is checked for congenital abnormality of the cleft palate. Milk may run from the nose when a calf with this defect tries to swallow (Fig. 5.14). The defect may be narrow and small or involve most of the roof of the mouth.

Teeth

The *teeth may be temporary or permanent* and inspection of the incisors will enable the age of the patient to be estimated (Fig. 5.13). Problems with the teeth are unusual but occasionally an incisor tooth is loosened by injury. Abnormal growth, wear and discolouration of the teeth may be seen in *fluorosis*. The cheek

Table 5.1 Bovine dentition

	Incisors	Premolars	Molars	Total teeth
Deciduous teeth				20
Upper jaw	0	3	0	
Lower jaw	4	3	0	
Permanent teeth				32
Upper jaw	0	3	3	
Lower jaw	4	3	3	

teeth can be inspected visually and tapped with a long pair of forceps. *The clinician's hands must **never** be inserted into the bovine mouth beyond the diastema in ungagged animals. The risk of injury to the clinician by the sharp premolar and molar teeth is very high.*

Bovine dentition
The arrangement of teeth in cattle is given in Table 5.1.

Age of eruption of the teeth in cattle
The first and second pair of temporary incisors are usually present at birth, with the third and fourth pair erupting either before birth or in the first 2 weeks of life.

The permanent incisors erupt as follows:

1st (central) pair	21 months
2nd (medial) pair	27 months
3rd (lateral) pair	33 months
4th (corner) pair	39 months

Tongue

The *tongue* is mobile and very muscular in cattle, and attempting to hold it still for examination can be difficult. Observation *without* restraining the tongue provides a good opportunity for assessment of mobility and evaluation of gross appearance. In the gagged animal the tongue can be palpated *in situ* without attempting to pull it forward. The caudal part of the tongue – the dorsum – is thicker than the more anterior part from which it is divided by a small transverse sulcus. Idiopathic *injuries to the tongue* including quite deep cuts are sometimes found on the dorsum of the tongue of young calves. If the tongue is infected or if a foreign body is present a foul odour may be detected in the mouth. In cases of *wooden tongue* caused by *Actinobacillus lignieresii* the tongue is very firm and inflexible to the touch; the animal is unable to advance it through the lips and excessive salivation may be seen. Inability to withdraw the tongue may be associated with damage to the 12th cranial (hypoglossal) nerve or with cerebral damage in areas of the brain which control hypoglossal function. *Paralysis of the tongue* is seen in cases of botulism. *Ulceration of the tongue* is seen in a number of diseases including foot-and-mouth disease (Fig. 5.15), malignant catarrh and mucosal disease.

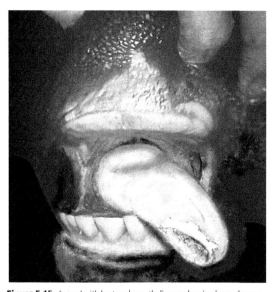

Figure 5.15 Animal with foot-and-mouth disease showing large ulcer on tongue.

CLINICIAN'S CHECKLIST – THE MOUTH

Ability to open the mouth
Ability to prehend, masticate and swallow food
Tongue – movements, texture and mucosal surface
Oral mucosa
Hard palate and dental pad
Teeth

Examination of the internal pharynx and larynx

Examination of the internal pharynx and larynx through the mouth can be achieved by manual palpation in the gagged and carefully restrained animal. A large rigid metal, rubber or plastic tube passed through the gagged mouth will allow a limited view, assisted by a good light, of the pharynx and larynx (Fig. 5.16). A detailed examination can be readily carried out endoscopically – the instrument is passed through the ventral meatus of the nasal passages. Using the *fibreoptic endoscope*, laryngeal function can be closely observed. Advancement of the endoscope allows examination of the *trachea* and *oesophagus*. Patency or obstruction of the oesophagus can be detected using a *nasogastric tube* or probang. The tube can alternatively be passed through the oral cavity, but even in the gagged animal risks being damaged by the sharp edges of the cheek teeth.

Endoscopy of the nasal passages, pharynx, larynx, trachea and oesophagus

Restraint and sedation of the patient
The patient should be placed in a crush with its head restrained by a halter. Sedation is not always necessary but should be used if the animal is at all fractious. Fibreoptic endoscopes are very expensive and easily damaged. They must always be used with caution and the exact whereabouts of the objective part of the instrument checked by frequent observation through the eyepiece. If this is not done the instrument may bend ventrally behind the soft palate before passing into the mouth where it can be seriously damaged by the teeth.

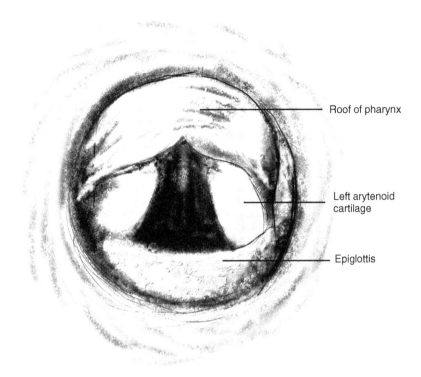

Figure 5.16 Bovine larynx viewed through a wide tube passed through the mouth.

Roof of pharynx

Left arytenoid cartilage

Epiglottis

The endoscope

In adult cattle a 1 metre long endoscope 11 mm in diameter can usually be passed along the ventral meatus of the nasal cavity. In smaller animals a human paediatric endoscope may be needed.

Introduction of the endoscope

Local gel anaesthetic is applied topically to both nostrils. The objective end of the endoscope is introduced quickly past the sensitive nasal mucosa. It is inserted as medially and as ventrally as possible into the ventral meatus. Once within the nasal cavity it appears to cause little discomfort. An assistant passes the endoscope slowly forward as the operator views the visible structures.

Nasal cavity The mucosa of the ventral meatus and the ventral turbinate bone is pink in colour. It may be thickened and inflamed in cases of upper respiratory infection. The endoscope may occasionally impinge on and be obstructed by the ethmoid bone in the caudal part of the nasal passage. If the endoscope is withdrawn slightly and redirected ventrally to the

ethmoid bone it can usually be passed towards the pharynx without difficulty. At other times vision may be obscured by the end of the endoscope making contact with the mucosa at any point during the examination. Slight withdrawal of the endoscope and flushing its end will usually allow its position and surroundings to be ascertained.

Pharynx This appears to be longer and less spacious than that of the horse. Swallowing movements by the patient further reduce the apparent size of the pharynx. The mobile soft palate forms the ventral floor of the nasopharynx and the two small openings of the Eustachian tubes are visible in the dorsolateral walls of the pharynx. Occasionally, signs of traumatic injury may be seen in the pharyngeal walls. The roof of the pharynx may be depressed by enlarged and infected retropharyngeal lymph nodes.

Larynx This may not be visible until the endoscope has passed well into the pharynx. The two arytenoid cartilages are very large in cattle and extend dorsally over the laryngeal aditus partially obscuring it (Fig.

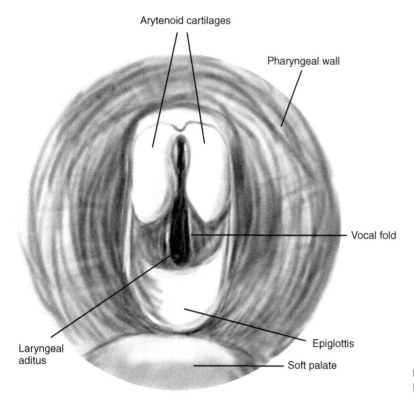

Arytenoid cartilages

Pharyngeal wall

Vocal fold

Laryngeal aditus

Epiglottis

Soft palate

Figure 5.17 Endoscopic view of bovine larynx.

5.17). The epiglottis is visible ventrally except when the animal swallows and the soft palate moves caudally to cover the larynx. The laryngeal aditus is quite small in cattle and the movements of the vocal folds which partially occlude the entrance are subtle. In cases of laryngeal paralysis one or both folds do not move laterally when the animal breaths in. When laryngeal paralysis is associated with *Fusobacterium necrophorum* infection, small quantities of green pus may be seen adhering to the laryngeal cartilages.

Trachea To enter this the endoscope is advanced towards the laryngeal aditus and then further advanced carefully but quite quickly under the arytenoid cartilages and between the vocal folds into the trachea. The trachea appears circular in outline and the inside of the cartilaginous tracheal rings are clearly visible (Fig. 5.18). In normal animals little mucus is present. Large amounts of mucopurulent material may be seen on the ventral floor of the trachea and possibly moving slightly with air flow in animals

with a respiratory infection. The endoscope is advanced further into the trachea. The entrance to the right apical lobe is seen, and further down the coryna is identified at the point where the trachea divides into two main stem bronchi. Just anterior to this point a tracheal wash can be taken using the endoscope.

Eesophagus This is entered from the pharynx by passing the endoscope over the top of the larynx aided by swallowing movements of the patient. The muscular oesophagus has a small lumen in its relaxed state. Folds of mucosa are seen passing longitudinally down towards the rumen (Fig. 5.19). These folds disappear if the oesophagus is inflated by passing air through the endoscope. Distension of the oesophagus by inflation allows better evaluation of the mucosa. The endoscope is gently advanced progressively along the oesophagus and is directed to view the mucosa checking for signs of injury or penetration. Small ulcers may be seen in cases of mucosal disease. In medium sized animals the endoscope can

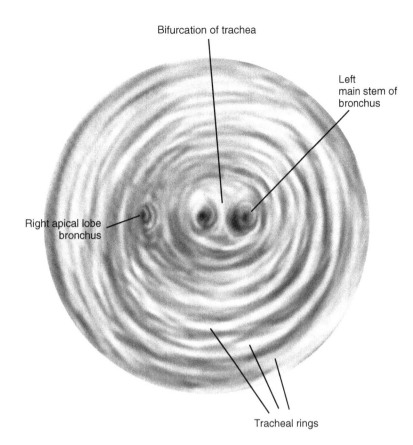

Bifurcation of trachea

Left
main stem of
bronchus

Right apical lobe
bronchus

Tracheal rings

Figure 5.18 Endoscopic view of bovine trachea.

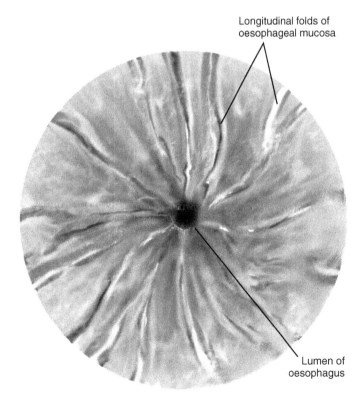

Longitudinal folds of
oesophageal mucosa

Lumen of
oesophagus

Figure 5.19 Endoscopic view of bovine oesophagus.

be advanced as far as the rumenal entrance. It then passes through the muscular cardia allowing green rumenal contents to be seen. Occasionally areas of ulceration may be seen in the distal oesophagus. Neoplasia of the oesophagus, oesophageal groove and rumen wall have been reported in some cases of bracken poisoning in cattle. Such lesions may be seen endoscopically.

CLINICIAN'S CHECKLIST – ENDOSCOPIC EXAMINATION

Nasal mucosa
Pharynx
Larynx – appearance and function
Trachea
Oesophagus
Cardia of rumen

Neck

Mobility

A further check of the neck's mobility can be made if observation of the animal suggested any problems with movement. The neck should bend sufficiently to the left and right to enable the animal to lick its withers, flanks and hind limbs. The head should be flexed and rotated to ensure that the atlanto-occipital and the atlantoaxial joints have normal pain-free movement (Fig. 5.20). Nodding movements are possible using the atlanto-occipital joint, and rotation along the long axis of the neck is possible using the atlanto-axial joint. Both movements are aided by the articulations of the 3rd–8th cervical vertebrae. Poor flexibility may indicate pain in the bones, joints or

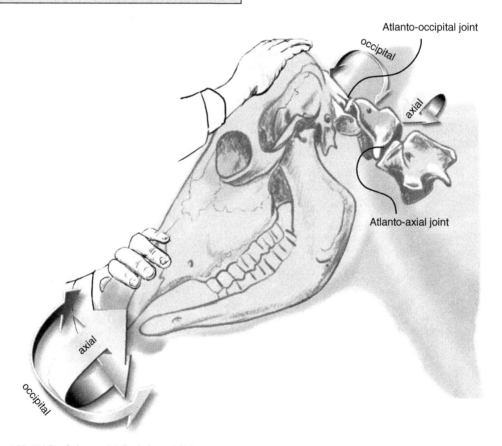

Figure 5.20 Mobility of atlanto-occipital and atlantoaxial joints.

muscles of the neck. Stiffness of the neck with reduced mobility can also be a sign of tetanus.

Swellings and scar tissue

Soft tissue swellings and scar tissue may be present if injections have been given either into the muscles of the neck or subcutaneously. Occasionally, subcutaneous nodules arranged linearly are palpable and are associated with so called 'skin TB' – non-specific *Mycobacterium* infection (Fig. 5.21).

Larynx

The larynx is firm and non-compressible to the touch. If the laryngeal aditus is compromised by infection, gentle external compression may produce vibration or stertor. In cases of severe obstruction, stertorous breathing may be present without palpating the larynx. Auscultation of the larynx and trachea reveals greatly increased sound levels in cases of laryngeal obstruction. Increased referred lung sounds

may also be present in such cases. The greatest intensity of sound is auscultated over the seat of obstruction in the larynx.

Pharyngeal cavity

The pharyngeal cavity lies dorsal to the larynx and can be readily compressed manually unless the retropharyngeal lymph nodes are infected and enlarged. A large pharyngeal foreign body, such as a potato, can sometimes be detected just dorsal to the larynx by external palpation.

Trachea

The trachea is readily identified by palpation of the tracheal rings as it passes down the ventral part of the neck. The trachea is not normally compressible unless some damage to the integrity of the tracheal rings has been sustained. Palpation of the trachea may occasionally provoke a single cough in a normal animal. In cases of upper respiratory infection and

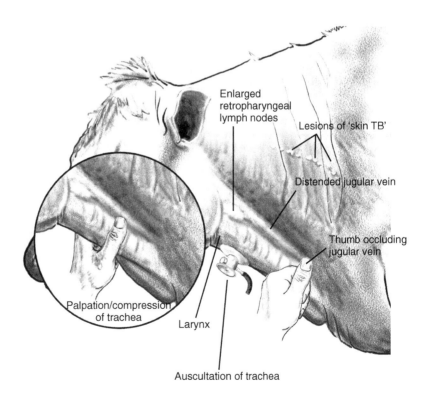

Figure 5.21 Lateral view of neck.

pneumonia gentle palpation of the trachea may produce paroxysmal coughing (Fig. 5.21). Increased tracheal sounds may be heard on auscultation.

Oesophagus

The muscular and softer oesophagus is less readily identified than the trachea as it passes down the ventrolateral neck. In normal animals with fine coats boluses of food can be seen in it passing down to the rumen. Boluses of cud pass up and down during rumenation. Eructation of gas can occasionally be seen and often heard as it passes up into the pharynx. Difficulty in swallowing – *dysphagia* – may occur if there is an inflammatory lesion in the pharynx or if the retropharyngeal lymph nodes are enlarged. The oesophagus may be obstructed by tumour masses in the mediastinum and heart base tumours.

Dilation and malfunction of the distal oesophagus may be caused as a result of malfunction of the 10th cranial (vagus) nerve. *Rupture of the oesophagus* may occur through careless administration of anthelmintic boluses. Dysphagia and local swelling around the injury are seen. Further investigation by endoscopy and contrast radiography can be used to confirm the presence of a penetrating injury.

Jugular vein

The jugular vein is readily visible in the jugular furrow on both sides of the neck. In healthy animals the vein should not be distended unless venous return is obstructed by manual pressure on the vein lower down the neck or in cases of right sided heart failure. For further evaluation see Chapter 6.

Clinical signs and diagnosis of choke in cattle

Obstruction of the oesophagus by a foreign body is termed 'choke' in cattle and usually occurs when cattle are eating unchopped root crops such as carrots and potatoes. The foreign body may lodge anywhere along the length of the oesophagus, but common sites include the pharynx, the thoracic inlet and over the base of the heart.

Initial signs of choke include discomfort, profuse salivation, coughing up of saliva and the development of rumenal bloat. Pharyngeal foreign bodies can sometimes be palpated externally and their presence confirmed by manual palpation of the pharynx with the clinician's hand advanced through the mouth of the gagged animal. Foreign bodies may be palpable within the cervical part of the oesophagus whilst those lower down may be located by careful passage of a stomach tube.

The tube is passed through the ventral meatus of the nose and into the oesophagus (Fig. 5.22). Its passage to the rumen is halted by the foreign body but in some cases it can be carefully pushed on into the rumen. The position of the obstruction can be determined by comparing the length of stomach tube which has passed into the oesophagus to the point of obstruction with the route of the oesophagus pictured outside the animal's body.

CLINICIAN'S CHECKLIST – THE NECK

Mobility
Soft tissue swellings
Larynx – external palpation
Pharynx – external palpation
Retropharyngeal lymph nodes
Trachea – auscultation and compression
Jugular vein – initial assessment

CLINICIAN'S CHECKLIST – CLINICAL SIGNS OF CHOKE IN CATTLE

Exposure to root crops
Unsuccessful attempts to swallow
Profuse salivation
Coughing up saliva
Distension of the rumen
Obstruction palpated in pharynx
Obstruction located by stomach tube

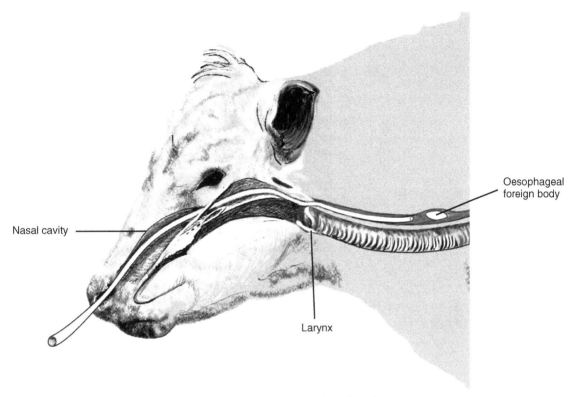

Figure 5.22 Passage of nasogastric tube in a cow to confirm and possibly treat an oesophageal foreign body.

PHYSICAL SIGNS OF DISEASE ASSOCIATED WITH THE HEAD AND NECK

Head
  Carriage
    Abnormal
    Tilt
  Shape
    Domed
  Symmetry and contour
    Abnormal

Salivary gland
  Region swollen
  Salivation excessive

Sinus
  Blow-fly strike

Pain on percussion
Purulent discharge
Unpleasant smell

Skin
  Circumscribed dry crusty lesions
  Fulminating lesions (warts)

Ear
  Drooping (unilateral)
  Purulent discharge
  Skin sunburnt
  Stiff (increased muscle tone)
  Swollen

Injury
Tremor
Deaf

Face
  Loss of sensation
  Paralysis (unilateral)
  Swelling
  Swelling over cheek(s)

Mandibles
  Crepitus/pain/deformation
  Discharging sinus
  Focal swelling
  Malocclusion

(*Continued on p. 50*)

PHYSICAL SIGNS OF DISEASE ASSOCIATED WITH THE HEAD AND NECK CONTINUED

Maxilla
  Shortened

Eye
  Vision
    Blind
  Eye reflexes
    Menace absent
    Palpebral absent
    Pupillary light response abnormal
  Eyelids
    Mass
    Blepharospasm
    Foreign body
    Ptosis
  Tears
    Epiphora
    Excessive
  Eyeball
    Prominent
    Sunken
    Abnormal position
    Nystagmus
  Conjunctiva
    Conjunctivitis
    Pale
    Yellow
    Blue
    Cherry red
    Bright red
    Brown
  Sclera
    Foreign body
    Petechial haemorrhages
    Yellow
  Intraocular pressure
    Increased
    Decreased
  Cornea
    Foreign body
    Oedema
    Keratitis
    Opacity

  Pannus
    Peripheral neovascularisation
    Staphyloma
    Ulceration
  Anterior chamber
    Hypopyon
    Hyphaema
  Pupil
    Abnormal constriction (miosis)
    Abnormal dilatation (mydriasis)
  Iris
    Iritis
    Synechia
  Lens
    Cataract
  Retina
    Incomplete
    Optic disc papilloedema

Muzzle
  Dry
  Papules
  Sunburnt

Nares
  Breath
    Ketones
    Unpleasant smell
    Obstruction of flow
  Nasal discharge
    Unilateral/bilateral
    Serous
    Purulent
    Haemoptysis
    Blood-stained
    Milk
  Mucosa
    Erosions
  Nasolachrymal ducts
    Non-patent

Mouth
  Swallowing

  Dysphagia
  Cough
    Productive
    Non-productive
  Cheeks
    Accumulation of food
    Diphtheritic membranes
  Dental pad
    Papules
    Vesicles
    Erosions
  Hard palate
    Cleft palate
  Teeth
    Missing
    Damaged
    Discoloured
  Tongue
    Flaccid paralysis
    Laceration
    Swollen
    Hard
    Painful
    Vesicles
    Erosions
  Pharynx
    Diphtheritic membranes
    Traumatic penetration
    Foreign body palpable

Neck
  Jugular vein
    Distended
    High pulse
    Slow emptying
    Abnormally warm
    Swollen
    Painful on palpation
  Swellings
    Foreign body palpable
    Soft tissue swellings
  Mobility
    Reduced

Clinical Examination of the Cardiovascular System

Introduction

Cattle are phlegmatic animals and rarely undertake strenuous exercise. As a result, signs of cardiac disease may not be recognised until the disease is at an advanced stage. Cardiac anomalies are not uncommon in calves. Affected calves may show signs of poor growth and, in advanced cases, heart failure. In mild cases there may be no external signs and the cardiovascular abnormality is only detected during a careful clinical examination. In severe and advanced cases of heart disease some external signs of illness, including those of heart failure, may be seen. Animals may lose condition and may show increased respiratory effort in an attempt to compensate for developing hypoxia. Exercise tolerance may be reduced. Specific signs of heart failure are described below.

Much of the cardiovascular system is deep within the body and cannot be directly examined. Abnormalities of cardiac function may be suspected when some specific signs are detected during observation of the patient. Since the cardiovascular and respiratory systems are physiologically interrelated it is important to decide whether either one or both systems are involved in the condition.

Applied anatomy

The heart lies in the anterior part of the thorax between the 3rd and 6th pair of ribs (Fig. 6.1). The base of the heart is situated approximately half way up the thorax. The heart is tilted in a craniocaudal direction in the thorax. The anterior extremity of the base of the heart where the great vessels originate is level with the 3rd rib. The posterior extremity is higher up in the chest and is level with the 5th rib. The apex of the heart is low down in the chest and level with the 6th rib.

Visual inspection and physical examination of the cardiovascular system

As part of the complete clinical examination the patient is inspected to see if there are any gross signs of cardiac disease or cardiac failure. The cardiovascular system is then carefully and methodically examined to determine whether any abnormalities are present. Abnormalities detected during the examination might be contributing to physical signs already present or which might cause signs at a later stage of the disease.

Signs of heart failure

These have been divided into those involving the right and left side of the heart and relate to the physiological functions of that part of cardiac activity.

Right-sided heart failure

The signs of right-sided heart failure are associated with congestion of the peripheral circulation. They include distension of the jugular veins, brisket and submandibular oedema, and less commonly distension of the abdomen by ascites (Fig. 6.2). The hypovolaemia of a failing peripheral circulation may result in reduced renal perfusion and lowered urinary output. Venous congestion in the portal system may result in enlargement of the liver, a reduction in hepatic activity and diarrhoea. Poor exercise tolerance may also be observed, and the animal may appear dull and depressed. Occasionally in cardiovascular disease cases, signs of collapse with temporary loss in consciousness (syncope) may be seen.

Left-sided heart failure

In left-sided heart failure there is increased

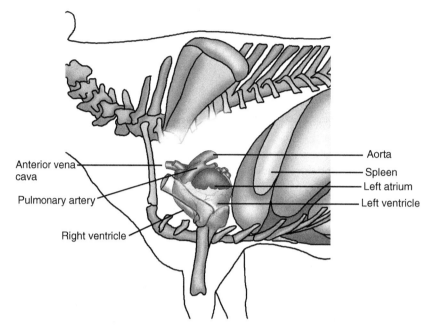

Figure 6.1 Position of the bovine heart and great vessels.

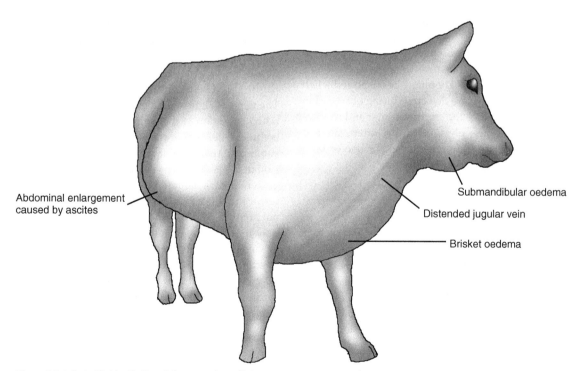

Figure 6.2 Bullock with right-sided heart failure. Note submandibular and brisket oedema, distended jugular vein and ascites.

pulmonary venous pressure causing oedema and decreased elasticity of the lung tissue. Breathing may appear laborious, and the rate and depth of respiration may increase. The animal may have reduced exercise tolerance, there may be cyanosis of the mucous membranes and the animal may occasionally have a cough. In advanced cases both sides of the heart are affected and signs of generalised congestive heart failure including diarrhoea may be evident.

Abnormalities associated with specific cardiac diseases including endocarditis, pericarditis and cardiomyopathy may also be observed. Some specific signs of these conditions are discussed in greater detail below.

Examination of the cardiovascular system

Peripheral pulse

The peripheral pulse may have been taken earlier on in the clinical examination but can be checked again. (See Chapter 2 for the sites at which the pulse may be taken.) The pulse is influenced by many factors and the significance of abnormalities in its rate, rhythm, strength and character must be interpreted with care and in relation to the other clinical findings. If a peripheral pulse cannot be easily and safely detected the pulse rate can be measured during cardiac auscultation. Pulse deficits – noted when the pulse rate is slower than the heart rate – are uncommon in cattle.

Pulse rate   Normal pulse rates are given in Table 6.1. The following terminology is used:

tachycardia – increased heart rate
bradycardia – decreased heart rate

Tachycardia may occur in nervous and stressed animals, and the patient should be allowed time to settle down before the pulse is taken. The pulse rate also rises in pyrexic animals and those which have undergone strenuous exercise or are experiencing pain. It

Table 6.1 Normal pulse rates in cattle

Adult 60–80 beats/min
Calf 100–120 beats/min

also rises when oxygen levels in the body fall or CO_2 levels rise. An increase in pulse frequently accompanies conditions such as cardiac disease, pneumonia and anaemia.

Bradycardia may occur in terminally ill animals and in some cases of vagal indigestion.

Rhythm, strength and character   The rhythm, strength and character of the peripheral pulse should also be assessed.

Irregularities of rhythm – dysrhythmias – are seen in some cases of chronic cardiac disease and also in some cases of metabolic disease such as ketosis. In the latter cases cardiac dysrhythmia returns to normal after the metabolic disease has been resolved. Dysrhythmia is also seen in cases where blood potassium rises, including some cases of calf diarrhoea and in downer cows with ischaemic muscle necrosis.

A hard bounding pulse is recognised by the strength with which it pushes against the clinician's fingers. It indicates a greater stroke volume by the heart. It occurs in response to pain, excitement and resistance to blood flow.

A weak soft pulse can be difficult to detect, especially if the animal is restless. It indicates a reduced cardiac output or a loss of blood volume. This type of pulse may also be seen in terminally ill animals, those with heart failure and following severe blood loss. A weak pulse may also be found in cows suffering from milk fever.

Cold extremities in an animal may suggest poor peripheral blood perfusion.

Ideally *the pulse should be assessed in a number of body locations* to check that it does not vary. The pulse may be affected by local inflammation and be strong in areas close to abscesses. Arterial thrombosis, fibrosis and local oedema can all reduce the strength of the pulse in an affected area.

Colour of mucous membranes

The colour of the mucous membranes should always be observed. Normally salmon pink in colour, the membranes may be cyanotic in cases of terminal heart failure or severe respiratory disease. Pale mucous membranes indicate poor peripheral perfusion. Anaemia may be caused by blood loss or by a failure in the production of blood. It may also develop in some cases of endocarditis and in calves with cardiac anomalies in which red blood cells are destroyed by a turbulence in blood flow. Primary anaemia, not associated with cardiac disease, may also give rise to signs of exercise intolerance, tachycardia and sometimes tachypnoea. Other causes of discolouration of the mucous membranes are discussed under the General Clinical Examination in Chapter 2.

Capillary refill time

This is a measure of effective cardiac function. Digital pressure on an area of non-pigmented mucosa of the lips, dental pad or vulval mucosa causes blanching of the mucous membranes. Colour should return quickly – in less than 2 seconds – after pressure is released. Prolonged capillary refill time of more than 5 seconds is indicative of a poor circulation. It can be caused by cardiovascular disease or by other abnormalities such as dehydration.

Apex beat of the heart

The apex beat of the heart, caused by the apex or point of the heart contacting the chest wall, may be palpable low down in the chest at the level of the 6th rib. The apex beat can often be seen and readily palpated in the new-born calf. Its presence in older animals may indicate a degree of cardiac enlargement.

Jugular pulse

Some pulsation of the jugular vein associated with closure of the left atrioventricular (mitral) valve is normally visible in the lower third of the jugular furrow on both sides of the body. It is associated with atrial systole. Compression of the vein in normal animals should lead to the disappearance of the jugular pulse as the vein empties. Pulsation extending up to the angle of the jaw is abnormal and may suggest incompetence of the tricuspid valve. In such cases compression of the vein does not result in a loss of the jugular pulse. The pulsation may be particularly obvious when the jugular vein is already distended by circulatory failure. If a normal animal's head is lowered – as for example when feeding – pulsation can often be seen throughout the length of the jugular veins. This pulsation disappears when the head is raised and is of no pathological significance. The normal jugular vein looks full when the head is lowered

and the vein is below the level of the heart. *False jugular pulsation* may be observed if pulsation of the carotid artery beneath the vein is displacing it.

Jugular filling

The filling and emptying of the jugular veins are important indicators of the efficiency of the cardiovascular system, especially in terms of venous drainage (return) and the ability of the heart to pump back blood from the peripheral and pulmonary circulations. Distension of the jugular vein can be a sign of right-sided heart failure and should not be present in normal animals. Blocking venous return in the jugular vein by pressing on the vein near the base of the neck causes rapid distension of the vein in a normal animal (Fig. 5.21). The distension should disappear as soon as pressure on the vein is removed. Release of digital pressure on a distended jugular vein does not result in it emptying in cases of congestive heart failure. Distension of the jugular veins may also be observed in animals in which there is a space-occupying lesion at the thoracic inlet. The large *external abdominal veins* ('milk veins') which lie below the level of the heart normally appear full of blood. In dehydrated animals or those suffering from shock the jugular veins may appear flat and empty. Pressure on the lower extremity of the vein may fail to produce any degree of filling.

CLINICIAN'S CHECKLIST – OBSERVATION OF THE CARDIOVASCULAR SYSTEM

Patient's willingness to walk and its exercise tolerance

Presence of rapid breathing – may indicate cardiac or lung disease

Visible cardiac apex beat

Position of the elbows

Brisket and submandibular oedema

Peripheral pulse – rate, rhythm, strength and character

Colour of mucous membranes

Capillary refill time

Presence of jugular pulse

Jugular filling and jugular vein refill time

Consequences of cardiac failure including renal dysfunction and diarrhoea

Auscultation of the heart

This is carried out on both sides of the chest between the 3rd and 6th ribs. As this area is covered by the triceps muscle it helps to pull the patient's foreleg forwards, a movement that may not be tolerated except in small or very quiet animals.

The observations made during auscultation are now described.

Normal heart sounds

Four heart sounds have been described in cattle: S1, S2, S3 and S4. S1 and S2 are normally heard without difficulty, but S3 and S4 may not be readily detected under noisy farm conditions. The events accompanying the normal heart sounds are as follows:

S1 – 'lub': closure of the atrioventricular valves in full systole

S2 – 'dup': closure of the aortic and pulmonary valves at the start of diastole

S3 – a dull thud sometimes audible immediately after S2: the ventricles fill with blood in early diastole

S4 – a soft sound, sometimes heard just before S1, which is associated with atrial contraction

Intensity of heart sounds

The bovine heart should be clearly audible through the stethoscope. In fat, heavily muscled animals the intensity of the heart sounds may be reduced, but in such animals there should be no other signs of heart failure. Pericardial effusion may result in reduction of the audible intensity of the heart sounds and may be accompanied by other signs of cardiac disease such as brisket oedema. Pericardial effusion may occur in early cases of pericarditis and in some cases of endocarditis. Heart sounds are usually equally intense on both sides of the chest, but may be slightly louder on the left side. The heart sounds may be very loud in cases of acute hypomagnesaemia when they may be audible without a stethoscope through the chest wall.

Cardiac rate and rhythm

The pulse of the animal has been taken already. The difficulties of finding a good pulse in a restless or aggressive animal make it important to assess the rate and rhythm of the heart by auscultation. *Bradycardia* is seen in some cases of vagal indigestion; *tachycardia* is seen in a number of clinical conditions including anaemia, fever, terminal heart failure and toxaemia.

Auscultation of the heart valves

The position of the heart valves is shown diagrammatically in Figs 6.3–6.5. In the living animal they can be located within the area bounded by a line drawn

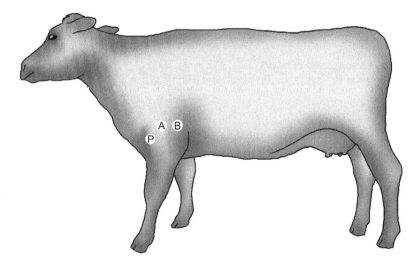

Figure 6.3 Position of the pulmonary (P), aortic (A) and bicuspid or mitral (B) heart valves. The stethoscope is advanced under the triceps muscle to get as close to the valves as possible.

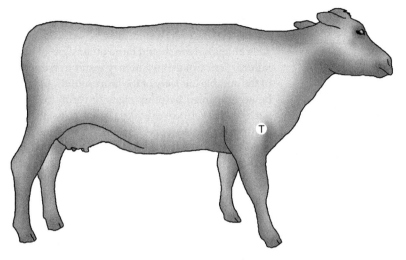

Figure 6.4 Position of the tricuspid (T) heart valve. See also Fig. 6.3.

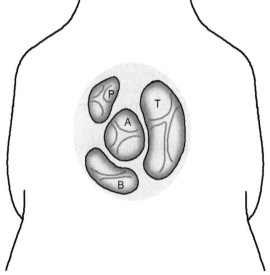

Figure 6.5 Positions of the cardiac valves looking down into the heart from above: P, pulmonary; A, aortic; T, tricuspid; B, bicuspid or mitral valve.

horizontally back from the shoulder joint and a line drawn vertically up from the elbow joint.

Abnormal heart sounds

Adventitious sounds – *cardiac murmurs* – are sounds which are superimposed over the normal heart sounds. They may be so loud that they mask normal heart sounds or so quiet that they are overlooked in a noisy environment. Murmurs are mostly caused by leakage of blood through closed but incompetent valves, or through congenital orifices between the chambers of the heart. Other murmurs are caused by the presence and movement of fluid within the pericardium. It is important to detect, by careful auscultation over a series of cardiac cycles, the nature and location of any cardiac abnormality which is causing the murmur. Small defects can produce quite loud murmurs. Murmurs are most likely to be heard in systole when blood within the heart is under the greatest pressure. It is important to be sure that audible murmurs are arising from the heart and not from the respiratory system. Friction rubs caused by pleural adhesions may be mistaken for abnormal heart sounds. Brief blockage of the nostrils will eliminate respiratory but not cardiac sounds.

Murmurs may be classified according to the part of the cardiac cycle over which they can be heard. A *pansystolic murmur* extends over the whole period of systole. Such a murmur may be heard in cases where there is incompetence of an atrioventricular valve. *Diastolic murmurs* are less common but may be audible, for example, where there is incompetence of the aortic valve: this allows blood to leak back into the heart with a resultant murmur when the valve is closed. In cases of patent ductus arteriosus (PDA) the murmur, which is of varying intensity, extends over the whole cardiac cycle.

In some cases the *audible pitch of the murmur* remains constant, in which case it is called a *plateau murmur.* If the pitch rises it is known as a *crescendo murmur.* If the pitch falls it is known as a *decrescendo murmur.* If it rises and falls it is known as a *crescendo–decrescendo murmur.*

Haemic murmurs may be heard during systole in the region of the tricuspid valve. They are sometimes present in anaemic animals, possibly as a result of cardiac dilation and reduced viscosity of the blood.

In some animals with cardiac defects where the patient is chronically hypoxic an increase in the number of circulating blood cells – *polycythaemia* – occurs as a compensatory mechanism.

Grading of abnormal heart sounds

Murmurs can be graded from 1 to 6 according to their intensity or loudness:

Grade 1 – very quiet, heard only with difficulty
Grade 2 – quiet but easily heard
Grade 3 – equal intensity with the normal heart sounds
Grade 4 – louder than the normal heart sounds
Grade 5 – very loud with a thrill (a vibration) that is palpable through the chest wall
Grade 6 – very loud and audible through a stethoscope held just off the chest wall

Point of maximum intensity (PMI) of a murmur

This point should be located by moving the stethoscope carefully around the area of the chest wall between the 3rd and 6th ribs. Murmurs may be audible on one or both sides of the chest with a PMI on either side.

Description of some common cardiac murmurs

Ventricular septal defect Murmurs are present on both sides of the chest: (i) on the right side a systolic, plateau murmur grade 3 to 6 with PMI over the tricuspid valve; (ii) on the left side a systolic crescendo–decrescendo murmur grade 3 to 6 with PMI over the pulmonary valve.

Patent ductus arteriosus Systolic and diastolic (continuous) murmur, grade 3 to 5 with PMI over the left side of the heart base which waxes and wanes. Sometimes described as a 'machinery murmur'.

Endocarditis Systolic, plateau murmur, grade 2 to 6 with PMI over the tricuspid (most common) or the mitral valve. The clinician may occasionally also hear a diastolic crescendo murmur, grade 1 to 5 with PMI over the aortic valve. The heart sounds may be muffled if a pericardial effusion is present.

Pericarditis Pansystolic tinkling sounds may be heard in early cases when free fluid is present in the pericardial sac. Later the pericardial fluid may solidify with purulent material and fibrin deposits. The murmur – a friction rub – may be quiet, loud or occasionally absent.

CLINICIAN'S CHECKLIST – AUSCULTATION OF THE HEART

Intensity of the heart sounds
Cardiac rate and rhythm
Detection of S1 and S2 (occasionally S3 and S4)
The cardiac valves
Abnormal heart sounds – location, pitch, grade and PMI

Further diagnostic tests

Percussion of the heart

This test can provide a useful indication of the size of the heart and whether it is enlarged. Pulling the foreleg forward helps expose the area for percussion on the chest wall. Cardiac percussion should normally be included with general percussion of the chest, since findings can be influenced by the presence of pulmonary abnormalities. The heart lies beneath the 3rd and 6th ribs on the right and beneath the 3rd and 5th ribs on the left; it extends approximately half way up the ribs on both sides. Percussion around and across this region indicates the area of cardiac dullness. The area may be more obvious on the left than on the right. Any increase in the size of the area of cardiac dullness can be caused by compensatory

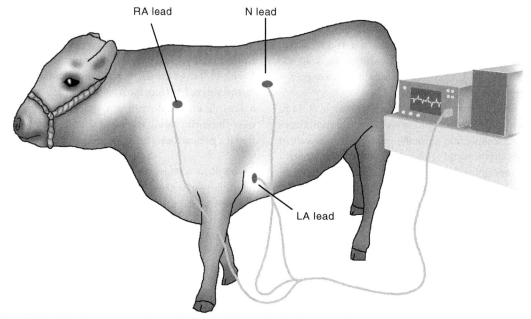

Figure 6.6 Recording a bovine electrocardiograph. The right arm (RA) lead is placed on the neck, the left arm (LA) lead is placed on the chest wall just above the sternum, and the neutral (N) lead is placed on the withers. See also Fig. 6.7.

enlargement of the heart in cases of chronic cardiac disease. It is also increased by the presence of a pericardial effusion. The area of cardiac dullness can be reduced by emphysema in the lungs. In cattle with pneumonia, ventral consolidation of the lungs can make identification of areas of cardiac dullness difficult.

Electrocardiograph

The ECG is of limited value in cattle but can be used to confirm abnormalities of rhythm. The extensive Purkinge network of the bovine heart makes it unlikely that changes in ventricular size can be inferred from an ECG recording. A three-lead system is used (Fig. 6.6) with the right arm (RA) lead attached to the thoracic wall over the base of the heart. The left arm (LA) lead is attached over the cardiac apex and the neutral (N) lead is attached to the skin over the withers. The P and T waves of the ECG trace are usually clearly visible as is the QRS complex (Fig. 6.7). In cases of atrial fibrillation including some animals with gastrointestinal disturbance, the normal P–QRS–T sequence in the trace is not visible. A series

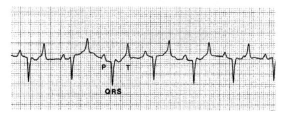

Figure 6.7 ECG from a normal animal recorded using the lead configuration shown in Fig. 6.6. Note the positive P and T waves and the negative QRS complex.

of abnormal F waves replace the P wave, with QRS complexes appearing at random.

Ultrasonographic (US) evaluation

This is useful to detect abnormalities around the heart and some details of its internal structure. Evidence of fluid within the pericardial sac may be seen as a black non-echogenic area surrounding the heart. If the contents of the pericardial sac are purulent, flecks of hyperechogenic material may be seen. The B-mode scanner can also be used to guide a needle

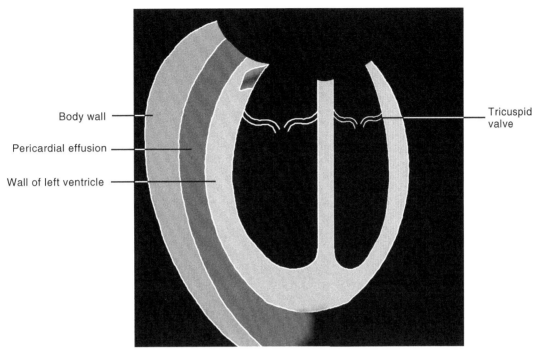

Body wall

Pericardial effusion

Wall of left ventricle

Tricuspid valve

Figure 6.8 Diagram of an ultrasonographic scan of an animal suffering from pericarditis showing the presence of a pericardial effusion.

into the pericardial sac to collect a sample of fluid for analysis. A 3.5 or 5 MHz probe is suitable for examining the heart in calves. For larger cattle, a 2.25 or 3.0 MHz probe, which gives greater penetration, is needed. Access for ultrasonography to the bovine heart may be difficult since in the lower thorax the ribs are wide and the space between them is very narrow. Quite good visualisation of the cardiac chambers can be achieved in calves using a basic linear array scanner. Such scanners can also be used to detect the presence and character of pericardial fluid (Fig. 6.8). Sophisticated but expensive scanners such as the Doppler flow sector scanner produce more information, including the direction and pressure of blood flow. This information is particularly helpful in cases of congenital cardiac abnormality.

Radiography

This is of limited value in assessing bovine cardiac morphology. The size and mass of the bovine heart prevent clear demonstration of the internal divisions of the heart. An outline of the heart can be delineated radiographically giving an approximate measure of size. Radio-opaque foreign bodies (such as wires) may be detected as they pass through the diaphragm from the reticulum to the pericardium.

Pericardiocentesis

This technique is used to collect and assess pericardial fluid. A 12 cm spinal needle of size 16 BWG (1.65 mm) is used. The needle is inserted through the chest wall into the pericardial sac and fluid is allowed to flow or is aspirated using a syringe. Local anaesthetic is injected into the skin and muscle layers of the space between the 5th and 6th ribs. The area is prepared aseptically and the needle with syringe attached is advanced carefully towards the heart. Fluid, which may be very foul smelling if infection is present, is aspirated for cytology, culture and drainage purposes. If ultrasonographic equipment is available the needle may be directed visually. If such equipment is not available care must be taken to avoid penetrating the myocardium with the needle (Fig. 6.9).

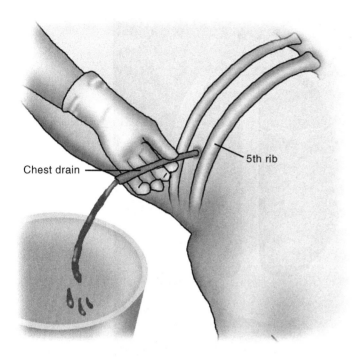

Chest drain

5th rib

Figure 6.9 Pericardiocentesis from an animal suffering from pericarditis. See text for details.

Blood culture

Blood for culture may be taken aseptically from the jugular vein. This can be useful in cases of endocarditis, but repeated samples may be needed as bacterial release from valve lesions may be intermittent.

CLINICIAN'S CHECKLIST – RESULTS OF SPECIAL DIAGNOSTIC TESTS IN SELECTED CASES

Percussion of the heart
ECG evaluation
Ultrasonographic evaluation
Radiography
Pericardiocentesis
Blood culture

Clinical signs of specific cardiac diseases

Endocarditis

Endocarditis usually involves the tricuspid valve in cattle and compromises cardiac function. Less frequently the mitral or the aortic valves may be involved. Valvular regurgitation occurs and cardiac failure follows in most cases. Initial signs may include intermittent pyrexia; later signs are exercise intolerance and thoracic pain. The animal may be anaemic following destruction of red blood cells by the turbulence associated with regurgitation of blood through the affected valve. A grade 2 to 6 systolic plateau murmur may be audible over the tricuspid valve. Heart sounds including the murmur may be slightly muffled in cases where a pericardial effusion is present. The ECG is normal and percussion may reveal evidence of cardiac enlargement. An ultrasonographic scan may demonstrate clear pericardial fluid and evidence of vegetative growths on the affected valve. In advanced cases signs of right-sided heart failure, including a distended jugular vein and brisket oedema, are present.

Pericarditis

This often follows the penetration of the reticulum by a sharp foreign body which passes through the diaphragm into the pericardial sac. Affected animals may lose weight, show a reluctance to move and become pyrexic. The animal often stands with its back arched, elbows abducted and grunts in pain if the withers are pinched or the chest is percussed. Initially a tinkling or 'washing machine' sound which is superimposed on the heart sounds may be audible on auscultation as fluid accumulates in the pericardium. As the case progresses the pericardium becomes filled with septic debris and then adherent to the heart. At this stage the heart sounds may become muffled and the fluid sounds disappear. A friction rub associated with cardiac movement is heard in some cases. As the heart becomes compromised by pericardial constriction, signs of right-sided failure develop. Pericardiocentesis may reveal quantities of foul smelling septic fluid. Ultrasonographic scanning may initially reveal evidence of a fluid filled pericardial sac surrounding the heart. The initially clear fluid is gradually replaced by debris and fibrin tags, and eventually the pericardium appears as a thickened dense layer surrounding the heart (Fig. 6.8).

Inherited cardiomyopathy

Affected animals may die suddenly or show signs of severe right-sided heart failure. Ultrasonographic scanning may show some clear pericardial effusion, and the movements of the heart muscle may appear less extensive than normal. Heart failure may also be seen in cases of white muscle disease and as a complication of foot-and-mouth disease.

Myocarditis

Myocarditis is seldom diagnosed in living cattle. Sudden heart failure in calves suffering from septicaemia may be the result of myocardial infection and compromise.

CLINICIAN'S CHECKLIST – SIGNS OF SPECIFIC CARDIAC DISEASE

Endocarditis
Pericarditis
Cardiomyopathy
Myocarditis

Diseases of the blood vessels

Most of the major blood vessels in cattle are situated deep in the body and are not directly visible. The jugular vein can be readily raised by pressure exerted on it low down in the jugular furrow. In heart failure the vessel is often already distended. Veins can be seen running subcutaneously on the limbs and other parts of the body surface. They are particularly noticeable in short coated animals and in warm weather. The large external abdominal veins ('milk veins') are readily visible in cows as they run subcutaneously forward from the udder on either side of the midline. Each vein passes through the abdominal musculature via a palpable orifice known as the milk well which is anterior and lateral to the umbilicus. Normal veins are readily compressible and can be occluded using digital pressure.

Venous thrombosis

Obstruction of the vein by a clot may follow local infection (*phlebitis*) of the affected vein. It can also follow the insertion of an intravenous catheter or the intravenous injection of an irritant solution such as calcium borogluconate. Venous thrombosis may also follow compression of the vein by a surgical tourniquet. *Thrombosis of the saphenous vein* in the hind limb may occur as a result of the severe pressure exerted on it by the leg lifting strap of a foot care crush. The affected vein may be swollen, warm and painful to the touch, signs which are also seen in phlebitis. Later the vein may become hard and non-compressible. Necrosis of the vein occasionally occurs and sloughing of the dead tissue may be seen. In these cases the necrotic end of the vein protrudes through the skin from which it may be pulled.

Embolus formation

This is another possible complication of venous thrombosis. Sections of the clot break off into the circulation and lodge in capillary beds elsewhere in the body. Sudden, severe and sometimes fatal dyspnoea may be seen in cases of *pulmonary embolism* in which fragments of the thrombus seed into the capillary bed of the lungs.

Local growth of a thrombus

This is also possible and is especially likely in the case of a jugular vein thrombus which develops after prolonged catheterisation of the vein. The thrombus may occlude the vein, often asymptomatically. Portions of the thrombus may break off and, if large, may completely occlude venous return to the heart with sudden fatal consequences.

Thrombosis of the caudal vena cava

This may give rise to specific clinical signs in affected cattle. Liver abscess formation may lead to phlebitis and thrombus formation in the caudal vena cava. Emboli pass to the lungs where they produce abscessation, chronic pneumonia and lesions in the pulmonary arterioles. Arteritis and thromboembolisms develop, and aneurysms (see below) form in the pulmonary artery. In suspected cases a thoracic radiograph may demonstrate abscess formation around the caudal vena cava. Affected cattle may cough frequently sometimes producing blood in their sputum (*haemoptysis*). They show signs of thoracic pain, pallor of the mucous membranes and increased lung sounds. Sudden death may occur in some cases following profuse pulmonary haemorrhage as aneurysms rupture. Large amounts of blood may be seen at the nostrils just before or after death. In milder cases melaena may be seen where blood has been swallowed and has passed through the gastrointestinal system.

Arterial thrombosis

This is uncommon in cattle. Evidence of the condition may be seen in some cases of septicaemia, including salmonellosis in calves. Affected animals may show necrosis of the digit or the ear tips in which arterial thrombosis has resulted in loss of blood supply.

Arterial aneurysm

This is also uncommon but can be a potential cause of sudden death, for example in the pulmonary arteries as a consequence of thrombosis of the caudal vena cava (see above). An *aneurysm in the middle uterine artery* may occasionally be detected during routine rectal examination of cattle. Sometimes the consequence of foetal pressure on the affected blood vessel, the aneurysm may be palpable within the broad ligament of the uterus in the postparturient animal. These aneurysms are often about the size of a hen's egg and arterial pulsation is detected over their entire surface if enclosed in the clinician's hand.

Dissecting aneurysms involving the common carotid artery

These have been reported in cattle. Affected animals showed respiratory distress and swelling in the laryngeal region. Further evaluation of the mass by ultrasonography may aid diagnosis.

CLINICIAN'S CHECKLIST – SIGNS OF BLOOD VESSEL ABNORMALITY

Visual evidence of venous thrombosis especially in the jugular, saphenous and external abdominal veins
Phlebitis
Arterial aneurysm

Blood clotting defects

Such defects should always be considered where blood clotting appears to be abnormal.

Haematoma formation

This is common in cattle. Most cases are the result of trauma (Fig. 4.8), but in rare cases there may be an underlying blood clotting defect. If a blood clotting defect is suspected it should be fully investigated by evaluation of the patient's haematological profile, blood clotting and bleeding times. In cases of platelet deficiency a bone marrow aspirate can be useful to evaluate thrombocyte production.

Diffuse intravascular coagulopathy (DIC)

The possibility of DIC should be considered in seriously ill animals in which unexpected haemorrhage is seen. DIC can occur in a wide variety of circumstances including the presence of endotoxins. Red blood cell damage, thrombocytopenia, reduced fibrinogen and an extended prothrombin time may be found in animals with developing DIC.

Blood clotting defects specific to cattle

A number of specific blood clotting defects have been described in cattle.

Idiopathic thrombocytopenia in calves

This can result in the sudden death of calves as a result of haemorrhage which is usually internal. Other animals may be found with signs of anaemia and evidence of profuse blood loss from the rectum. Petechial haemorrhages may be seen in the mucosae and also the sclera. Multiple bleeding points may be present on the skin, and free blood may be found within joint capsules. The blood profile reveals evidence of severe anaemia with very few platelets. Bone marrow aspirates may reveal very few megakaryocytes which are not producing platelets.

Bone marrow aspirate   This is collected from the sternum in calves and a rib or the ilium in older cattle. The area over the selected bone is prepared aseptically and local anaesthesia is instilled. A heavy duty trocar and cannula approximately 4 cm long is introduced into the marrow cavity using a screwing motion. Advancing the trocar and cannula through the cortical bone encounters considerable resistance which disappears as the marrow cavity is entered. Once in the marrow cavity the trocar is removed and marrow is aspirated through the cannula using a syringe. Harvested marrow is spread on a slide and stained with Giemsa for examination.

Factor XI deficiency

This has been reported in Holstein cattle. Affected animals may show prolonged bleeding from injection sites or after surgical interference. The presence of factor XI can be genetically determined.

CLINICIAN'S CHECKLIST – BLOOD CLOTTING DEFECTS

Visible signs of haemorrhage
General signs of blood loss
Abnormal findings on bone marrow biopsy

PHYSICAL SIGNS OF DISEASE ASSOCIATED WITH THE CARDIOVASCULAR SYSTEM

N.B. Some of these physical signs are also associated with diseases of other body systems and regions.

Posture
  Back arched
  Collapse
  Syncope
  Recumbent

Demeanour
  Dull
  Depressed
  Lethargic
  Reluctant to move

Behaviour
  Grunting
  Bruxism

Condition
  Loss of weight
  Poor growth
  Poor condition
  Exercise tolerance reduced

Appetite
  Depressed

Mucous membranes
  Pale
  Haemorrhages (petechial, echymoses)
  Slow capillary refill time
  Cyanotic

Respiratory signs
  Depth increased
  Effort increased

Rate increased
  Dyspnoea
  Elbow abduction
  Cough
  Thoracic pain
  Haemoptysis

Oedema
  Submandibular
  Intermandibular
  (Ascites)

Heart rate
  Bradycardia
  Tachycardia

Heart rhythm
  Dysrhythmias

Heart intensity
  Sounds loud
  Sounds soft

Abnormal sounds
  Washing machine sounds
  Frictional squeaks (pericardial)
  Tinkling sounds, pansystolic
  Murmur

Murmur
  Diastolic
  Systolic

Murmur: point of maximal intensity
  Right
    Tricuspid/other
  Left
    Mitral/pulmonary/aortic/other

Murmur character
  Pansystolic
  Crescendo–decrescendo
  Plateau

Jugular veins
  Distended
  Abnormally high
  Refill time increased

Veins
  Swollen, warm, painful to touch and necrosis

Arteries
  Focal enlargement

Liver
  Enlargement

Extremities
  Extremities cold
  Necrosis (digits, ears, tail)

Pulse
  Bounding
  Weak, soft
  Missed pulse

Temperature
  Pyrexia

Clotting defects
  Haematomata
  Haemarthrosis
  Frank haemorrhage
  Disseminating intravascular coagulation

Faecal quality and quantity
  Diarrhoea

Clinical Examination of the Respiratory System

Introduction

Respiratory disease is common in cattle. Conditions affecting the respiratory system may be acute, chronic, mild or severe. Some of these conditions are sporadic whereas others may have a high morbidity. The economic losses and the animal welfare implications of respiratory disease associated with pulmonary disease can be severe and should not be underestimated. In particular, pneumonia and lungworm may have a high morbidity and can be clinically severe.

Examination of the upper respiratory tract has been described in Chapter 5. This chapter will focus on the lower respiratory tract.

Applied anatomy

The lower airway is composed of the trachea and the right and left lungs. The lung lobes are shown in Fig. 7.1. The *left lung* is composed of three lobes, the apical (cranial) lobe, the cardiac (middle) lobe and the diaphragmatic (caudal) lobe. The *right lung* is composed of four lobes, the apical (cranial–cranial part) lobe, the intermediate (cranial–caudal part) lobe, the cardiac (middle) lobe and the diaphragmatic (caudal) lobe. The lungs lie within the thorax which is bounded by 13 pairs of ribs, 13 thoracic vertebrae, the sternebrae and the diaphragm. In addition to the lungs, the chest contains the heart, the major blood vessels, the oesophagus, the pleura and the thymus. The topographical relationships of the lungs are shown in Figs 7.2–7.4.

The *thoracic lung fields* in cattle are relatively small and are illustrated in Fig. 7.5; they are triangular in shape with a ventral border, a dorsal border and an anterior border. On the left chest the *ventral border* of the left thoracic lung field extends posteriorly from a point just above the caudal border of the elbow at the 6th costochondral junction. The ventral border is demarcated by an imaginary curving line passing through the middle of the 9th rib to the most proximal part of the 11th intercostal space.

The *dorsal border* extends anteriorly from the 11th intercostal space along a line just below the transverse processes of the thoracic vertebrae to the caudal musculature of the scapula and the triceps muscle. The *anterior border* extends from this point ventrally to the 6th costochondral junction. The right thoracic lung field occupies a comparable position on the right side of the thorax. The internal surface of the diaphragm is convex in shape and extends forward to the level of the 8th rib. There is an additional lung field which is located just in front of the scapula on each side of the thorax. This is called the *prescapular lung field*. The inner thoracic wall is covered by the parietal pleura and the lungs are covered by the visceral pleura. The pleural cavity is the space between them.

Normal breathing

In normal cattle there is relatively little movement of the rib cage during respiration. Some movement of the abdominal muscles is usually seen just behind the rib cage during each inspiration, and this should be symmetrical. The normal respiratory volume in the adult is 3 to 8 litres. In healthy cattle breathing is normally costoabdominal, with a small thoracic component and a small abdominal component. The ratio of the duration of inspiration to expiration in cattle is 1.0:1.2, with a short pause at the end of expiration.

The normal resting respiratory rate in cattle is 15 to 35 breaths per minute and in calves it is 20 to 40 breaths per minute. Counting breaths by observation of rib movements at the costal arch and the flank from a position behind and to one side of the animal is the

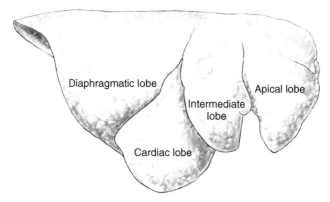

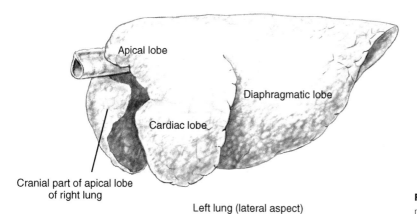

Figure 7.1 Left lung (lateral aspect) and right lung (lateral aspect).

most reliable way to obtain the respiration rate. It is preferable to have the animal in the standing position, as abnormalities can be modified by recumbency and may be missed. On a cold winter's day the respiratory rate can be counted accurately by observing the plume of condensation from the nostrils on expiration.

Conditions causing respiratory disease

Conditions of calves

These may include enzootic pneumonia, infectious bovine rhinotracheitis (IBR), parainfluenza 3 (PI3), respiratory syncytial virus (RSV), bovine viral diarrhoea (BVD), mycoplasmas, *Pasteurella* and foreign body pneumonia.

Conditions of growing cattle

These may include IBR, RSV, lungworm, *Pasteurella* and *Haemophilus*.

Conditions of adult cattle

These may include chronic suppurative pneumonia, caudal vena caval syndrome, tuberculosis, fog fever, diffuse fibrosing alveolitis (bovine farmer's lung), pasteurellosis and lungworm.

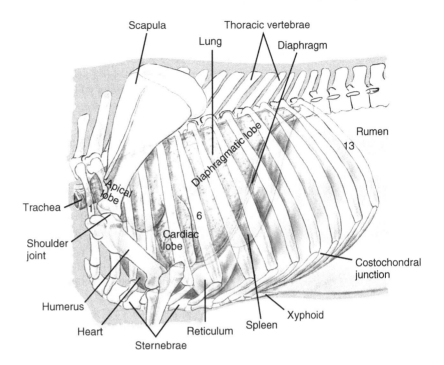

Figure 7.2 Left lung *in situ*.

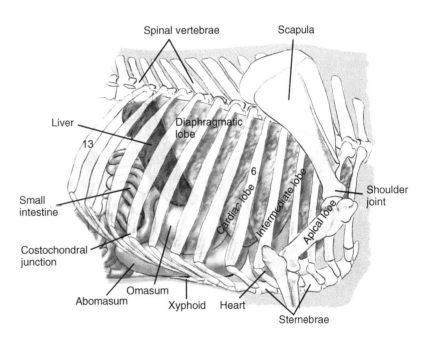

Figure 7.3 Right lung *in situ*.

Manifestations of respiratory disease

The clinical signs seen in respiratory disease are not

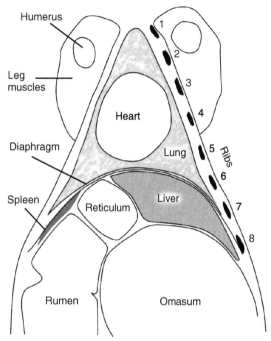

Figure 7.4 Horizontal section of the thorax at the level of the proximal humerus.

all unique to respiratory disease and may be caused by diseases in other body systems and regions.

Severely affected animals adopt a characteristic posture, standing motionless with elbows abducted, neck extended, head lowered and extended with the mouth open and the tongue protruding. This posture maximises the airway diameter and minimises the resistance to air flow. Other clinical signs include depression, frothing at the mouth, increased respiratory rate, mouth breathing, dilation of the nostrils, puffing of the cheeks, purulent nasal discharge, epiphora, roughened staring coat, ears drooping, abdominal breathing, laboured breathing, cyanosis, coughing, recumbency, increased heart rate, dehydration, anorexia, loss of weight, grunting and pyrexia. Some of the *clinical signs observed in pulmonary disease* are illustrated in Fig. 7.6.

History

The prevalence of pneumonia in housed calves and growing cattle is highest in November–December and February–March in the UK. *Farm records* may indicate recent outbreaks of pneumonia, the groups affected, the calf mortality and current treatment regimes.

In the current outbreak the group(s) affected, the signs observed, date of onset, duration, number

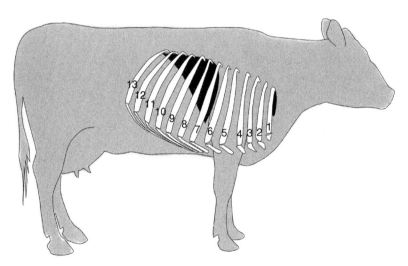

Figure 7.5 Position and extent of the prescapular and thoracic lung fields on the right side.

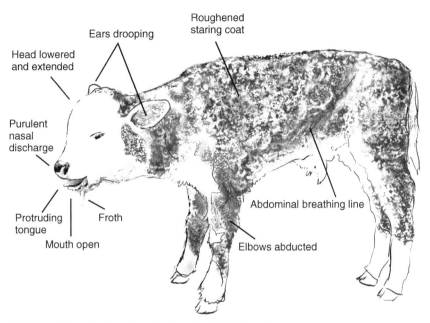

Figure 7.6 Some clinical signs which may be observed in cattle with severe respiratory disease.

affected and number of deaths should be ascertained. The history may suggest the severity and chronicity of the outbreak.

Predisposing risk factors

The presence or absence of predisposing risk factors should be established, some of which are listed below.

Calf pneumonia

Stress – Large diurnal temperature fluctuations, failure of passive transfer, weaning, housing, transport, disbudding, castration

Vaccination – Vaccine(s) used, date administered, age of calf, method of administration and protocol used

Age – Common in housed calves 1 to 4 months of age

Source of infection – Bought-in calves, mixing calves of different ages, common air space, pens in contact

Growing cattle/adult cattle pneumonia

Stress – Large diurnal temperature fluctuations, housing, transport, mixing, markets

Vaccination – Vaccine(s) used, date administered, method of administration and protocol used

Source of infection – Bought-in animals, return from show, common air space, pens in contact

Biosecurity – Non-compliance with protocols

Lungworm – Vaccination and anthelmintic programmes, recurrent problem on farm

Fog fever – Adult cattle grazing with unlimited access in the aftermath of haymaking

Infectious bovine rhinotracheitis (IBR) – A dairy herd in which IBR is present may show reduced milk yield.

Examination of the environment

If the outbreak occurs during the housing period, careful inspection should be made to identify predisposing risk factors. These include poor ventilation, high humidity, overcrowding, poor quality bedding, large groups, common air spaces and mixing animals of different ages.

Observations at a distance

Observations at a distance are very important in respiratory disease to establish which animals in a group may be affected and the severity of the condition. Many respiratory disease clinical signs can be detected by observation. The affected group should first be observed at rest. Severely affected animals are often recumbent with mouth breathing. The amount of coughing and which individuals are coughing should be noted. If the group is being fed, animals slow at rising and not feeding are likely to be ill. Moving slowly towards a recumbent resting group stimulates the animals to stand. Animals slow to rise can be noted and examined in detail. The exercise tolerance of the animals can then be assessed by driving them gently in a circular manner around the house. Affected animals will have more pronounced clinical signs, including coughing and respiratory distress, following exertion.

General clinical examination

This should precede the examination of the respiratory system so that major clinical signs of other body regions and systems can be detected. In some outbreaks all the animals in the group have their temperatures taken to identify grossly normal but pyrexic animals for early treatment.

Abnormal breathing

Abnormal breathing may not be related to pulmonary disease but may be in response to acid/base disorders, cardiovascular disease, excitement, systemic toxaemias, pain, neurological conditions or changes in the oxygen-carrying capacity of the blood.

It is important to observe the rate, depth, character and rhythm of respiration. As a result of hypoxia due to the reduced capacity for pulmonary gaseous exchange, breathing may become laboured (dyspnoeic) with increased thoracic and abdominal wall movements. There may be an increase in the rate of breathing (tachypnoea). This can also occur with excitement, pain and fear, as well as disease.

Increased effort on inspiration may suggest upper airway obstruction. Increased expiratory effort, with the possible accompaniment of a grunt, may indicate severe lower respiratory disease. A reduction in the respiratory rate (oligopnoea) can be caused by a metabolic alkalosis. A complete absence of breathing (apnoea) may occur in meningitis or severe acidosis, and is episodic. An increase in the depth of breathing (hyperpnoea) may accompany pulmonary disease, metabolic acidosis or a toxaemic state. A decrease in the depth of respiration may indicate thoracic or anterior abdominal pain.

Thoracic asymmetry with restricted movements on one side may indicate collapse or consolidation of one lung. Predominantly thoracic breathing may indicate abdominal pain (traumatic reticulitis, perforated abomasal ulcer) or increased abdominal pressure (bloat). Predominantly abdominal breathing may indicate thoracic pain (pleuritis) or severe pulmonary disease (severe pneumonia).

Audible abnormal respiratory sounds

Coughing

This may be non-productive and may indicate tracheal irritation such as in IBR. Alternatively, coughing may be productive resulting in the removal of excess mucous, inflammatory products or foreign material.

Sneezing

Sneezing is not common in cattle but can occur in cases of allergic rhinitis.

Upper airway noise

Stridor heard on inspiration and caused by a reduction in the cross-sectional area of the larynx is sometimes heard in cases of laryngeal calf diphtheria. A louder noise known as *snoring* may be heard with retropharyngeal abscessation causing external pressure on the larynx or upper airway.

Expiratory grunting

This is indicative of thoracic pain and may be heard in cases of severe pneumonia and pleuritis. Inspiratory and expiratory grunting may also occur in severe cases of anterior abdominal pain, e.g. traumatic reticulitis.

Physical examination

Physical examination of the thorax includes *palpation*, *auscultation* and *percussion*.

Palpation

Chest palpation can be useful to identify thoracic pain which may be caused by rib fractures and pleuritis. Gentle pressure should be applied to the thorax using the palm of the hand and the animal observed for a pain response. The entire thorax should be explored in a systematic manner to identify focal areas of pain. In addition to pain, subcutaneous emphysema may be detected as a spongy sensation which may be accompanied by crackling noises. This clinical sign is sometimes seen in outbreaks of respiratory syncytial virus (RSV) and is caused by rupture of emphysematous bullae in the lungs.

Auscultation

A good stethoscope with a phonendoscope diaphragm is necessary to evaluate the breathing sounds and detect abnormal sounds within the chest. It is important to try to *reduce or eliminate background noises*, such as tractor engines or milking machines, which are common on most farms.

During auscultation the stethoscope should be moved systematically to cover the whole of thoracic lung fields with the aim of identifying any abnormal sounds present, their location and their occurrence in relation to the respiratory cycle. The location of an abnormal sound is deduced from the position of maximal intensity. Particular attention should be given to the apical lobe if bacterial pneumonia is suspected, or the diaphragmatic lobe if lungworm is suspected.

Hyperventilation

This can be used to increase the loudness of normal and abnormal sounds which may not be clearly audible on auscultation if the animal is breathing normally. Hyperventilation can be achieved by using a rebreathing bag in small or docile animals. A rebreathing bag can be constructed by securing a long-arm plastic rectal glove over the mouth and nostrils using a large elastic band. The glove is kept in position for 30 to 60 seconds. This is shown in Fig. 7.7.

Normal breathing sounds

These are produced by air movement through the tracheobronchial tree, the intensity of the breath sounds varying directly with airflow velocity. Air movement in the terminal airways is inaudible. Normal breathing sounds are loudest over the base of the trachea and quietest over the diaphragmatic lobes of the lung. The sounds are louder on inspiration, which is an active process, than on expiration which is passive. Thin animals have louder normal breathing sounds on auscultation than fat animals. In healthy cattle at rest the breathing sounds are quiet and can only be heard by auscultation of the chest.

Extraneous sounds

These can be produced by regurgitation, eructation, rumination, muscular tremors, teeth grinding, movement of the animal causing hair rubbing, and by normal and abnormal heart sounds.

Identification and interpretation of abnormal breathing sounds

Referred sounds   Care is required in the interpretation of sounds heard upon auscultation. Sounds may not relate directly to the area of the lung field under the stethoscope but may be referred sounds. Sounds emanating from the larynx can be heard over the chest lung field, and tracheal auscultation must be carried out to rule out referred sound from the upper airway. The point of maximum intensity is greatest over the source of the sound.

Increased loudness of the breathing sounds   This can occur in normal physiological states (e.g. exer-

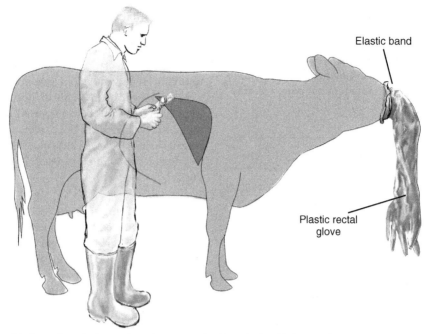

Figure 7.7 Rebreathing bag can be used to increase the respiratory rate and to aid auscultation of the lung sounds.

cise, excitement) or due to pathological states (e.g. pyrexia, pneumonia with lung consolidation). Louder or abnormal sounds are produced by increased air velocity through narrowed airways. Sound is transmitted more efficiently by denser material, and louder breath sounds can be caused by an increase in the density of the tissue through which the sound is being transmitted. Pneumonia with lung consolidation and atelectasis are examples.

Abnormal inspiratory sounds These indicate upper airways abnormalities. In conditions which cause narrowing of the upper airways, such as a retropharyngeal abscess or laryngeal calf diphtheria, abnormal respiratory sounds such as *stridor* may be heard on inspiration. This noise may radiate throughout the trachea and the lung fields. It is produced by an increase in the airflow velocity through the narrowed upper airway. Narrowing of the airway is most pronounced on inspiration because of the lower pressure in the trachea at this stage of the respiratory cycle. During expiration there is a higher positive pressure in the airway which tends to open it up.

Abnormal expiratory sounds These indicate lower airway abnormalities. In conditions which cause narrowing of the lower airways within the thorax, such as bronchopneumonia, the breath sounds are louder during expiration and quieter during inspiration. During inspiration, the diameter of lower airways within the thorax is increased by the outward movement of the chest wall and decreased during expiration by compression of the chest. The airflow velocity is therefore greatest during expiration.

In cattle with tachypnoea and hyperpnoea there is an increase in the airflow velocity on both inspiration and expiration, with an increase in the loudness of both sounds.

Decreased loudness of breath sounds The reasons may be physiological (e.g. a very fat animal) or pathological (e.g. pleural effusion, pneumothorax, space-occupying lesions). These conditions insulate

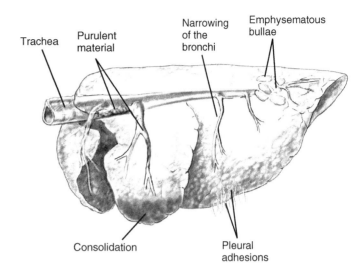

Figure 7.8 Example of lung pathology which may cause abnormal lung sounds.

the sounds produced with a consequent reduction in loudness.

Abnormal lower respiratory sounds   These include clicking, popping or bubbling sounds, crackling sounds, wheezes, pleuritic friction rubs and extraneous noises. *Clicking, popping* or *bubbling sounds* are associated with the presence of exudate and secretions causing pressure fluctuations as the airway becomes blocked and unblocked. *Crackling sounds* are associated with interstitial pulmonary emphysema (RSV, fog fever, husk). *Wheezes* are continuous whistling squeaking sounds due to narrowed airways. *Pleuritic friction rubs* produce a high pitched squeak during the respiratory cycle and indicate adhesions or other pathological changes which increase the friction between the the parietal and visceral pleurae. These changes result in pain during respiratory movements and may be accompanied by grunting. Sometimes it is difficult to distinguish whether the source of the abnormal rubbing sounds is pericardial or pleural. The breathing sounds can be eliminated by covering the nose for 15 seconds which will eliminate the sound if it is pleural in origin but not if it is pericardial. This is very easy to do in calves, but is often impossible in adult cattle.

Some examples of lung pathology which may cause abnormal lung sounds are shown in Fig. 7.8.

Percussion

In percussion the body surface is tapped. *The audible sounds produced vary with the density of the tissue set in vibration.* As with auscultation it is only possible to percuss a portion of the lung region because much of the anterior lung field is covered by the forelimb.

There are *four methods of percussion* available.

(1) *Tapping the thoracic wall with the fingers held slightly flexed.* This method is simple and easy to perform and is illustrated in Fig. 7.9.
(2) *Placing the fingers flat against the chest wall and tapping the fingers with the fingers of the other hand vigorously.* This can be quite painful to the operator, particularly on a cold winter morning.
(3) *Placing a flat oblong piece of plastic such as a plastic ruler (the plexor) flat against the body wall and hitting it with small rubber hammer or spoon (the pleximeter).* This is a useful method, although it may startle the animal at the beginning of the procedure; it is illustrated in Fig. 7.9.
(4) *Transthoracic percussion.* One side of the chest, for example the left side, is repeatedly percussed at a single location over the left dorsal lung field whilst the entire right lung field is systematically auscultated. As the stethoscope is moved over

73

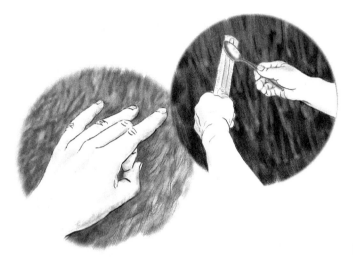

Figure 7.9 Two methods of chest percussion.

the right lung field any changes in resonance of the right lung field will be detected. The sides percussed and auscultated are then reversed This method can be most usefully performed on calves.

To compare the sounds produced from different topographical areas *the strength and position of the percussion must be consistent*. For example, over the thorax either the ribs or the intercostal spaces should be used, but not both, during an examination. Percussion must also be performed systematically, covering the whole of the lung fields of the chest as in auscultation.

The sounds produced on percussion can be classified as resonant, tympanitic and dull. *Resonant sounds* are produced by organs containing air, such as the lungs. Increased resonance may indicate emphysema or a pneumothorax. Reduced resonance may occur in cases of pulmonary oedema. *Tympanitic sounds* are drum-like noises which are produced when an organ containing gas under pressure, such as the rumen, is percussed. *Dull sounds* are emitted by solid structures during percussion. Dull sounds are normal over the heart and liver. However, dull sounds may be caused by disease such as a consolidated lung, or less commonly by pleural effusions or a space-occupying lesion. The most common abnormal finding on percussion is dullness over the cranioventral chest consistent with apical lung lobe consolidation found in some cases of pneumonia.

In the healthy animal there is a gradual decrease in the resonance from the dorsal lung field to the ventral lung field. Percussion over the heart produces dullness and this area is known as the area of *cardiac dullness*. There are important differences in the sounds produced by horizontal percussion of the chest on the left and right sides. As percussion proceeds caudally on the left side there is a sudden transition from the resonant lung field to the *tympanic gas cap of the dorsal sac of the rumen*. On the right side there is a sudden transition from the resonant lung field to an area of dullness over the liver known as the area of *hepatic dullness*.

CLINICIAN'S CHECKLIST – THE RESPIRATORY SYSTEM

History of the farm and patient
Observation at a distance
   Identify the animals affected
      At rest
      Rising
      Feeding
      Exercise tolerance
      Take temperatures of animals in group affected
   Clinical signs observed
General clinical examination
Examination of the respiratory system
   Upper or lower respiratory condition?
   Severity of disease (pathophysiological assessment)
      Breathing abnormalities
      Palpation
      Abnormal breath sounds on auscultation
      Percussion
Further investigations
   Aetiological agent
      Bronchoalveolar lavage (BAL)
      Paired serum samples
      Nasal swabs
      Faeces
      Saliva
      ELISA test for lungworm
   Lesions
      Ultrasonography
      Radiography
   Pathology
      Lung biopsy
      Thoracocentesis
   Pathophysiology
      Pulse oximetry
      Acid/base blood gas analysis

Further investigations

A complete physical examination including auscultation and percussion may be sufficient to characterise respiratory disease. Sometimes additional investigations may be helpful. *The additional costs must be considered carefully.* Bronchoalveolar lavage (BAL) is particularly helpful in cases of calf pneumonia in which the identification of the aetiological agent is required. Further investigations may include serology, nasopharyngeal swabs, sampling for lungworm larvae, fibreoptic endoscopy, radiography, ultrasonography, blood gas analysis, thoracocentesis and lung biopsy.

Bronchoalveolar lavage (BAL)

This is a simple technique and enables a bronchalveolar sample to be obtained which can be used for the rapid identification of viral antigens by indirect fluorescent antibody tests (IFAT), bacteriological culture and cytology. Sampling of severely affected animals should be avoided because of the added stress caused by the procedure. New acute cases are ideal. This technique is usually used when there has been an outbreak of pneumonia with high morbidity and vaccination programmes are being contemplated. In order to obtain an accurate profile of the aetiological agent it is best to select up to five animals for sampling.

Although this technique can be performed through a fibreoptic endoscope, more rudimentary equipment can successfully be used. The equipment required is a 50 ml catheter tip syringe, disposable gloves, a sterile 90 cm long flexible tube of small (6 mm) diameter, 20 ml of warm sterile saline, viral transport medium and topical local anaesthetic gel.

The technique is illustrated in Fig. 7.10. Local anaesthetic gel is applied to the inner surface of a nostril; 2 minutes are allowed for anaesthesia. The distances to the larynx and the base of the neck are both measured and marked on the tube. The tube is gently passed intranasally via the ventral meatus to the larynx. Once the larynx is reached the tube is pushed quickly forwards on inspiration to gain entry to the trachea through the glottis. If successful, breathing will be felt and heard at the end of the tube accompanied by some mild coughing. Getting the tube into the trachea and not the oesophagus may require repeated attempts; if entry to the trachea has not been successful the tube may have to be withdrawn a few centimetres and advanced again. When it is in the trachea, the tube is then advanced to the base of the

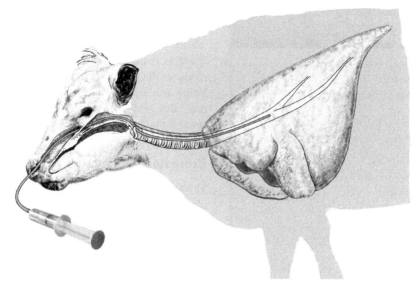

Figure 7.10 Bronchoalveolar lavage.

neck until there is resistance: the tube is now at the bifurcation of the major bronchi (the coryna) of the trachea. The 50 ml catheter syringe containing 20 ml of warm sterile saline is attached to the proximal end of the tube and the saline is injected. Suction is immediately applied to the syringe to withdraw as much of the injected saline as possible. About 10 ml is usually retrieved. Gross examination may reveal cellular debris, suggesting inflammatory changes in the trachea and bronchi, and occasionally lungworm larvae may be observed.

Some of the refluxed saline should then be decanted into the viral transport medium and some placed in a sterile tube for bacterial culture. A further aliquot should be placed in EDTA for cytological examination. Analyses may include IFAT for PI3, RSV, IBR and BVD, and bacterial culture for *Pasteurella* and *Haemophilus*.

A modification to the technique to avoid contamination of the sample by nasopharyngeal commensels is to place a short wider bore 8 mm tube through the ventral meatus to the entrance of the glottis and feed the 6 mm collection tube through the wider bore tube, thus avoiding contamination of the collecting tube.

Diagnosis of lungworm

Lungworm infestation is an important disease affecting all ages of cattle. *Examination of faeces, bronchoalveolar samples and oral saliva samples for larvae may confirm a diagnosis of lungworm.* Exposure to lungworm can also be confirmed by an ELISA test on the patient's serum.

Acute and convalescent sera

Rising serological titres may give a retrospective indication of the possible causal agent(s) of an outbreak of viral pneumonia. Serological samples are taken from five affected animals at the time of the outbreak followed by repeat samples from the same animals 4–6 weeks later. *A rising titre from weaned animals indicates recent antigenic exposure.*

Nasopharyngeal swab

Bronchoalveolar samples are better than nasopharyngeal swabs in identifying the aetiological agents of pneumonia in cattle, although nasophyrangeal swabs have been used successfully to identify PI3 and IBR infections.

Pasteurella isolates may be commensals. Long-handled sterile swabs are used. Swabbing must be vigorous to obtain samples of mucosal cells required for virus isolation. Early clinical cases are preferable. Material for virus analysis from the swabs must be placed in viral transport medium.

Fibreoptic endoscopy

Endoscopy is covered in Chapter 5.

Radiography

Radiography is of limited value, especially in older animals, and in many cases alternative investigative procedures have proved more diagnostic.

In cattle the presence of the heart just anterior to the elbow and the rumen caudal to the diaphragm prevents reliable interpretation of the area of lung overlying or adjacent to these structures. The interstitium of the lungs is normally prominent and is not a sign of interstitial pneumonia.

In the adult animal the increased thickness and size of the thorax result in magnification of the normal and abnormal making interpretation difficult and unreliable. Heavy musculature of the shoulder overlying the thorax restricts diagnostic imaging to the caudal lobe. In addition, powerful radiographic equipment is required and is usually only available in referral centres.

Radiography in calves can be quite rewarding, although to increase the examination of the anterior lobes the forelimbs have to be pulled well forward. Chemical restraint of compromised patients may lead to an unacceptable risk.

Radiography has been used to assist the diagnosis of reticular wires which have penetrated the thorax, fractures of the ribs, lungworm, enzoootic calf pneumonia, diffuse fibrosing alveolitis, pulmonary abscessation, tuberculosis, emphysematous bullae, pneumothorax, pleural effusions and pleural adhesions.

Ultrasonography

This is a non-invasive technique that can provide useful diagnostic information, although some experience is required to interpret the images correctly.

The pleura and pulmonary surfaces of both lung fields can be examined through the intercostal spaces between the 7th and the 11th ribs. Sector transducers are the most useful, but linear transducers are more readily available. The highest resolution is obtained with a high frequency transducer (usually 7.5 MHz) the and the greatest depth of penetration obtained with a low frequency transducer (usually 3.5 MHz). To obtain diagnostic images the hair over the lung field has to be clipped and contact gel applied. Structural changes and changes in lung density such as those found in pneumonia can be detected. Free fluid, although rare in cattle, can be detected. Focal abscesses can be identified.

Blood gas analysis and packed cell volume (PCV)

Blood gas analysis needs to be performed rapidly and is usually only available in referral centres. Hand-held cow side machines are available but are expensive.

Blood gas analysis can be helpful in defining the severity of an hypoxia or characterising acid/base disorders. Arterial samples are the most useful, and the auricular artery or coccygeal artery are usually used.

The percentage oxygen saturation of arterial heamaglobin can be measured using a pulse oximeter. Oxyhaemaglobin and deoxyhaemaglobin differ in their absorption of red and infrared light. Pulse oximeters measure the absorption of red and infrared light in non-pigmented skin. The degree of light absorption is a function of the saturation of the arterial haemaglobin. Pulse oximeters with protective sheaths to block out extraneous light sources have been used in calves. The sensors were attached to shaved non-pigmented skin of the tail, the non-pigmented areas of the scrotum or the vulva. Pulse oximeters are portable, non-invasive, easy to use, inexpensive and can be used with success in field conditions.

Evidence of polycythaemia from an elevated PCV may indicate chronic hypoxia.

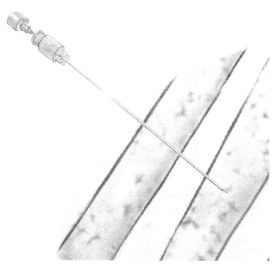

Figure 7.11 Thoracocentesis: lumbar spinal needle penetrating the thoracic wall.

Thoracocentesis (Fig. 7.11)

This technique is rarely performed in cattle as accumulation of large amounts of fluid in the pleural cavity is rare in cattle.

Samples of fluid from the pleural cavity can be obtained by inserting a spinal needle or a catheter into the pleural cavity under local anaesthesia via an intercostal space using strict asepsis. Guidance with ultrasound is useful but not essential. Without ultrasound it is best to select a ventral site caudal to the heart.

Equipment required includes hair clippers, an 18 BWG (1.20 mm) 9 cm lumbar spinal needle, skin disinfectant, alcohol, swabs, EDTA tube and plain tube.

The side of the thorax to be sampled is selected by auscultation and percussion. The distal 5th intercostal space within the lung field is the site of choice as it is the most ventral accessible point of the pleural cavity. However, care is needed to avoid cardiac puncture, and ultrasound guidance is recommended. In the absence of ultrasound guidance the preferred site is the 6th or 7th intercostal space within the ventral border of the lung field.

Whichever site is used, the area is clipped and surgically prepared. Sedation and local anaesthesia may be required. Local anaesthesia is achieved by using 1–2 ml of lignocaine 2% subcutaneously and intramuscularly. An 18 BWG (1.20 mm) 9 cm spinal needle with stylet is used. The needle is pushed carefully through the skin and intercostal muscles into the pleural cavity at the prepared site. The stylet is then removed and a syringe attached and negative pressure applied to assist the withdrawal of any pleural fluid. Care is required to avoid cardiac puncture if the 5th intercostal space is used. Any sample obtained should be examined grossly for abnormalities and samples collected in a plain tube for bacteriology and into EDTA for cytology.

Lung biopsy (Fig. 7.12)

Lung biopsies may be useful to identify pathological changes within the lung but should be reserved for cases of respiratory disease in which less invasive techniques have failed to establish a diagnosis.

A limitation to this technique is that the area of the lung lobe biopsied may not contain abnormalities found elsewhere in the lung. It is a technique that is of most value in conditions that are generalised throughout the pulmonary system. In addition, the dangers of fatal haemorrhage in animals with pulmonary hypertension and the formation of pneumothorax should be carefully considered. However, percutaneous lung biopsy has been used safely in cattle using a Tru-cut needle.

Equipment required may include 10% buffered formalin, surgical scrub, alcohol, lignocaine 2%, needles and syringes, a Tru-cut biopsy needle, sterile disposable gloves, antibiotics and tetanus antitoxin.

The biopsy can be performed in the standing animal or in the sedated animal in lateral recumbency. Common sites for the biopsy are the 6th, 7th, 8th or 9th intercostal space in the mid-lung field. The hair is shaved or clipped over the proposed site and the site aseptically prepared. 1–2 ml of lignocaine 2% local anaesthetic is injected subcutaneously and then a further 1–2 ml of lignocaine 2% is injected intramuscularly slightly more caudally into the intercostal muscles. A cutaneous stab incision is made with a scalpel blade into the anaesthetised skin. The skin is then moved caudally and the Tru-cut needle thrust through the cutaneous stab incision and through the intercostal muscles and pleura into the stroma of the

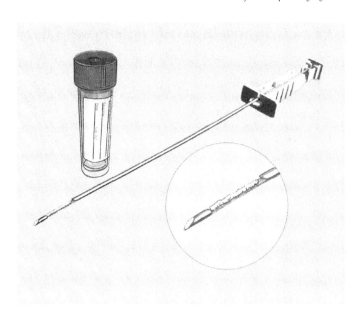

Figure 7.12 Lung biopsy: a Tru-cut needle with a liver sample.

lung lobe. This ensures that the skin incision will not directly overlie the deeper wound and helps to minimise the possibility of pneumothorax. The cutting stylet of the Tru-cut needle is then advanced to cut the sample and the cover is advanced over the cutting stylet to retain the biopsy sample. The Tru-cut needle is then removed. The biopsy is placed in 10% formal-saline and submitted for histopathology analysis. Consideration should be given to prophylactic antibiosis and tetanus antitoxin administration.

PHYSICAL SIGNS OF DISEASE ASSOCIATED WITH THE RESPIRATORY SYSTEM

N.B. Some of the signs may be encountered in diseases of other systems and regions.

General condition
    Staring coat
    Loss of weight

Milk yield
    Decreased

Appetite
    Decreased
    Absent

Demeanour
    Depression
    Dull

Posture
    Recumbent
    Elbows abducted
    Slow to rise
    Neck extended
    Head lowered
    Head extended
    Ears drooping

Breathing
    Laboured breathing/increased effort
    Shallow breathing
    Increased depth of breathing

(Continued on p. 80)

PHYSICAL SIGNS OF DISEASE ASSOCIATED WITH THE RESPIRATORY SYSTEM CONTINUED

Absence of breathing
Thoracic asymmetry during breathing
Predominantly thoracic breathing
Predominantly abdominal breathing

Audible sounds
  Coughing
    Productive
    Non-productive
  Grunt

Respiratory rate
  Increased
  Decreased

Temperature
  Increased

Heart rate
  Increased

Mucous membranes
  Pale
  Cyanotic

Hydration status
  Dehydrated

Eyes
  Ocular discharge
    Serous
    Purulent
    Unilateral/bilateral
  Epiphora
  Sunken

Nares
  Nasal discharge
    Serous

Purulent
Unilateral/bilateral
Haemoptysis
Dilated

Nasal mucosa
  Inflamed
  Ulcerated

Mouth
  Tongue protruded
  Mouth breathing
  Frothing

Cheeks
  Puffed out

Chest palpation
  Pain
  Subcutaneous emphysema

Upper respiratory sounds
  Snoring
  Stridor

Lower respiratory sounds (auscultation)
  Increased loudness of breath sounds
  Decreased loudness of breath sounds
  Increased inspiratory sounds
  Increased expiratory sounds
  Clicking, popping, bubbling
  Crackles
  Wheezes
  Pleuritic friction rubs
  Grunts

Percussion
  Abnormal thoracic areas of dullness

Clinical Examination of the Gastrointestinal System

This chapter describes the clinical examination of the gastrointestinal system, the peritoneum, the umbilicus and the liver. Examination of the mouth, pharynx and oesophagus is decribed in Chapter 5. Examination of the adult and calf are described separately.

Applied anatomy

The gastrointestinal system within the abdomen is composed of the forestomachs, the small intestine and the large intestine. The forestomachs are composed of the reticulum, rumen, omasum and abomasum. These structures are shown in Fig. 8.1. The development of the newborn calf from a functional monogastric animal to a ruminant is illustrated by the increase in volume of the rumen relative to the abomasum with age as shown in Table 8.1. The adult pattern of ruminal movement is established between 6 and 8 weeks of age. The oesophageal groove crosses the reticulum and when closed forms a tube which enables ingesta to bypass the rumen. The forestomachs in adult cattle have a volume in the region of 150 litres with the relative proportions being rumen 70 to 80%, reticulum 5%, omasum 8% and the abomasum 7 to 15%. In the normal adult the rumen fluid has a pH of 5.5 to 7.0 depending upon the diet. Cattle fed high levels of concentrates will have a lower pH than animals fed on a roughage diet. The abomasum has a normal pH range of 2.0 to 4.0. The small intestine is composed of the duodenum, the jejunum and the ileum. It enters the large intestine at the ileocaecocolic junction. The large intestine is composed of the caecum, colon (ascending, spiral and descending) and rectum. Other structures in the abdomen are the lesser omentum, greater omentum, liver, spleen and urogenital system.

The rumen and reticulum after feeding occupy the entire left part of the abdominal cavity, extending from the diaphragm at about the 7th rib to the pelvis.

The reticulum lies medial to the 6th to 8th ribs on the left side with the anterior wall at about the level of the elbow. The spleen lies on the anteriolateral aspect of the left side of the rumen beneath the last four ribs; this is shown in Fig. 8.2. The omasum lies in the lower part of the right anterior abdomen between the reticulum and anterior rumen to the left and the liver on the right, opposite ribs 7 to 11. The abomasum lies largely on the abdominal floor at about the midline or just to the right side, with the pylorus at about the level of the ventral end of the 11th or 12th rib. The liver is situated on the right side of the anterior abdomen against the diaphragm opposite the upper part of the last three ribs. The rest of the right side of the abdomen is occupied by the small and large intestines within the omentum. These structures are shown in Fig. 8.3. The left kidney is displaced by the rumen to the right side of the sublumbar region beneath the 3rd to 5th lumbar vertebrae. The right kidney is anterior to the left and lies ventral to the last rib and first two lumbar transverse processes, with the anterior pole surrounded by the liver.

Normal behaviour and physiology

In calves, a balanced diet regarding the quantitiy and quality of fibre and concentrate is required to ensure normal anatomical and functional development of the rumen. Proliferation of the mucosal tissue and ruminal pupillae is dependent upon the production of butyric acid and to a lesser extent propionic acid. Roughage stimulates the growth in volume of the reticulum and rumen and the development of the muscle layers. Incorrect diet can result in a dysfunctional rumen.

Adult cattle ruminate for a total of 8 hours daily: there are between four and 24 ruminating periods, with each period lasting 10 to 60 minutes. There are 360 to 790 regurgitated boluses produced a day with

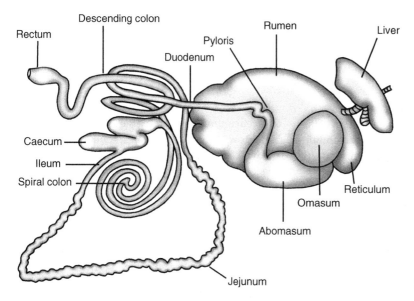

Rectum

Descending colon

Duodenum

Pyloris

Rumen

Liver

Caecum

Ileum

Spiral colon

Reticulum

Omasum

Abomasum

Jejunum

Figure 8.1 The gastrointestinal tract.

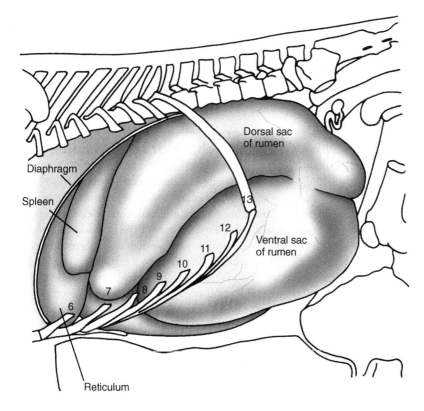

Dorsal sac
of rumen

Diaphragm

Spleen

Ventral sac
of rumen

Reticulum

Figure 8.2 Abdominal viscera *in situ*.
Left lateral view.

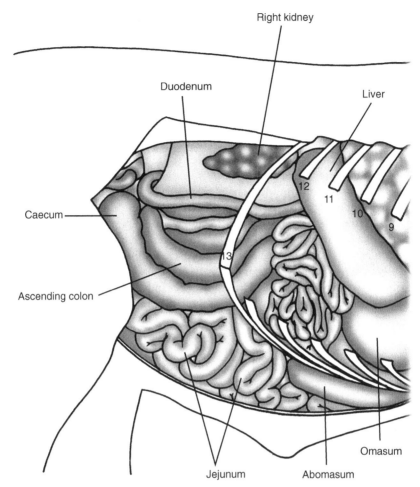

Figure 8.3 Abdominal viscera *in situ*. Right lateral view with the greater omentum removed.

Table 8.1 The ratio of the rumen volume to abomasal volume with age

Age	Rumen	Abomasum
4 weeks	0.5	1.0
8 weeks	1.0	1.0
12 weeks	2.0	1.0
Adult	9.0	1.0

each weighing 80 to 120 g. The boluses are chewed 40 to 70 times over a period of 60 seconds. Rumenal fermentation may produce up to 600 litres of gas a day which is removed by eructation. On a hay diet there may be 15 to 20 eructations an hour, whilst on a grass diet this increases to 60 to 90 eructations an hour.

Adult cattle defaecate 10 to 24 times daily, producing 30 to 50 kg of faeces. The passage time of faeces is 1.5 to 4 days. Cattle generally pass some faeces every 1.5 to 2.0 hours, and an absence of faeces for 24 hours is abnormal.

Rumen movements are controlled by the vagus nerve and have four functions: mixing ingesta, moving ingesta, eructation and regurgitation for rumination. Functionally, rumen movements can be classified into primary (A) cycles, secondary (B) cycles and regurgitation movements. The primary (A) cycle mixes the ingesta within the rumen and occurs every 1 to 2 minutes. The A cycle begins with a diphasic contraction of the reticulum followed by a monophasic contraction of the dorsal sac and then the ventral sac. This results in mixing of reticular-rumen contents and assists the passage of the rumen contents into the omasum. The B cycle results in eructation and occurs at intervals of 1 to 2 minutes. Movement is confined to the rumen and consists of a rumen dorsal wall contraction followed by a contraction of the ventral sac. This movement causes gas to be displaced from the dorsal sac of the rumen to the cardia and eructated. Eructation contractions are independent of the mixing contractions and their rate is dependent upon the pressure of the gas in the rumen. Regurgitation results from an additional ruminal contraction interposed between normal mixing movements of the rumen. Ruminal movements keep the oesophageal cardia flooded with reticular fluid. A voluntary inspiratory effort is made with the glottis closed, the negative pressure of the thorax is greatly increased and the reticular fluid carrying some floating ingesta is carried up to the pharynx.

Conditions occurring in adult cattle

Reticulum – actinobacillosis/actinomycosis infection of the oesophageal groove, neoplasia of the oesophageal groove, reticular abscess, reticuloperitonitis

Rumen – secondary free gas bloat, frothy bloat, ruminal acidosis, cold water ruminal atony, neoplasia of rumen, rumen collapse syndrome, rumen foreign body, rumen impaction, vagal indigestion

Omasum – omasal impaction

Abomasum – right abomasal dilatation (RDA) and torsion, abomasal rupture, left abomasal displacement (LDA), abomasal impaction (dietary), abomasal ulceration, abomasal neoplasia

Small intestine – Johne's disease, salmonellosis, winter dysentery, bovine virus diarrhoea, gut tie (intestinal strangulation), foreign body intestinal obstruction, intussusception, neoplasia of small intestine, prolapse of the intestines through the mesentery, torsion of the root of the mesentery, small intestine rupture post calving, spasmodic colic

Large intestine – caecal dilatation and torsion

Rectum – rectal perforation, rectal prolapse

Abdomen/peritoneum – ascites, uroperitonium, fat necrosis, focal or diffuse peritonitis, acute pnemoperitonium

Liver – abscessation, hepatitis, cholangitis.

History

Vaccination and anthelmintic protocols may be related to the current problem. The farm or practice records may indicate a recurrent problem. Recent outbreaks of disease such as salmonellosis may be ongoing. Some diseases may be endemic, such as Johne's disease. Some conditions are diet related, and recent changes in diet or management may be implicated. Inappropriate nutrition may be the cause of pot bellied calves. Onset of disease may be related to the introductions of new replacement stock or heifers joining the milking herd. In this regard biosecurity protocols should be reviewed. The group affected should be etablished. The time of onset, the duration, number affected and the severity and the signs of disease observed. Sudden changes in condition scores, sudden drop in milk yield, or a reduction in apppetite and food consumption, may be disease indicators. Calving date and stage of lactation may be significant. Left displacement of the abomasum is most commonly diagnosed in the the first 3 weeks post-calving in dairy cows. Poor management practices around calving time may result in colostrum deprivation, with a high incidence of neonatal diarrhoea and umbilical infections.

Signalment

Many gastrointestinal conditions are age related. *Mycobacterium johnei* causes clinical (Johne's) disease in older adult cattle, whereas rotavirus may cause diarrhoea in calves. The class of animal and the production level may be disease associated. High-yielding dairy cows have an increased incidence of primary ketosis.

Examination of the environment

Sudden access to legume-rich pastures may result in frothy bloat. Breaking into maize fields, food stores or orchards may be related to an outbreak of ruminal acidosis.

Mouldy feed may contain mycotoxins. Overcrowding and floor feeeding are associated with outbreaks of coccidiosis in growing animals.

Observations at a distance

Behavioural manifestations of abdominal pain include kicking at the abdomen, reluctance to get up and down, and movements made with care. Grunting may be audible. Animals may adopt abnormal postures such as lowering the back and stretching the forelegs forwards and the hind legs backwards. This is called the rocking horse posture and is seen with intussception. Grinding of teeth or bruxism may be observed. The animal may appear depressed. Straining in attempts to defaecate (rectal tenesmus) may be apparent and can be confused with urinary tenesmus. The rate of eructation, regurgitation and cudding may be reduced. In chronic conditions there may be a low body condition score and loss of weight. Dropping of the cud may indicate pathology of the cardia. Ruminal tympany may cause dyspnoea. Sunken eyes may indicate dehydration or cachexia. An increased respiratory rate may indicate compensation of a metabolic acidosis. Recumbency may occur due to weakness or pain. Appetite may be reduced or there may be anorexia. There may be a reduction in the quantity and a change in the composition of the faeces. The production and passage of faeces may be confirmed by defaecation or the presence of faeces on the floor. Jaundice may be observed in non-pigmented areas of the skin such as the udder, and neurological signs may be present in hepatic encephalopathy.

Distension and changes in the silhouette of the abdomen may be caused by distension of the rumen, distension or displacement of the abomasum, distension of the intestines, uterine enlargement, or fluid accumulations within the peritoneum. Expansion of the rumen can be caused by free gas bloat, frothy bloat and excessive fibre fill. Displacement and distension of the abomasum may be caused by right side abomasal dilatation, displacement and torsion. Distension of the intestines may be caused by caecal dilatation and/or torsion and torsion of the greater mesentery. Enlargement of the uterus occurs in normal pregnancy and hydrops amnion/allantois. Fluid accumulation in the peritoneal cavity may be caused by ascites in congestive heart failure or urine from a ruptured bladder.

Observations of the abdominal silhouette should be made from a distance of several metres from behind the animal to get an overall impression of its shape. Viewing each side from an oblique angle can be useful to highlight changes in the lateral contours. The abdomen should be approximately symmetrical, having a pear shape when viewed from behind (Fig. 8.4). Regional changes can assist in identifying the organ affected and the underlying condition. For observational purposes the abdomen can be split into four quadrants, left dorsal, left ventral, right dorsal and right ventral. Abnormalities of contour within each quadrant should be noted. In some conditions the changes can be very subtle and further confirmation of the diagnosis will be required. The left costal arch is sometimes 'sprung' or pushed outwards by a left displaced abomasum. Great care is required to detect this minor change in abdominal silhouette. Profound changes are more easily recognised. Animals suffering from ruminal bloat have a distended left dorsal quadrant (Fig. 8.5). Right-sided abomasal dilatation causes a distension of the right dorsal quadrant. Pneumoperitoneum may cause bulging of the left and right dorsal quadrants (Fig. 8.6) Cattle with vagal indigestion will develop distension of the left dorsal quadrant and the right ventral quadrant. This has been called a 'ten to four' or a 'papple' profile. The papple shape refers to the pear shaped contour on the right side and an apple shaped contour on the left (Fig. 8.7). Hydrops uteri and accummulations of fluid in the peritoneum can cause gross distension of the right and left ventral quadrants (Fig. 8.8). Bulging of the right ventral quadrant, and to a lesser extent the left ventral quadrant, occurs in late pregnancy in the normal animal.

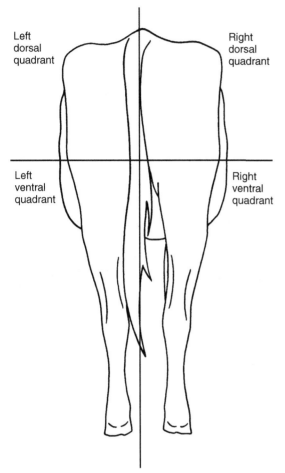

Figure 8.4 Normal silhouette of the lateral contours of the abdomen. Posterior view.

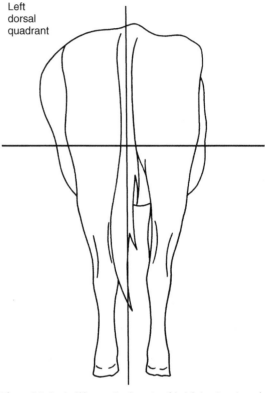

Figure 8.5 Ruminal bloat causing distention of the left dorsal quadrant of the abdomen. Posterior view.

Physical examination

Examination of the left abdomen

Examination of the left side of the abdomen is primarily concerned with the assessment of the rumen and reticulum and to check for evidence of a left displaced abomasum.

Rumen and reticulum

The rumen can be palpated through the abdominal wall at the left sublumbar fossa. An impression can be obtained of the size and fullness of the rumen. In the normal animal the contents of the upper part of the rumen have a doughy consistency, but digital pressure should not leave a lasting impression once palpation ceases. In vagal indigestion there may be rumen overfill with fibre and an impression of a fist pushed into the sublumbar fossa will remain follow-

---

CLINICIAN'S CHECKLIST – OBSERVATIONS AT A DISTANCE

Signs of abdominal pain
Posture
Systemic signs associated with conditions of the abdomen
Body condition
Passage of faeces or faecal staining
Lateral abdominal silhouette
    Left dorsal quadrant
    Left ventral quadrant
    Right dorsal quadrant
    Right ventral quadrant
Ventral abdominal silhouette

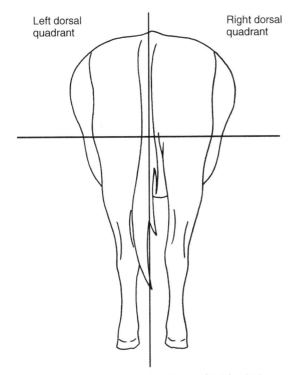

Figure 8.6 Pneumoperitoneum causing distention of the left and right dorsal quadrants of the abdomen. Posterior view.

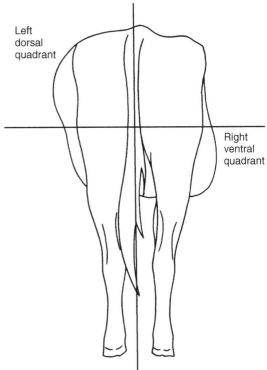

Figure 8.7 Vagal indigestion causing distention of the left dorsal and right ventral quadrants of the abdomen. Posterior view.

ing withdrawal. The rumen is much reduced in size but never empties completely in inappetent or cachexic animals. The reticulo-omasal orifice is situated on the medial wall of the reticulum a few centimetres from the floor and this prevents residual emptying of the rumen and reticulum. In some cattle that have been anorexic for several days, the dorsal sac of the rumen may collapse and cannot be palpated; this can be confirmed by rectal examination.

Rumen movements can be detected and measured by observation of the sublumbar fossa, palpation of the rumen and auscultation of the rumen. *Observation of rumen movement at the left sublumbar fossa* is only possible in good light and in animals that have a short coat. The moving rumen can be detected indirectly by observing the lateral displacement of the body wall.

Palpation of the rumen is achieved by exerting pressure on the rumenal wall via the left sublumbar fossa using a clenched fist. As the wave of movement passes beneath the hand the hand can be felt to be pushed gently outwards. *Auscultation* of the rumen movements by stethoscope is the most sensitive of the three methods. The phonendoscope diaphragm is placed in the sublumbar fossa and directed downwards towards the rumen (Fig. 8.9). The loudness, character and duration of sounds can vary. It is not a discrete single sound. The sound has been described as a rasping or crushing sound or as crackling crescendo–decrescendo rolling thunder. The noise may persist for 5 to 8 seconds. Using this method, weak contractions can be detected that may be missed by the other techniques. Percussion of the left abdominal wall will produce resonance over the gas in the dorsal sac of the rumen. As the percussion proceeds ventrally the resonance declines over the fibre and fluid sectors of the rumen.

Changes in rumen motility are indicators of disease. Hypomotility (less than one movement every

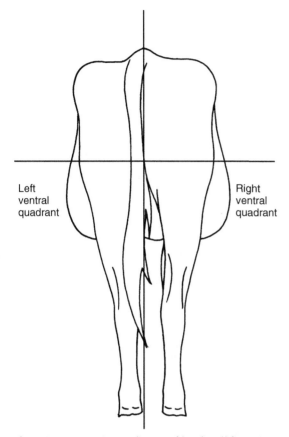

Figure 8.8 Ascites causing gross distension of the right and left ventral quadrants of the abdomen. Posterior view.

Left
ventral
quadrant

Right
ventral
quadrant

sometimes be detected. A rumbling sound followed by a liquid pouring sound may be heard. Palpation of the left abdominal wall may enable pain to be localised, although reactions by fractious animals may be misleading.

Pneumoperitoneum caused by intraperitoneal gas may cause mild distension of the right and left sublumbar fossae. This may occur following abdominal surgery. Pneumoperitoneum is usually less tympanic, and the normal rumen can be palpated through the left sublumbar fossa. A diagnosis of ruminal bloat can be supported if hyper-resonance is present on percussion of the distended left sublumbar fossa. Differentiation between frothy and free gas bloat can only be achieved by attempts at decompression. Decompression can be attempted either by using a large 16 BWG (1.65 mm) 5 cm needle inserted into the tympanic dorsal sac of the rumen through the flank, or by passing a stomach tube into the rumen *per os* (Fig. 8.10) or *per nasum*. Free gas bloat can easily be decompressed. Frothy bloat simply blocks the tube without decompression. In cases of ruminal acidosis, the fluid volume of the rumen will increase due to osmosis into the hypertonic rumen. Ballottement of the rumen may reveal sloshing sounds caused by the excess fluid.

Rumen fluid collection and analysis when pyloric obstruction, ruminal acidosis or poor rumen function are suspected may provide useful additional information. The collection and analysis is described under 'Further investigations'.

There are several tests and signs that may support a diagnosis of *traumatic reticulitis*. The animal may be reluctant to move and stand with an arched back (Fig. 8.11); it may be anorexic and pyrexic. Animals that have progressed to a traumatic reticulopericarditis may have additional cardiovascular signs, including signs of congestive heart failure. The animal may grunt when it moves or breathes due to pain induced by parietal peritoneal irritation. The grunt is produced by forced expiration against a closed glottis. Grunts may be produced by thoracic as well as abdominal pain. The detection of a grunt is improved by auscultation with a stethoscope placed against the trachea. A condition should not be ruled out if a grunt is absent, but if a grunt is present this indicates there is anterior abdominal pain.

2 minutes) or rumenostasis may cause a free gas bloat and is associated with a number of conditions including milk fever, carbohydrate engorgement (ruminal acidosis) and painful conditions of the abdomen. Hypermotility (more than five movements every 2 minutes) is less common and conditions include the development of frothy bloat, vagal indigestion and Johne's disease.

Differentiation of the A and B waves can only reliably be made by detecting eructation. This can be done by observation, listening or by auscultation with a stethoscope over the trachea. External palpation and observation of the reticulum is not possible. Auscultation of reticular contractions can sometimes be achieved by stethoscope auscultation over ribs 6 or 7 ventrally on the left side. A diphasic contraction every 40 to 60 seconds at the start of the A cycle can

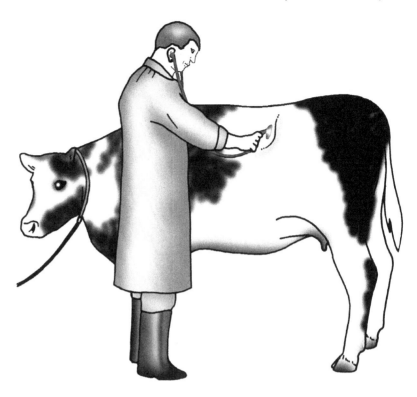

Figure 8.9 Auscultation using a stethoscope of the ruminal movements at the left sublumbar fossa.

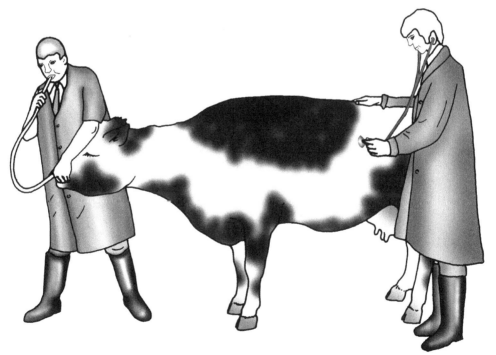

Figure 8.10 Passing a stomach tube into the rumen *per nasum* with auscultation at the left sublumbar fossa.

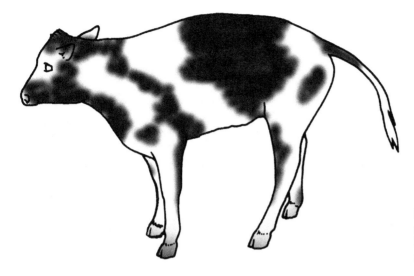

Figure 8.11 Traumatic reticulitis. The animal is reluctant to move, has an arched back and grunts while defaecating with a raised tail.

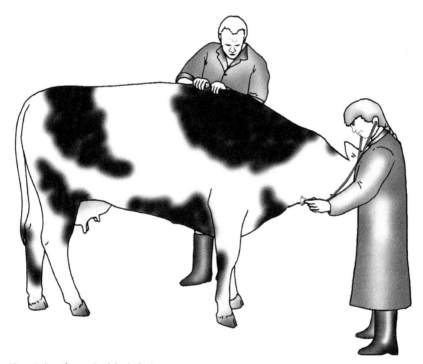

Figure 8.12 The withers pinch test for anterior abdominal pain.

Physical tests for the anterior abdominal pain which is usually associated with traumatic reticulitis are the withers pinch test, the bar test, the knee test and the Eric Williams' test.

Withers pinch test – The withers pinch test is performed by grasping a fold of skin over the withers (Fig. 8.12). This will cause the animal to dip the spine. If there is a penetrating foreign body which

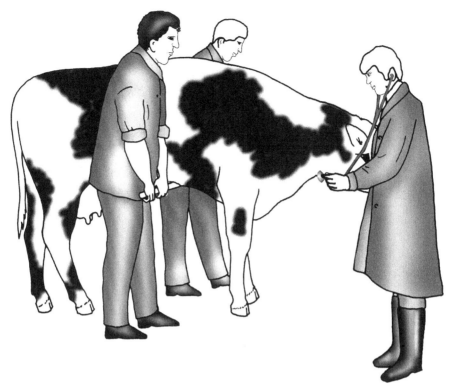

Figure 8.13 The bar test for anterior abdominal pain.

causes irritation of the parietal peritoneum during the test, the animal will resent making this movement and will usually grunt. The bar test and the knee test involve upward pressure on the xiphoid area to check for discomfort and associated grunting.

Bar test – In the bar test an operator stands either side of the animal. A padded metal or wooden bar is placed beneath the animal and positioned just behind the xiphisternum. Each operator slowly raises the bar and then lowers it quickly. The veterinary surgeon should place a stethoscope over the trachea in the ventral midline of the neck and auscultate for a grunt (Fig. 8.13). In an animal with an acute traumatic reticulitis this sudden movement will often elicit discomfort and a grunt.

Knee test – This test involves applying a sudden upward force with the knee in the area of the xiphisternum. A grunt with resentment is expected if the animal has anterior abdominal pain. Localisation of the pain can sometimes be achieved by regional palpation or percussion of the anterior abdomen. (Fig. 8.14).

Eric Williams' test – The Eric Williams' test is a more subtle technique for the early detection of the condition. If there is ruminostasis the test cannot be performed. A stethoscope is placed over the trachea and a hand placed in the left sublumbar fossa to detect ruminal movement. A quiet and otherwise ordinarily inaudible grunt may be heard via the stethoscope just before the commencement of the ruminal component of the A wave. The grunt is caused by the pain elicited by the double reticular contraction causing the penetrating foreign body to produce parietal peritoneal irritation.

Further investigations which may be useful include sampling of the peritoneal fluid by peritoneal tapping, radiography, examination using a metal detector and laparotomy/rumenotomy. These techniques are decribed under 'Further investigations'.

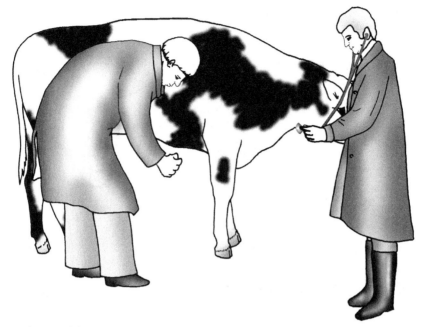

Figure 8.14 Percussion for anterior abdominal pain.

A compass can be used to indicate the presence of a prophylactic magnet in the reticulum. If a magnet is found to be present, indicated by the movement of the compass needle, traumatic reticulitis is less likely to be the cause of the illness.

No physical examination of the left side of the body is complete without checking for a left displaced abomasum (Figs 8.15 and 8.16). Left displacement of the abomasum is a very common condition in high yielding dairy cows and is usually recognised during the first few weeks after calving. Milk yield and appetite are depressed. Ketosis is invariably present and can be identified by a 'pear drop' smell on the breath or by the presence of ketones in urine, milk or saliva. Rothera tablets or the ketone patch on a urine test stick can be used to confirm the presence of ketones. The Rothera reagent turns purple in the presence of ketones. Concurrent conditions such as mastitis or endometritis are common.

The presence of a left displaced abomasum must always be checked for during the examination of the abdomen of adult cattle. In this condition the fluid and gas filled displaced abomasum is between the left abdominal wall and the rumen. Characteristic sounds are pro-

duced by rising bubbles of gas and by the gas–fluid interface within the displaced abomasum. The *musical tinkling sounds* produced by escaping gas bubbles can sometimes be heard by simple auscultation using a stethoscope and are probably produced in response to adjacent ruminal movements. Alternatively, gentle ballottement of the abdomen using a clenched fist or by gentle rocking may evoke them. *High pitched resonant pings* can be produced by percussion of the displaced abomasum. The pings may be heard in association with the musical tinkling sounds of escaping gas by simultaneous auscultation using a stethoscope. The ping sounds like a basketball being bounced upon a concrete floor or a steel drum being hit.

The position and size of the displaced abomasum are variable. It is suggested that clinical evaluation should be focused along a line drawn from the left elbow to the left tuber coxae, although it can be found much higher or lower than this. In general, clinical evaluation from the 9th to the 13th rib along this line is often the most rewarding (Fig. 8.17). The resonance produced by the gas cap of the rumen can sometimes be misleading. This can usually be discounted by

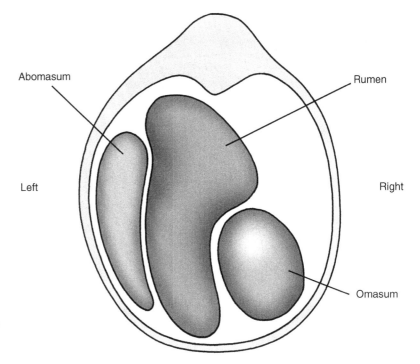

Figure 8.15 A left displaced abomasum. A posterior transverse view at the level of the 13 th rib.

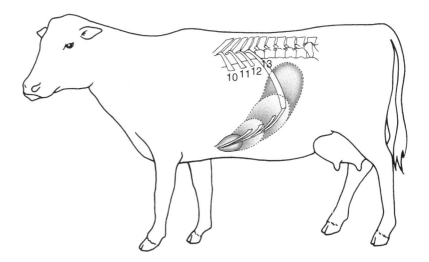

Figure 8.16 The progressive development of a left displaced abomasum: a left lateral view.

passing a stomach tube and decompressing any gas that may be present. The clinical evaluation is then repeated. A collapsed dorsal sac of the rumen can produce a ping with a lower pitch. The rumen movements may be normal or reduced in amplitude and frequency.

Further confirmation can be achieved by abomasocentesis. To perform an abomasocentesis, the skin in the intercostal space over the ping is antiseptically prepared and a lumbar-spinal needle quickly inserted. A sample of abomasal fluid is withdrawn by syringe. The pH of the sample can then be measured

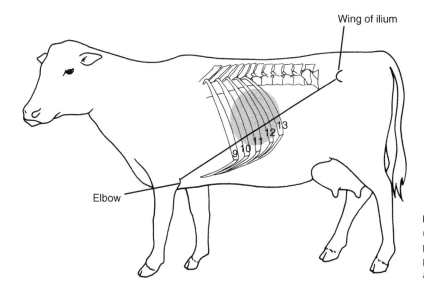

Wing of ilium

13
9 10 11 12

Elbow

Figure 8.17 The topographical location of abnormal pings that may be produced by percussion and auscultation in the presence of a left displaced abomasum: a left lateral view.

using pH papers. If the pH is between 2 and 4 this usually confirms the diagnosis if the clinical presentation is consistent. If it is impossible to obtain a fluid sample, a section of damp pH paper can be held close to the hub of the needle in the stream of escaping gas from the abomasum. The indicator paper should register a low pH if the abomasum has been punctured. Ultrasonography can be used to identify the displaced abomasum as the folds of the abomasal mucosa contrast with the papilliform mucosa of the rumen. However, experience is required to differentiate these two structures. Alternatively, if the abomasum can be identified by ultrasonography in the normal position just to the right of the ventral midline, a diagnosis of left displaced abomasum can be ruled out. Laparoscopy or surgical laparotomy will allow direct visualisation to rule in or rule out a left displaced abomasum.

CLINICIAN'S CHECKLIST – EXAMINATION OF THE LEFT SIDE OF THE ABDOMEN

Detailed examination of any distension of the rumen
Assessment of rumen contents
Assessment of rumen motility by palpation and auscultation
Rumen fluid collection and analysis if required
Auscultation and percussion for a left displaced abomasum
Tests for anterior abdominal pain

Examination of the right side of the abdomen

Examination of the right side of the abdomen is performed to assess the gravid uterus, the abomasum, the intestines and the liver.

Abomasum, intestines and the gravid uterus

Abnormal contours identified earlier should be explored in more detail. Distension of the right sublumbar fossa may be seen with right-sided abomasal or caecal dilatation and/or torsion. A distended lower right flank is normal in the last trimester of pregnancy. Other causes include distension of the rumen in vagal indigestion, omasal impaction and abomasal impaction.

The technique of *simultaneous percussion and auscultation* is used to explore the right side of the body. Pings produced by percussion and auscultation represent abnormal accumulations of fluid and gas within abdominal structures. The right body wall should be examined by percussion and auscultation dorsal and ventral of a line from the elbow to the tubae coxae. Conditions producing pings include abomasal dilatation, caecal dilatation or torsion, gas in the rectum and pneumoperitoneum. The topographical locations of the organs producing the pings are shown in Fig. 8.18.

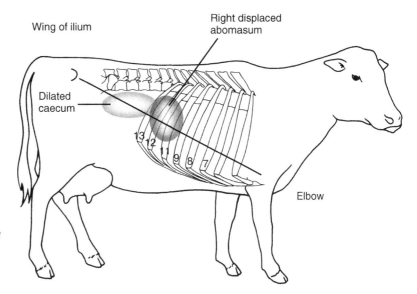

Figure 8.18 The topographical location of abnormal pings that may be produced by percussion and auscultation in the presence of a right displaced abomasum and a distended caecum: right lateral view.

Normal intestinal sounds called *borborygmi* can be heard intermittently in the right ventral quadrant; these normally occur every 15 to 30 seconds but may be inaudible. Repeated peristaltic sounds may indicate intestinal hypermotility. Splashing sounds caused by excessive fluid in the intestines may be detected by ballottement and succussion. These sounds may be detected in association with an enteritis, ruminal acidosis or intestinal obstruction.

Ultrasonography of the small intestines is possible, and peristaltic movements can be observed easily in the normal animal. The contents of the intestines can also be imaged.

Ballottement of the lower flank in late pregnancy will cause the foetus to impact on rebound on the ballotting hand. Sometimes large lumps of fat present in fat necrosis and impactions of the abomasum may also be detected in this way.

Pain tests should be performed on the anterior ventral quadrant of the abdomen by pressing the knee or a clenched fist quickly and firmly into the abdomen. Alternatively, percussion with a pleximeter can be used. A sharp pain may indicate a focal peritonitis secondary to a perforated abomasal ulcer. This usually occurs in high yielding dairy cows during early lactation.

Liver

Commonly used methods of diagnosis of liver disease in cattle include

- clinical signs
- palpation and percussion
- clinical pathology and liver function tests
- ultrasonography
- liver biopsy.

Additional techniques include radiography, laparoscopy, exploratory laparotomy and post-mortem examination.

Clinical signs of liver disease

These may include the following:

- weight loss
- diarrhoea
- heamorrhage
- hepatic encephalopathy
- photosensitisation
- ascites
- jaundice.

Prehepatic causes of jaundice, such as haemolytic anaemia, are more common in cattle.

Palpation and percussion

The liver lies beneath the costal arch and cannot normally be palpated. If it is grossly enlarged or displaced posteriorly it may be palpated by pushing the fingers behind the right costal arch. The liver may be enlarged in chronic liver fluke infestation and congestive heart failure. The exact location of the liver can be confirmed by percussion.

Ultrasonography

Using ultrasonography, the size, position and consistency of the liver can be characterised and the presence of abscesses may be confirmed. The *gall bladder* lies on the caudal border of the liver but is seldom involved in pathology, although it may be enlarged in some cases of salmonellosis. The gall bladder can be visualised using ultrasonography.

Clinical pathology and liver function tests

Liver function This can be assessed by using the bromosulphophthalein (BSP) clearance test and the gluconeogenic test using propionic acid. These tests are described under 'Further investigations'.

Clinical pathology This may be used to identify liver disease. Biochemical changes such as hypoproteinaemia occur in some types of liver disease. In disease, the enzyme aspartate aminotransferase (AST) may be elevated in the liver, but it is also produced by other tissues including cardiac and skeletal muscle. Sorbitol dehydrogenase (SDH) and glutamate dehydrogenase (GLDH) are liver specific and are elevated in the acute phase of disease. Gamma glutamyltransferase (γGT) is a good indicator of bile duct damage and is raised in liver fluke infestations. Bile salts may be elevated in hepatic pathology. Conjugated bilirubin increases with bile duct obstruction and unconjugated bilirubin increases in haemolytic anaemia. Indirect measures of liver function in cows with fatty liver syndrome have been used including non-esterified fatty acids, glucose levels and AST levels.

Liver biopsy

A *liver biopsy* can be useful to characterise liver pathology such as fatty liver syndrome and ragwort poisoning in addition to trace element analysis, for example for copper. The risks of severe iatrogenic haemorrhage during and following this procedure must be considered. This technique is described under 'Further investigations'.

Examination of the contents of the peritoneum

Detection of excessive fluid in the abdomen by physical means is difficult unless accumulations are large. Distension of the abdomen due to ascites is uncommon. The results of ballotting for a fluid thrill are difficult to interpret because of the fluid content of the ventral rumen. Abdominocentesis or ultrasonography are usually more rewarding, and these techniques are described under 'Further investigations'.

Some characterisation of the fluid is possible with ultrasonography. Transudates or urine in the peritoneum can be identified as non-echogenic fluid images. Floating leaves of oedematous omentum may be present with a ruptured bladder. Peritonitis may produce hyperechogenic tags of fibrin. Peritoneal samples can be assessed by gross examination or sent for laboratory analysis and bacteriological culture. Interpretations are provided under 'Further investigations'.

CLINICIAN'S CHECKLIST – EXAMINATION OF THE RIGHT SIDE OF THE ABDOMEN

Detailed examination of any contour abnormalities

Palpation and auscultation of the right body wall for abnormal pings

Auscultation and succussion to assess intestinal motility and content

Ballottement to identify normal and abnormal structures

Test for pain in the right ventral anterior quadrant

Check for enlargement of the liver by palpation

Liver clinical pathology

Assessment of the peritoneal cavity contents

Rectal examination

Rectal examination can be used to identify conditions of the gastrointestinal and urogenital tracts. The latter is described in Chapters 10 and 11. Rectal examination is usually limited to cattle over 12 months of age and, to avoid creating a pneumorectum and tenesmus which may confuse abdominal auscultation and percussion, is the last part of the clinical examination.

Rectal examination of the gastrointestinal tract can be used to detect a viscus which is displaced or enlarged. The rectal examination is particularly useful in palpating a grossly distended rumen, caecal dilatation and torsion, gut tie, and intestinal intussusception. The gas or fluid content of the abnormal viscus can be assessed. Indicators of peritonitis such as adhesions and a sandy grating sensation may be palpable. The quantity and composition of the faeces can be assessed.

Method

Examination *per rectum* requires care and patience with good restraint. It is best performed in the standing animal, although it is possible in the recumbent animal. In the recumbent animal the abdominal contents are displaced caudally, which makes palpation difficult unless the animal is placed in lateral recumbency. The safety of the operator should be considered if the animal is likely to rise. Fingernails should be short and well manicured; watches and rings should be removed; the gloved hand should be well lubricated. The tail has to be elevated to enable access to the rectum. It is likely that a rectal prolapse will have been detected before this point in the examination, either by observation or by the presence of tenesmus. However, on raising the tail a rectal prolapse will present with inflamed oedematous rectal mucosa protruding through the anus.

The rectal examination proceeds by coning the fingers and gently pushing through the anal sphincter. Sometimes a small rotatory movement of the hand helps to facilitate entry. Palpation is performed with the open hand. If the rectum is full of faeces, manual evacuation of the faeces will be required. This must be done slowly and carefully to avoid the entry of air into the rectum. If air is allowed to enter the rectum the wall may balloon and make palpation of internal structures impossible. Gentle backwards stroking of the ventral rectal mucosa may facilitate a peristaltic wave which may decompress the rectum so that palpation can continue. Peristaltic waves should be allowed to pass over the arm and active palpation suspended. If blood is seen on the glove, bleeding of the mucosa may be suggested and the examination should be curtailed.

The rectal examination

The contents of the posterior abdomen should be checked in a set order to avoid missing any organ. The examination area may be divided into quadrants or conducted by body system. Alternatively, a combination of both approaches can be used. Each quadrant examination area is palpated and the organs present assesed or noted if unexpectedly absent. Under normal conditions the omasum, abomasum and liver cannot be felt. Parts of the small intestine and large intestine can be felt but are not discrete structures.

In the normal animal it is possible to palpate the caudal surface of the dorsal sac of the rumen to the left of the pelvic brim. The degree of filling and nature of the contents should be assessed. In vagal indigestion the rumen is often packed with undigested fibre. The absence of the dorsal sac usually indicates a collapsed dorsal sac. A left displaced abomasum cannot be felt *per rectum* unless the gas-filled viscus is displaced very high and caudal in the left flank, which is exceptional. A right displaced and/or dilated abomasum may be felt at arm's length laterally on the right as a tense gas-filled viscus. Intussusceptions usually occur at the ileocaecal junction. The invagination of one part of the intestine into another can sometimes be felt as a large hard sausage-like structure on the right. A distended caecum can be palpated on the right as a tense gas-filled sausage-shaped balloon with the blind end caudally. If displacement has also occurred, the blind end of the caecum may have been rotated cranially out of reach. In gut tie a tense band may be felt ensnaring the intestine on the right side. This is caused by peritoneal adhesion of the remnant of the spermatic cord following castration. Abdominal masses, such as the large focal fat deposits in fat necrosis, may be palpated. Thickening of the intestine may be detected in Johne's disease, but this is highly subjective. Nonspecific referred pain or focal pain responses may be elicited on rectal examination. Referred pain may arise from a peritonitis or traumatic reticulitis. Focal pain may be provoked on palpation of an intussusception. Smears prepared from rectal mucosal scrapes, and ileum and ileocaecal lymph node biopsies using a right-sided laparotomy, may be useful in confirming *Mycobacterium avium* subsp. *panatuberculosis* infection.

Examination of the faeces

The presence of *faeces* in the rectum or voided onto the floor indicates active gut motility. An absence of faeces is abnormal. The volume, consistency, colour, fibre length (comminution), mucous covering and odour should be noted. The comminution of the undigested fibre in the faeces is an indication of the degree of mastication and rumen function. Poor comminution indicates poor rumination or accelerated passage through the forestomachs. The consistency of the faeces is diet dependent. Animals on fresh spring grass at turn out may have very watery faeces, while dry cows on a straw-based diet may have very stiff faeces that will support a stick if placed vertically into a pat. Cattle faeces are usually the consistency of a thick milk shake, although it is always more meaningful to compare the faeces of a sick animal with the other healthy cows in the group.

Slow passage through the gut or dehydration results in the faeces becoming dry, dark brown and ball shaped with a shiny surface due to the covering of mucus. In haemolytic anaemia there is an increase in the bile salts which produces faeces of a dark green colour. Reduction in the bile content of the faeces produces a paler olive green. A foetid smell may be present in salmonellosis. Normal cattle fed on unprocessed grain have undigested grains in their faeces. Faeces may be absent, indicating gut stasis. Dysenteric faeces occur in salmonellosis, mucosal disease and winter dysentery, and are composed of a mixture of undigested blood, mucus and watery faeces, usually with an offensive smell. Fibrin may appear as casts or as pieces of yellow-grey material, sometimes with sheets of sloughed mucosa. Melanic faeces are black on gross appearance. This type of faeces is caused by the presence of digested blood. Digestion of the blood occurs in the abomasum and proximal intestinal tract. The source of the blood may be direct from the gut (e.g. haemorrhagic abomasal ulceration) or swallowed blood from the lungs (e.g. posterior vena caval syndrome) or from the pharynx

(e.g. bracken and/or papilloma induced tumours). Firm dry faeces covered in excessive mucus indicate a slower than normal passage through the gastrointestinal tract. Bleeding from the large intestine produces fresh blood or clots of blood in the faeces; coccidiosis and bleeding following rectal examination are examples. Plentiful pasty faeces may be observed in Johne's disease. Scant and pasty faeces usually indicate prolonged passage through the forestomachs. Diarrhoea may indicate an enteritis or an osmotic pathophysiology such as ruminal acidosis following carbohydrate engorgement. Faecal samples can be colleced for laboratory analysis which may include bacteriology, virology and examination for parasitic gastroenteritis, fascioliasis, coccidiosis and *Cryptosporidium*.

CLINICIAN'S CHECKLIST – THE RECTAL EXAMINATION

The quantity and composition of faeces should be noted

Palpate the dorsal sac of the rumen for size, content and presence

Palpate the right side to check for

Dilated and distended loops of bowel (caecum, large and small intestine)

A solid intussusception

A dilated abomasum

Abdominal masses

Gut tie

An enlarged liver

Fibrous adhesions or peritoneal roughness

Conditions occurring in the calf

Rumen – chronic recurrent ruminal bloat, putrefaction of milk in rumen, chronic ruminal acidosis, ruminal impaction with fibre (pot bellied calves), ruminal hairballs (trichobezoars)

Abomasum – abomasal hairballs (trichobezoars), abomasal ulceration, abomasal displacement, abomasal bloat and/or dilatation

Small intestine – intussusception, torsion of the root of the mesentery, atresia of small intestine

Large intestine – caecal torsion, atresia coli

Rectum – atresia ani

Umbilicus – omphalophlebitis, omphaloarteritis, patent urachus, umbilical hernia, diaphragmatic hernia.

Examination of the calf

The general examination may have already identified systemic signs caused by abdominal conditions. These may include dehydration, tachycardia, endotoxaemic shock and pyrexia or hypothermia. The detailed examination begins with observations of the calf from a distance and is followed by a physical examination of the abdomen to assess the developing rumen, abomasum, intestines, umbilicus and peritoneum. A digital rectal examination and faecal evaluation then follow.

Observations

As in the adult, careful observation of the *contours of the abdomen* is important. Conditions affecting the rumen, abomasum and intestines may cause *symmetrical distension of the abdomen* and differential diagnosis can be difficult. These conditions include atresia ani, atresia coli, mesenteric torsion, rumen fibre fill and abomasal bloat. Calves with atresia ani will present with progressive bilateral abdominal distension without passage of faeces. Torsion of the greater mesentery and abomasal bloat cause recumbency, severe pain and shock. The animal deteriorates rapidly.

Recently weaned calves with *pot bellies* are common. They have a poorly adapted rumen or abnormal, usually incoordinate, rumen movements. In these calves the dorsal quadrants of the abdomen appear sunken and the *ventral quadrants appear disproportionately large*. They may also present with *chronic recurrent distension of the left dorsal quadrant* caused by free gas bloat. Predominantly *right-sided distension* may indicate dilatation and displacement of the abomasum and caecum in addition to intestinal obstructions.

Inspection of the *ventral abdominal contour* from the lateral aspect is important. In neonatal calves bleeding may sometimes be observed from the umbilical stump. If a patent urachus is present, urine may be seen at the umbilicus. Swellings in this region may indicate an umbilical hernia or an omphalitis with possible infection of intra-abdominal congenital remnants.

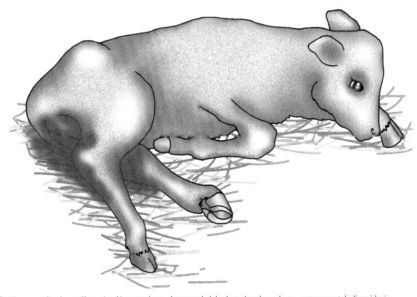

Figure 8.19 Calf with severe diarrhoea. The animal is recumbent, depressed, dehydrated and may have a severe metabolic acidosis.

Calves with severe diarrhoea may be recumbent and reluctant to stand (Fig. 8.19). Faecal staining may be pronounced around the tail and perineum. The calf may appear depressed with drooping ears. The animal may have a gaunt, hunched up appearance with a staring coat. It may have tenesmus and void copious quantities of watery diarrhoea, the character of which can be appreciated by observation. *Faeces may be absent* in calves with atresia ani, atresia coli, obstructions of the intestines and intestinal ileus.

Signs of abdominal pain include kicking at the belly, paddling of the feet, and teeth grinding. The animal may be reluctant to stand or periodically get up and down. With an intussusception the animal may adopt a characteristic posture with the hind legs extended backwards and the forelegs placed forwards – the 'rocking horse' posture.

Physical examination

Palpation of the abdomen is possible in young calves both in the standing position and in lateral recumbency. It is extremely useful in trying to identify the presence of abdominal pain, and tensing of the abdomen on palpation can readily be appreciated. Although it is often impossible to accurately identify which part of the gut is distended, localisation of the resentment or distension by gas can be informative. *Percussion/ballottement/succussion with auscultation of the abdomen may indicate a tympanic gas and fluid filled viscus* such as ruminal bloat, abomasal bloat, a left displaced abomasum, or intestinal obstruction or torsion.

Left flank

Auscultation of the rumen at the left sublumbar fossa may reveal some rumen activity in calves from 3 to 6 weeks of age before weaning. These movements are indistinct in character. Deep palpation may reveal the presence of hairballs or overfilling of the rumen with fibre (Fig. 8.20). A tympanic area high on the left flank may indicate a *rumen free gas bloat* (Fig. 8.21). This condition can be confirmed by *passing a stomach tube* into the rumen, which may also confirm the presence of putrefying milk. Rumen fluid can usually be

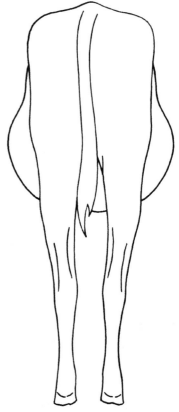

Figure 8.20 A pot bellied calf with abnormal rumen fibre fill. Posterior view showing distention of the right and left ventral quadrants of the abdomen.

obtained by passing a stomach tube. A low pH will confirm a ruminal acidosis. The activity of the anaerobic bacteria can be measured using the methylene blue dye reduction test. In an anorexic calf or a calf with a poorly adapted rumen the anaerobic bacterial activity will be low. If a left dorsal quadrant tympany is not relieved by stomach tube the distension is likely to be caused by a *left displaced abomasum*.

Tinkling sounds and pings following percussion and auscultation of the left abdominal wall are highly suggestive of a left displaced abomasum. Visualisation of the displaced abomasum is possible using ultrasonography. Rolling the animal may or may not relieve these sounds dependent upon the presence of adhesions preventing anatomical correction. Confirmation may be obtained by abomasocentesis

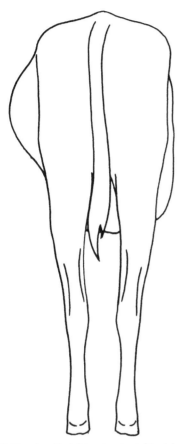

Figure 8.21 Distention of the left dorsal quadrant of the abdomen in a calf with chronic recurrent bloat: posterior view.

through the left flank. Abomasal fluid has a pH of less than 6 (the normal rumen pH of calves should be higher than this) and a chloride concentration greater than 90 mmol/l (the normal rumen has a chloride concentration of less than 25 mmol/l).

Right flank

Palpation may indicate abomasal impaction with hairballs. A rapidly developing abdominal distension of the right flank may indicate an abomasal bloat in a milk-fed calf. Abomasocentesis to decompress and confirm abomasal bloat can be achieved by placing the animal in dorsal recumbency and inserting a 16 BWG (1.65 mm), 5 cm needle into the distended

viscus approximately in the ventral midline. In abomasal ulceration, pain may be localised to the abomasum on the right ventral abdomen by palpation.

In the normal animal *intestinal peristaltic movements* may be heard on *auscultation of the right side of the abdomen*. These sounds are increased when enteritis is present. Abnormal fluid and gas accumulations may be detected by ballottement or succussion and auscultation using a stethoscope. In small valuable calves *radiology can be useful to identify abnormalities of the gastrointestinal tract* including displacement, abnormal fluid and gas content and obstructions. *Laparotomy may be required for diagnosis* and surgical correction, especially if the animal is severely ill and in rapid decline. Torsion of the greater mesentery and abomasal bloat usually present with a rapidly deteriorating patient. *Other systemic signs caused by gastrointestinal conditions* may include a metabolic acidosis, endotoxaemia, dehydration and haemorrhage.

Examination of the peritoneum

A *sample of peritoneal fluid* obtained by abdominocentesis may indicate a focal or generalised peritonitis. A midline site just anterior to the umbilicus in the standing calf is used. Ultrasonography can detect signs of peritonitis and abnormal accumulations of fluid within the peritoneal cavity.

Examination of the rectum and faeces

The presence of an anus can be easily established by lifting the tail. Atresia coli may be detected by contrast radiography using a barium enema. A *faecal sample* can be obtained by gentle digital evacuation from the rectum and the faecal quality examined. A high content of poorly digested plant fibres indicates poor rumen function. The sample may be diarrhoeic, dysenteric, or there may be an absence of faeces. The colour of *normal faeces* in the first week of life is yellow to light brown with a semisolid consistency once the greenish black muconium has been passed. On milk substitutes the colour is yellow to grey with a semisolid consistency. Increasing the ingestion of fibre darkens the faeces and makes them slightly more solid.

Constipation may be associated with a pyrexia or dehydration and may result in pelleted faeces. *Diarrhoeic faeces* can have an offensive odour, be pale in colour and may contain some intermittent streaks of blood. Diarrhoea caused by enterotoxigenic *Escherichia coli* is very watery and voluminous with or without undigested milk constituents. Rotavirus or coronavirus may produce watery green diarrhoea with undigested milk particles. Overfeeding or incorrectly mixing milk substitute powder so that the concentration is too high may produce a *fermentative diarrhoea* that is malodorous with a bubbly or foaming appearance. The normal pH of calf faeces is 7.0 to 8.5. In fermentative diarrhoea the pH is 5.0 to 6.0. Other causes of diarrhoea in which absorption of nutrients is reduced in the small intestine may cause a fermentation diarrhoea. Salmonellosis may produce *dysenteric faeces* which are composed of blood, mucus and fibrin. In advanced cases of intussusception, bloody mucoid material may be passed. *Melaena* may be present with haemorrhagic abomasal ulceration. *Bloody faeces* may be seen in salmonellosis, coccidiosis and necrotising enteritis of beef suckler calves. *Persistent chronic pasty diarrhoea* in combination with poor growth rates and poor body condition may be seen in persistent periweaning calf diarrhoea. This type of faeces may also be seen in calves with a poorly adapted rumen.

In severe outbreaks *identification of the aetiological agent* is important so that specific preventative and control measures can be implemented. Ideally, five sick calves and five healthy calves should be sampled from the infected group. With cost constraints, combined samples are usually analysed for infectious causes of diarrhoea.

Haematology, biochemistry and acid–base measurements

Haematology, biochemistry and acid–base measurements may provide useful additional clinical information in the calf. Metabolic acidosis is commonly found in diarrhoeic calves, although this may be more severe in calves over 6 weeks of age. Hyponatraemia, hypochloraemia, hyperkalaemia or hypokalaemia, and hypoglycaemia may also be present in these calves. Low packed cell volumes may indicate a haemorrhagic abomasal ulcer or a bleeding navel. High fibrinogen levels and differential leukocyte counts with a leukopenia or a leukocytosis will confirm an inflammatory process.

Umbilicus

Ventral abdominal masses are common in calves (Fig. 8.22).

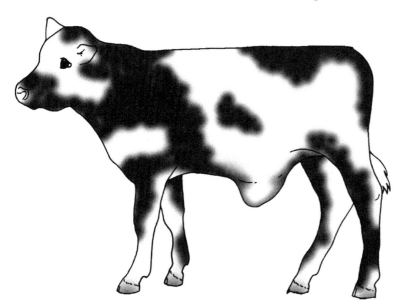

Figure 8.22 Umbilical swelling in a calf. Lateral view.

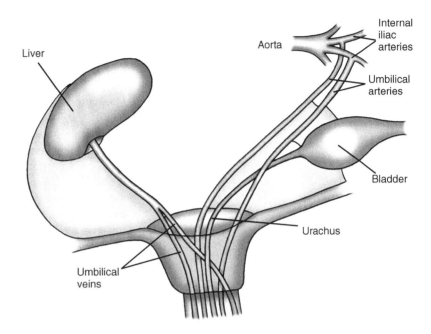

Figure 8.23 Congenital structures of the umbilicus.

Palpation of a ventral umbilical mass may indicate an umbilical hernia, the contents of which may be reducible or non-reducible on palpation. A non-reducible hernia may be strangulated with attendant systemic signs, but more usually adhesions are responsible. Normally it is the abomasum that is within the hernia rather than the intestines. Strangulation with ischaemic necrosis is accompanied by increasingly severe systemic signs. The margins of the hernial ring can usually be defined by careful palpation. The swelling may be a simple umbilical abscess or omphalitis which may be confirmed by needle aspirate. However, there may be involvement of deeper internal structures. With the calf in lateral recumbency it is sometimes possible to palpate abnormal congenital umbilical structures such as an omphaloarteritis. The umbilical structures of the neonatal calf are shown in Fig. 8.23. Infections of these internal structures may result in a discharging sinus with purulent material exuding.

Defining the abnormal structures can be attempted using a dog catheter to establish the direction of the tract internally, but the dangers of causing a peritonitis were the probe to rupture the wall of the structure should be considered. Ultrasonography can be extremely useful if available. Infected congenital umbilical remnants can be identified by the enlargement of the structures due to the accumulations of intraluminal hyperechogenic material. These include the umbilical vein, the umbilical arteries and the urachus. If there is a thrombophlebitis with extension to the liver, this can be identified. An infected urachus may be accompanied by cystitis, and cytology of the urine may indicate the presence of infection. It can also be used to investigate intestinal movement, distension and fluid content.

CLINICIAN'S CHECKLIST – EXAMINATION OF A CALF

Feeding history

General physical examination

Observations at a distance
  Faecal staining
  Behaviour
  Systemic signs
  Posture
  Signs of abdominal pain
  Caudal contour of animal
  Lateral contour of animal

Palpation
  Localisation of pain
  Intra-abdominal masses
  Fibre fill of rumen

Auscultation
  Rumen movement
  Peristalsis

Percussion
  Localisation of pain

Auscultation and percussion or ballottement or succussion
  Pings
  Tinkling
  Fluid sloshing sounds
  Tympanic resonance

Rumen stomach tubing
  Decompression
  Rumen fluid sample

Presence of anus, assessment of faeces, collection and examination of faecal samples

Laparotomy/rumenotomy

Investigation of umbilical enlargement

Further investigations

Further investigations

Clinical pathology

Haematology, biochemistry and acid–base measurements may provide useful additional clinical information. Metabolic acidosis may occur in carbohydrate engorgement or endotoxaemias. Metabolic alkalosis can occur in abomasal diplacements due to sequestration of hydrogen ions and in urea poisoning. Bicarbonate deficits can be estimated in the field using the Harleco apparatus. Hand-held biochemical and acid–base analyses are available but are expensive. Electrolyte measurements may indicate hypochloraemia and hypokalaemia, which may be present in left displaced abomasum. A low PCV may indicate a haemorrhaging abomasal ulcer, and a raised PCV may indicate dehydration. A leukocytosis with a relative neutrophilia may indicate an inflammatory process; alternatively a leucopaenia and a neutropaenia may be found in severe cases due to sequestration. Hypoproteinaemia may be a feature of a protein losing enteropathy, such as Johne's disease, or a reduction in hepatic production. A high concentration of fibrinogen is a useful indicator of inflammation.

Rumen fluid collection

A sample of rumen fluid may be obtained using a nasogastric tube or an oral stomach tube, or by performing a rumenocentesis. Use of a nasogastric tube avoids the dangers of placing a mouth gag, and the rumenocentesis method avoids the possibility of contaminating the rumen fluid sample with saliva which can increase the pH of the sample. The sample should be kept relatively warm by placing it close to the body, and the analysis is best performed within an hour of collection.

To obtain a rumen fluid sample using a *nasogastric tube* some local anaesthetic gel is applied to the ventral mucosa of one nostril. Two minutes are allowed for the gel to anaesthetise the area. The length of the tube required to reach the larynx and the rumen from the nose is marked on the tube. The nasogastric tube is advanced slowly and a finger is used to guide the tube into the ventral meatus. The tube is advanced to the larynx. The tube is further advanced at the pause following expiration. On passage through the larynx the animal is usually observed to swallow. If there is coughing and breathing sounds are detected at the end of the tube, it should be withdrawn into the nostril and advanced again. If the tube passes down the oesophagus into the rumen, gas may escape which has a characteristic odour if the end of the tube is smelled. To confirm that the tube is in the rumen, an assistant should blow forcefully down the tube and the veterinary surgeon should auscultate the rumen at the left sublumbar fossa for bubbling sounds as the gas penetrates the rumen fluid. To obtain a sample of rumen fluid negative pressure is applied to the end of the tube with a stirrup pump or by sucking the end of the tube. Free fluid may flow through the tube and be collected. If this fails, the tube should be bent and withdrawn and a sample decanted from the rumen fluid in its distal end. A sample can be collected into a universal sample pot. The only difference between using a *stomach tube* and a nasogastric tube is that the tube is advanced through the gagged mouth to the larynx.

The equipment required to perform a *rumenocentesis* includes clippers, surgical antiseptic, alcohol and a 9 cm 18 BWG (1.20 mm) spinal needle with a stylet. The rumen contains a dorsal gas cap, a fibrous raft and fluid in the ventral sac. A small area of skin in the left ventral quadrant of abdomen is surgically prepared. To protect the operator, a tail kinch or an anti-kick bar can be applied. The lumbar spinal needle is thrust up to the hilt through the skin of the prepared site into the fluid contained within the ventral sac. A syringe is attached to the needle and a sample withdrawn. Sometimes the needle can get blocked by solid material and may have to be cleared by injecting air. Once a sample has been obtained the needle is withdrawn.

Rumen fluid analysis

Care with sampling is required as saliva contamination increases the pH of the rumen sample. The sample should be evaluated as soon as possible because cooling and exposure to air alter protozoan and bacterial activity.

Colour

Normal rumen fluid is usually olive green or greenish brown. In ruminal acidosis the fluid may appear milky grey.

pH

The *rumen fluid pH* can be measured in the field by using pH papers with a range of 3.0 to 9.0. The rumen fluid pH is normally 6.0 to 7.0 in cattle on a roughage-based diet and 5.5 to 6.5 in cattle on a concentrate-based diet. In ruminal acidosis (carbohydrate engorgement) the pH will be 5.0 or less. In anorexic cattle, because of the constant production of saliva which has an alkaline pH and a lack of substrate for the rumen flora to produce volatile fatty acids, the pH will be alkaline and usually in the range 7.5 to 8.0. Higher pH values can occur with urea poisoning.

Sedimentation/flotation

This test is an indirect measure of the activity of the microflora; it must be performed within a short time following collection of the sample otherwise it may not be an accurate measure of their activity within the rumen. The sample of rumen fluid is placed in a measuring cylinder. The time is measured for complete sedimentation and flotation of solid particles. The finer particles sink and the coarser particles float supported by gas bubbles of fermentation. In healthy cattle the normal time for sedimentation and floatation is 4 to 8 minutes. Inactive microflora results in rapid sedimentation with little floating material. Chronically anorexic cattle would give this result.

Redox potential (methylene blue reduction time)

This test is a measure of the reduction–oxidation activity of the ruminal microflora and reflects anaerobic fermentation by rumen bacteria. It must be performed within a short time following collection of the sample to produce an accurate result. One ml of 0.03% methylene blue is mixed with 20 ml of rumen fluid and the colour compared with a control of rumen fluid only. The time taken to decolourise the methylene blue is measured. Rumen fluid from healthy cattle on a concentrate and hay diet will decolourise in 3 minutes or less; rumen fluid from cattle on a hay only diet will decolourise in 3 to 6 minutes. A time of 15 minutes to decolourise would indicate poor microbial activity.

Protozoal activity

Rumen fluid from normal healthy cattle contains high numbers of large and small protozoa with ciliate and flagellate forms. They are highly active. The sample should be agitated to resuspend the organisms. A drop of the sample should be placed on a warm glass slide and covered with a coverslip. The protozoan activity can be observed using the low power ×10 objective lens. Large protozoa are more sensitive to disturbances. All protozoa are killed when the pH drops below 5. There are reduced numbers in samples with low fermentation activity.

Gram staining

Gram stained smears from rumen fluid samples can be prepared. There are mainly Gram negative bacteria in normal rumen fluid, but in ruminal acidosis Gram positive streptococci and lactobacilli predominate.

Rumen fluid chloride concentration

This can be measured by most laboratories on request. In healthy cattle, rumen fluid has a chloride concentration of less than 30 mmol/l. Concentrations above this level are considered abnormal and may be caused by reflux of abomasal ingesta into the rumen. High levels also occur in ruminal acidosis and severe anorexia.

Exploratory laparotomy and rumenotomy

Exploratory laparotomies can be extremely useful in confirming and correcting some conditions of the abdomen. Laparotomies are carried out on either the right side, the left side or the midline, depending upon which conditions are suspected. A left-sided laparotomy may include a rumenotomy. Left-sided laparotomies enable the following structures to be palpated: the rumen, the reticulum, the spleen, the left border of the liver, part of the diaphragm, the apical beat of heart, the left kidney through peritoneal fat, the path of ureters, the bladder, the uterus, the right and left ovaries, and the descending colon. Adhesions of the reticulum to the parietal peritoneum may be palpable in traumatic reticulitis. A left displaced abomasum can also be confirmed. A rumenotomy can be performed during a left-sided laparotomy and can confirm the presence of an obstructive foreign body, such as ingested plastic bags or hay nets. The reticulum, rumen, oesophageal groove, reticularomasal orifice and cardia can be examined. The reticulum should be very carefully examined for penetrating foreign objects, abscesses and *Actinobacillus* infections of the oesophageal groove. A right-sided laparotomy gives access to the omasum, the abomasum, the spiral colon, the duodenum, the jejunum, the ileum, the caecum, the liver and gall bladder. Surgery will enable confirmation of a dilated caecum or torsion of the caecum, a right displaced abomasum, an intussusception and torsion of the root of the mesentery.

Abdominocentesis and peritoneal fluid analysis

Analysis of peritoneal fluid can be diagnostically useful to rule in or rule out abnormalities within the abdomen. It is useful in diagnosing peritonitis in conditions such as traumatic reticulitis, abomasal ulceration and intussusception; uroperitoneum in conditions such as a bladder rupture or a ureteral rupture; gut contents in the peritoneum caused by an intestinal rupture; haemorrhage into the peritoneum caused by abdominal tumours, hepatic and spleenic ruptures, and ascites caused by right-sided heart failure.

Abdominocentesis

Abdominocentesis is easy and inexpensive to perform, and requires little equipment. In normal healthy cattle there is usually only 15 to 20 ml of peritoneal fluid in the peritoneal cavity. As a consequence a sample is not always obtained and the lack of a sample should not be interpreted as abnormal. The only exception to this is during late pregnancy when the volume increases markedly. Abnormal peritoneal fluid, particularly in cases of local peritonitis, may be confined to a small area of the peri-

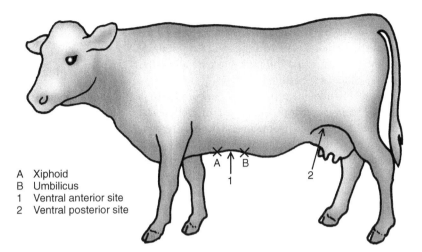

A   Xiphoid
B   Umbilicus
1   Ventral anterior site
2   Ventral posterior site

Figure 8.24 Sites at which to perform an abdominocentesis.

toneum and may not always be sampled during abdominocentesis.

There are several potential sites at which to perform an abdominocentesis (Fig. 8.24). A common site is in the *ventral anterior abdomen* midway between the xiphisternum and the umbilicus in the midline. This site is easy to identify and carries no risk of accidentally puncturing the milk vein. An alternative site in the anterior abdomen is 5 cm caudal to the xiphisternum and 5 cm to the left or right of the midline. Care is required to ensure that the milk vein is not punctured if close to the site. Other sites are on the *left or right posterior abdomen* just anterior to attachment of the mammary gland to the body wall.

The *preparation and the procedure are the same at each site*. Ideally, hair is clipped or shaved at the site and the skin aseptically prepared. Restraint using a kinch or an antikick bar can improve operator safety. A 5 cm 19 BWG (1.10 mm) needle is gently pushed into the peritoneal cavity of the abdomen through the skin, musculature and parietal peritoneum. If no peritoneal fluid is obtained the needle can be rotated and the degree of penetration increased. In ventral sites the rumen is sometimes penetrated and a dark gritty sample obtained. If no sample is obtained a new site should be selected. Applying a syringe to the barrel of the needle and applying gentle suction may be useful. Samples should be collected into plain tubes for bacteriology and EDTA tubes for cytology.

Peritoneal fluid analysis

Examination of the sample includes assessment of the volume, colour, viscosity, turbidity, cell number and type, specific gravity and protein concentration, preparation of stained smears for visualisation of bacteria and bacterial culture. Samples can be sent off to the laboratory for detailed analysis, but useful information can be obtained inexpensively from gross examination of the sample and simple microscopy.

The *volume* of a sample obtained from healthy cattle ranges from 0 to 5 ml. Volumes of 10 ml or above may indicate a pathological process unless the animal is in late pregnancy.

The *colour* of normal peritoneal fluid is clear, straw coloured or yellow. If the sample is *green* in colour this suggests the presence of food material and may indicate a gut rupture or that a gut sample (a rumen sample being the most common) has inadvertently been obtained. Repeating the abdominocentesis at a different site may help confirm the result. If the sample is an intense *orange-green* colour this indicates rupture of the biliary system, but this is very rare. A *pink to red* sample indicates presence of haemoglobin and/or red blood cells which may indicate the iatrogenic penetration of a blood vessel, a gut infarction or perforation. A *red-brown* colour indicates necrosis of the gut wall. A sample consisting of frank blood indicates haemorrhage into the peritoneum (haemoperitoneum) which may be pathological but may have been caused by the abdominocentesis procedure puncturing a blood vessel during sampling. Repeating the procedure at a different site may allow the two possibilities to be differentiated.

A *turbid sample* indicates an increased protein and cellular content. Large quantities of yellowish-coloured turbid fluid (sometimes with fibrin tags) suggest acute diffuse peritonitis. *A sample that forms a generous stable froth after vigorous shaking* indicates the presence of intra-abdominal inflammatory processes caused by the increased protein content of the peritoneal fluid. *Clotting of the sample* indicates an increase in the viscosity of the peritoneal fluid due to inflammatory processes.

More detailed laboratory analysis may include measurements of specific gravity and protein content. A *high specific gravity and high protein content* suggest vascular damage and leakage of plasma proteins in peritonitis or ischaemic necrosis of the bowel. *Microscopy* may indicate the presence of particulate food material from a ruptured bowel. *Cytology* may indicate an increased white blood cell (WBC) count of the peritoneal fluid with increased polymorphonuclear cells (PMN) which indicates inflammation (sterile or infectious), the presence of degenerative PMNs which suggests infection, and increased monocytes which suggests the presence of a chronic inflammatory process.

Table 8.2 provides a classification of normal, transudate, modified transudate and exudate peritoneal fluids. A *transudate* may be present in Johne's disease as a result of hypoproteinaemia. A *modified transudate* may be observed in lymphosarcoma of the gastrointestinal tract or congestive heart failure. An *exudate* may be septic or non-septic. Conditions causing a septic exudate include a ruptured infected uterine metritis and a traumatic reticuloperitonitis. A condition causing a non-septic exudate is a ruptured bladder.

Radiography

Radiography of the anterior abdomen may be useful in the diagnosis of traumatic reticulitis caused by a penetrating wire. However, powerful machines are required that are usually only available in referral centres. It can be useful in young valuable calves.

Metal detectors

Metal detectors have been used to rule out the presence of metal in the structures of the anterior abdomen. However, many normal cattle give positive results due to the presence of harmless metal fragments present in the reticulum. Examples are the ends of anthelmintic boluses and nuts and bolts.

Ultrasonography

Ultrasonography is non-invasive and is useful for investigating conditions of the umbilicus, gastrointestinal tract and liver. The equipment required includes a 5 or 3.5 MHz linear transducer, clippers and contact gel. The hair is removed using clippers. Liberal quantities of contact gel are applied to the clipped area of skin to ensure contact. The presence of fluid and adhesions in the abdomen can be detected. The abomasum and reticulum can be visualised using ultrasonography.

Infections of the *umbilicus*, the umbilical arteries, the umbilical veins and urachus are relatively common in calves. A patent urachus may also be present. Ultrasonography is very useful in identifying gross abnormalities of these structures. The hair of the ventral abdomen must be clipped and liberal amounts of contact gel applied to ensure a contact. It is best to begin the ultrasonography over the umblicus. Any abnormal structures can then be traced cranially (the umbilical vein(s)) or caudally (the umbilical arteries and urachus). It is important to scan the ventral abdomen from the umbilicus to the liver and the umbilicus to the bladder systematically, otherwise abnormalities may be missed. Enlarged and pus filled structures can be readily identified. The contents of umbilical hernias can also be evaluated.

The liver can be identified through the intercostal spaces 6 to 12 on the right side. Liver enlargment and liver abscessation may be detected. The caudal vena cava may be examined between ribs 11 and 12, and the gall bladder between the 9th, 10th or 11th intercostal spaces.

Table 8.2 Classification of normal, transudative, modified transudative and exudative peritoneal fluid

Type	Colour/volume	Total protein (g/l)	Specific gravity (g/cm³)	WBC × 10⁶/l	Differential WBC
Normal	Amber, clear 1–5 ml	<25 Does not clot	1.005–1.015	<1000	PMN : monocytes 1 : 1
Transudate	Pale straw, clear 10–20 ml	>25 Does not clot	>1.018	<1000	Non-degenerate PMN
Modified transudate	Clear, straw 10–20 ml	>25 Does not clot	>1.018	<5000	Non-degenerate neutrophils
Exudate Non-septic	Amber to pink, turbid	>25 Clots	>1.018	>5000	Non-degenerate PMN
Septic	Pink to red, turbid	28–58 Clots	>1.016	>5000	Degenerate PMN

PMN, polymorphonuclear cells.

Liver biopsy

Prophylactic antibiosis and tetanus antitoxin should be considered. Checking the prothrombin time before proceeding may be a wise precaution. The equipment required is 10% buffered formalin, a Tru-cut biopsy trocar, local anaesthetic, scalpel blade, syringe, needle, antiseptic and alcohol. The site of the biopsy is 15 cm below the transverse processes in the 11th right intercostal space. The site is also defined by imaginary lines from the wing of the ilium to the point of the elbow and the point of the shoulder. The site is the area of the 11th intercostal space enclosed by these lines (Figs 8.25 and 8.26). The hair is clipped and aseptically prepared. Local anaesthetic is infiltrated subcutaneously and more deeply into the intercostal mucles beneath. A stab incision is made through the skin at this site. The biopsy needle is pushed through the skin incision and aimed towards the opposite elbow. The needle is then pushed into the stroma of the liver. Ultrasonography can be used to guide the placement of the biopsy needle. The passage of the needle through the edge of the diaphragm and the liver gives a slight grating sensation. A biopsy is then taken and the needle withdrawn. The sample can then be placed in 10% formal-saline for histopathology, or the fresh sample can be used for specific gravity tests and chemical analysis for lipid content. Liver pathology such as fatty liver syndrome and a fibrotic liver from ragwort poisoning can be detected.

Bromosulphophthalein (BSP) and propionate liver function tests

BSP function test

The performance of the BSP function test is contraindicated if there is hypoalbuminaemia or high bilirubin levels present. It is now rarely performed. BSP is a dye that is injected intravenously as a bolus at a dose rate of 2 mg/kg. A healthy control animal is useful for comparison, although not essential in view of current UK legislation. Blood samples should be taken after 5, 10, 15, 30 and 45 minutes. In most normal cattle the dye has been cleared from the blood after 30 minutes. The half-life of the dye can be calculated. In normal cattle the half-life is less than 5 minutes. In cattle with liver dysfunction the dye is still present after 45 minutes. At 30 minutes, the interpretation of the liver dysfunction serum concentration as a percentage of the dye concentration at the start of the test is as follows: 5 to 10% mild, 10 to 25% moderate and more than 25% severe.

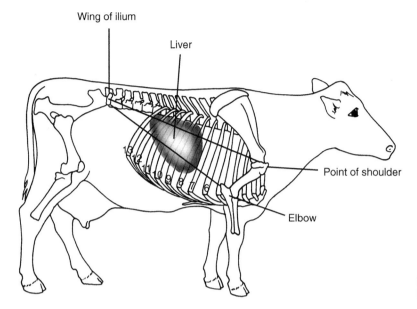

Figure 8.25 Topographical markers for a liver biopsy in a cow. Lateral right side.

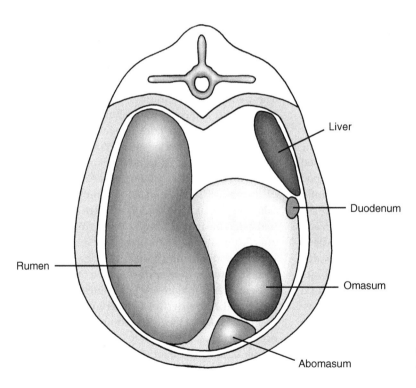

Figure 8.26 A posterior transverse view at the level of the 11th intercostal space.

Propionic loading

Propionic loading may be used to assess liver function. In a healthy liver this will cause a rise in blood glucose following increased hepatic gluconeogenesis. Sodium propionate at a dose rate of 3.0 mmol/kg is administered intravenously. In healthy animals there will be a rise in blood glucose of at least 2.0 mmol/l after 30 minutes. Values less than this indicate a reduced liver function.

Atropine test

Bradycardia (40 to 60 beats/minute) caused by an increase in the vagal tone (vagotonia) has been recognised in vagal indigestion, cattle deprived of food, and bovine spongiform encephalopathy. This can be confirmed by an increase in the heart rate following the administration of atropine. Disturbance should be minimal. Atropine is administered slowly by the intravenous route or subcutaneously. If the intravenous route is to be used an indwelling catheter should be placed sometime before the administration to avoid the tachycardia induced by stress. The dosage of atropine administered subcutaneously is 0.06 mg/kg or 30 mg for a 500 kg animal; the dosage given by slow intravenous injection is 0.02 mg/kg or 10 mg for a 500 kg animal. A rise in heart rate of 20 beats/minute is highly suggestive. The response following intravenous administration is usually observed within 2 minutes and persists for up to 30 minutes. Using the subcutaneous route the response is usually seen within 10 minutes.

PHYSICAL SIGNS OF DISEASE ASSOCIATED WITH THE GASTROINTESTINAL SYSTEM, LIVER AND UMBILICUS

N.B. Some of these physical signs are also associated with diseases of other body systems and regions.

Demeanour
  Dull
  Depressed
  Weak
  Lethargic

Condition
  Loss of weight
  Low condition score
  Sunken eyes

Appetite
  Reduced
  Anorexic

Posture
  Reluctant to rise and/or lie down
  Recumbent
  Rocking horse posture
  Arched back

Abnormal actions
  Tenesmus
  Kicking at the abdomen

Dropping of the cud
Grunting
Grinding of the teeth

Abdominal silhouette
  Papple (10 to 4)
  Pear shaped
  Distension of
    Left dorsal quadrant
    Right dorsal quadrant
    Left ventral quadrant
    Right ventral quadrant
  Sprung left costal arch
  Symmetrical distension

Rumen function: rate reduced/absent
  Regurgitation
  Cudding
  Eructation rate

General states
  Dehydrated
    Loss of skin turgidity

(*Continued on p. 112*)

PHYSICAL SIGNS OF DISEASE ASSOCIATED WITH THE GASTROINTESTINAL SYSTEM, LIVER AND UMBILICUS *CONTINUED*

Sunken eyes
Ketosis

Temperature
   Pyrexia

Heart rate
   Increased
   Decreased

Respiration
   Increased rate
   Increased depth
   Increased effort

Rumen
   Rate
      Stasis
      Hypomotile
      Hypermotile
   Contents
      Fibre filled
      Collapsed dorsal sac
      Tympanic bloat
      Hairballs
      Foreign body

Pain tests
   Anterior abdominal pain
   Left ventral anterior abdominal pain
   Right ventral anterior abdominal pain

Pings/tinkling sounds
   Left flank
   Right flank
      Anterior
      Posterior

Intestinal sounds (right flank)
   Hypermotile
   Absent
   Splashing

Abdomen
   Mass felt on ballottement
   Fluid thrill

Rectum and anus
   Anus absent
   Rectal prolapse
   Viscus enlarged right side
   Displaced viscus right side
   Sausage shape right side
   Pain on palpation
   Dorsal sac of rumen
      Enlarged
         Gas filled
         Fibre filled
      Collapsed

Faeces
   Faecal soiling of tail and perineum
   Absent
   Long fibre length (poor comminution)
   Dry ball shaped, dark, covered in mucous
   Foetid smell
   Dysenteric
   Frank blood
   Malaenic
   Diarrhoea
   Plentiful and pasty
   Contains mucous

Liver
   Palpable at right costal arch
   Jaundice
   Ascites
   Photosensatisation
   Convulsions (hepatoencephalopathy)

Umbilicus
   Swollen
   Sinus
   Purulent discharge
   Cyst
   Dripping urine
   Hernia
      Reducible
      Non-reducible
         Strangulated
   Painful on palpation

Clinical Examination of the Urinary System

Introduction

Effective function of the urinary system is essential to maintain good health and homeostasis in cattle. The incidence of diagnosed urinary system disease in cattle is quite low. Diseases such as pyelonephritis are specific to the urinary system. The system can also be damaged by generalised disease conditions such as septicaemia and by exposure to toxic substances including some heavy metals. It is also interdependent on other body systems and may malfunction as a result of the failure of these systems.

Malfunction of the urinary system

Malfunction may be prerenal, renal or postrenal. Circulatory failure (a prerenal problem) through heart disease or dehydration can have an adverse effect on renal function. Kidney damage though diseases such as pyelonephritis may severely compromise renal function. Inflammation of the bladder (cystitis) with the production of abnormal urine is an example of postrenal urinary disease. The effects of renal disease on other body systems can be serious. Compromise of renal function can result in disturbances of fluid balance and the accumulation in the body of substances, such as urea, which are normally excreted through the kidneys. The accumulation of these substances in the body can lead to reduced activity or malfunction of many body systems. Uraemia may give rise to clinical signs such as diarrhoea or neurological disturbance that do not appear to be directly related to the urinary system. The genital system in both sexes is closely related anatomically to the urinary system and concurrently involved with it in some diseases.

Passage of urine

The passage of urine is the main external sign of renal function. Increase or decrease in the frequency of urination, difficulty in urination and in the quantity of urine produced can all suggest malfunction of the urinary system.

Discolouration of urine

This may be an indication of prerenal, renal and postrenal diseases. Specific colour changes are discussed under urinalysis below. Urinalysis may reveal the presence of substances such as ketone bodies which indicate metabolic disease, but which do not cause discolouration of the urine.

Appraisal

Appraisal of the urinary system must include a careful clinical examination of the whole animal which takes into account its wide-ranging influence in the body.

Applied anatomy

Kidneys

The left kidney lies beneath the 3rd to 5th lumbar vertebrae, suspended in a fold of mesentery. It is pushed towards the midline or to the right of the midline by the dorsal wall of the distended rumen (Fig. 9.1). The right kidney lies beneath the 12th thoracic to the 3rd lumbar vertebrae and is immediately in front of the left kidney. Both kidneys are lobulated and are not normally palpable through the body wall. The caudal pole of the left kidney is palpable, and some gross abnormalities may be detected on rectal examination. Further evaluation of this part of the kidney is possible using ultrasonography *per rectum*. A scan through the right abdominal wall of the anterior pole of the right kidney is also possible where it lies in a notch on the caudal border of the liver.

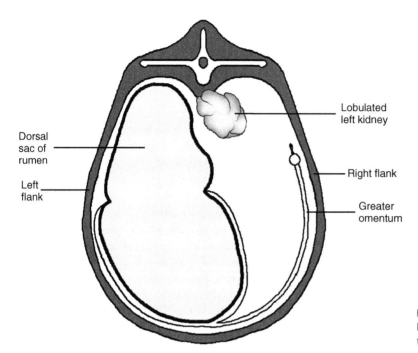

Dorsal
sac of
rumen

Left
flank

Lobulated
left kidney

Right flank

Greater
omentum

Figure 9.1 Diagram to show how the left kidney of the cow is displaced to the right by the dorsal sac of the rumen.

Ureters

These carry urine from the renal pelvises to the neck of the bladder. They are normally not palpable on rectal examination as they run, enclosed in a fold of peritoneum, down the lateral walls of the pelvis. They enter the ventral wall of the bladder at the trigonum vesicae. When chronically inflamed, the ureters may be enlarged and have a hard and roughened surface (Fig. 9.2). In cases of distal urinary obstruction the ureters may be distended with urine. They are rarely obstructed by urinary calculi.

Bladder

When empty the bladder often lies completely within the pelvis. When distended it lies within the peritoneal cavity just anterior to the pelvic brim. In female animals it lies beneath the uterus. In the male it lies beneath the rectum. The distended bladder is normally readily palpable as a tense, rounded viscus. In the pregnant cow it is found beneath and may be partially obscured by the uterus. In cases of cystitis the bladder may have a thickened wall and be tender

to the touch on rectal examination. The bladder and its contents can be readily assessed by a rectal (and sometimes by a transabdominal) ultrasonographic scan. In female animals the lining of the bladder may be viewed using a paediatric endoscope passed through the urethra.

Urethra

Heifers and cows

In heifers and cows the urethra is short, running from the bladder to the external urethral orifice which lies in the vaginal floor above the pubis. The entrance to the urethra has a sphincter protecting it. There is a small blind suburethral diverticulum arising from the caudal border of the external urethral orifice. This may cause some difficulty when attempting to catheterise the urethra.

Male cattle

In male cattle the urethra extends from the neck of the bladder to the anterior end of the penis (Fig. 11.1). It runs caudally back from the bladder along

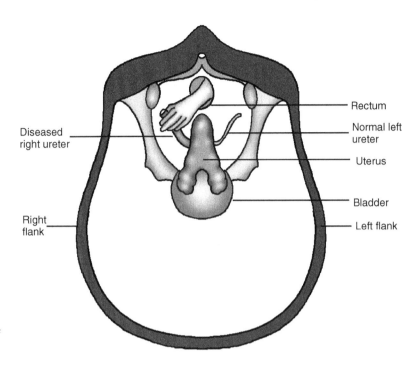

Figure 9.2 Diagram to show palpation of diseased right ureter at rectal examination.

the pelvic floor where it is surrounded by the disseminated part of the prostate gland. The urethra is readily palpable *per rectum* as a firm, muscular tube approximately 1.5 cm in diameter in the midline of the pelvic floor. Pulsations are felt in the urethra when the animal is either passing or attempting to pass urine, or ejaculating. In some animals pulsation is induced by palpation of the urethra. The two ampullae of the vas deferens enter the dorsal wall of the urethra near the neck of the bladder (Fig. 11.8). Leaving the pelvis, the urethra passes through the muscular root of the penis and ventrally downwards in the midline of the perineum. It is enclosed within the ventral part of the penis, follows the route of sigmoid flexure and terminates just caudal to the anterior tip of the penis.

Passage of urine

Cattle normally pass urine 8 to 12 times per day. They produce approximately 1 ml of urine per kilogram of body weight per hour. The average cow passes 6 to 12

litres of urine per day, the exact amount being influenced by many factors including her weight, diet, fluid intake and the ambient temperature. Urine is normally passed with ease and often after a resting animal gets to its feet. *Cows and heifers* arch their backs and stand with their hind feet apart whilst urinating. The bladder is emptied in 10 to 15 seconds. *Male cattle* pass urine less frequently and more slowly. Urine is passed either in a steady stream or in a pulsatile manner whilst the animal maintains a normal standing posture.

Collection of urine samples

Gentle tickling of the perineum around the vulva with a piece of straw or the fingers may encourage a cow or heifer to urinate. In some male animals similar handling of the prepuce may be followed by urination. This is only possible and safe in quiet animals.

Once collected, the urine sample should be inspected, smelled and its contents tested.

Collection of urinary samples by catheter

Cows and heifers

In cows and heifers a sterile, rigid metal or plastic catheter approximately 0.5 cm in diameter and 40 cm long may be passed into the bladder. The vulva is carefully wiped clean with mild disinfectant. A gloved forefinger is placed into suburethral diverticulum and the catheter passed over the finger into the urethra. Slight resistance is experienced as the catheter passes the sphincter just within the external urethral orifice. Urine may flow freely from the bladder, but it may be necessary to aspirate urine from the bladder via the catheter into a sterile syringe.

Bulls

Catheterisation is seldom possible in the bull. It is very difficult to extrude the penis from the prepuce in a non-anaesthetised animal. It is impossible in the prepubescent calf in which the penis is normally closely adherent to the prepuce.

Catheterisation of the anterior portion of the urethra in the bull is possible in the anaesthetised or heavily sedated patient. A catheter 3 to 4 mm in diameter is used, but it is extremely difficult to pass it further along the urethra. The tight bends of the sigmoid flexure and the curved route taken by the urethra as it leaves the pelvis make passage of the catheter difficult and hazardous. A small urethral diverticulum on the dorsal wall of the male urethra in the perineal region further complicates urethral catheterisation.

Urinalysis in cattle

An initial appraisal of the urine can be made by inserting a dipstick which may indicate the qualitative presence of blood, haemoglobin, ketones or bile pigments; an indication of the amount of protein present in the urine can also be obtained. Further quantitative analysis and culture in the laboratory can be arranged as required. Red and white blood cells and sediment can be detected by direct microscopy. A sediment of cells is present in haematuria but not in haemoglobinuria, although the urine is coloured red in both cases.

Quantity – approximately 6 to 12 litres per day. Measurement of the exact quantity is difficult. Cattle produce approximately 1 ml urine per kilogram body weight per hour.

Colour – normally golden and clear. Red discolouration may indicate the presence of red blood cells (haematuria) or haemoglobin (haemoglobinuria). A brown or yellow discolouration may indicate the presence of myoglobin or bile pigments, respectively. Urine may appear cloudy if pus or blood is present.

Odour – foetid if infected or retained. The odour of ketones may be detected in ketotic animals.

Specific gravity – 1.02 to 1.045.

pH – 7 to 8. Alkalinity may increase with urolithiasis. The urine is acidic in some infections.

Viscosity – normal urine is free flowing with a low viscosity. The viscosity increases in concentrated urine and in the presence of pus and blood.

Protein – high content if glomerular damage or amyloidosis are present.

Glucose – uncommon, but is occasionally present after stress such as a long journey. It is also seen in the rare condition of diabetes mellitus.

Porphyrins – congenital erythropoietic abnormality.

Abnormalities of urination and urinalysis

Dysuria

This is the frequent passage of small amounts of urine with pain during urination. It is seen in cystitis, urethritis, early urolithiasis and vaginitis.

Polyuria

There is an increase in the amount of urine produced. Causes include the following:

Diabetes insipidus – deficiency of antidiuretic hormone. This is very rare.

Diabetes mellitus – very rare.

Osmotic diuresis – increase in solutes in glomerular filtrate beyond the resorptive capacity of tubular epithelium. This is seen, for example, in chronic renal failure, mercury poisoning and the recovery (diuretic) phase of acute renal failure.

Idiopathic polydypsia – the calf drinks and urinates excessively and gets in the habit of drinking greatly in excess of its needs; it is able to concentrate its urine.

Damage to tubular epithelium – this can occur in some cases of renal disease or damage by heavy metal poisoning; in these conditions the animal is unable to concentrate its urine.

The water deprivation test is helpful in determining whether polyuria is permanent or reversible (see below).

Anuria

Anuria mostly occurs in cases of complete urethral obstruction, e.g. urolithiasis. It may also occur in terminal disease, complete renal failure and severe shock.

Oliguria

Oliguria may be prerenal, renal or postrenal. Causes include the following:

Prerenal – severe dehydration, shock, chronic heart failure
Renal – acute nephrosis, glomerulonephritis
Postrenal – ureteral or urethral obstruction.

Proteinuria

Causes include

- glomerulonephritis
- renal infarction
- nephrosis
- amyloidosis.

Haematuria

This may be renal or postrenal. Examples include the following:

Renal – severe glomerulonephritis, sulphonamide poisoning, renal infarction

Postrenal – pyelonephritis, cystitis, urolithiasis (early), enzootic haematuria (bleeding bladder tumours).

Haemoglobinuria

This is the result of rapid intravascular haemolysis of the blood. Causes include the following:

- isoerythrolysis – rare in cattle
- babesiosis
- leptospirosis
- postparturient haemoglobinuria
- bacillary haemoglobinuria – *Clostridium haemolyticum.*

Myoglobinuria

Causes include severe myopathy, especially calves with vitamin E and/or selenium deficiency, and downer cows.

Bile pigments

The presence of bile pigments in the urine suggests liver dysfunction and jaundice. A yellow froth is seen if a urine sample containing bile pigments is shaken.

Further tests of renal function

Estimation of blood urea and *creatinine* are useful indicators of the efficiency of renal function: the levels of both substances rise in cases of renal failure. *Low levels of plasma protein* are seen in a number of conditions, including severe renal damage.

Water deprivation test

This test is a useful indication of the patient's ability to concentrate its urine to preserve the water content of the body. Urine samples are collected before and after a period of 12 hours during which the animal's water supply is withheld. In normal animals the specific gravity of the urine rises to at least 1.030 after water deprivation. In animals with renal damage the specific gravity does not rise. The test should be used

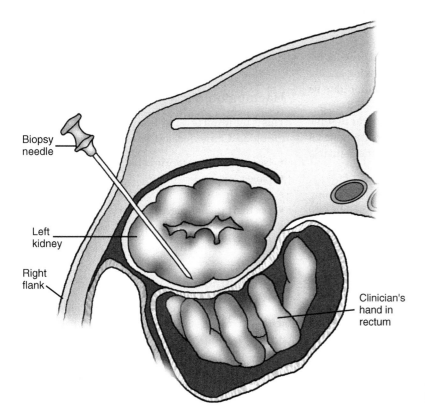

Figure 9.3 Technique for biopsy of the left kidney. See text for details.

with great caution in animals which are already dehydrated, and should not be performed in uraemic patients.

Fractional clearance of electrolytes

In cattle, creatinine is excreted by glomerular filtration. It is neither secreted or reabsorbed by the renal tubules following glomerular filtration. An index of renal tubular function for an electrolyte can be obtained by measuring the fractional clearance. The fractional clearance of an electrolyte A can be obtained by concurrently measuring the concentration of creatinine in serum (S_C) and in urine (U_C) and the concentration of electrolyte A in serum (S_A) and in urine (U_A). The percentage clearance is given by

$$\text{Percentage clearance of electrolyte A} = ((U_A/S_A)/(U_C/S_C)) \times 100$$

Normal mean percentage clearance values in heifers 11 to 14 months old have been reported as follows:

sodium, 1.97%; potassium, 49.3%; chloride 3.16%; phosphorus, 15.6%; and calcium, 1.38%.

Renal biopsy

A needle biopsy of left kidney can be taken through the right sublumbar fossa of the animal, preferably guided by ultrasound. The left kidney is pushed towards the right abdominal wall by manual pressure exerted *per rectum*. Using strict aseptic precautions, a Tru-cut 14 BWG (2.00 mm) biopsy needle of length 15.2 cm is guided through the abdominal wall and into the kidney (Fig. 9.3).

History of the case

The general history of the case will have been considered at an earlier stage in the process of diagnosis. Although some diseases of the renal system such as pyelonephritis are sporadic, other conditions such as urolithiasis may affect several members of the herd.

Some specific points of history may be of particular interest in the investigation of urinary disease. Both the immediate and past history of the patient should be investigated. The owner may have observed some difficulty or discomfort in the passage of urine. Straining with arching of the back may be seen before, during or after urination, but this may be mistaken by owners as a sign of constipation. Changes in diet and an interruption of the water supply may predispose to urolithiasis. The water consumption of individual animals provides useful information, but may not be known unless the patient is in isolation. Discoloured urine may have been seen sometimes, with possible evidence of blood or pus.

Animals with severe renal dysfunction, including uraemia, may show few specific signs other than anorexia, lethargy and depression. Animals with urolithiasis may show an unexpected improvement and freedom from pain when rupture of the bladder or urethra occurs. Such improvement is temporary and the animal's condition usually deteriorates again as the consequences of leakage of urine become apparent. Loss of bodily condition is observed in some, mostly chronic, cases of renal disease.

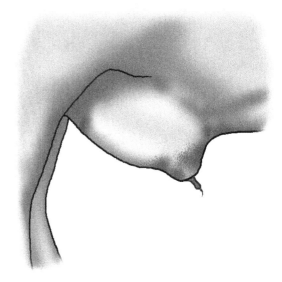

Figure 9.4 Male calf with ruptured urethra with leakage of urine around prepuce 'water belly'.

domen, frequent changing of position, straining, bruxism and bellowing in discomfort may be seen. Abdominal distension may be seen in animals in which rupture of the bladder has caused urine to accumulate in the abdomen. Swelling around the prepuce extending along the ventral abdominal wall may be seen in animals with rupture of the urethra (Fig. 9.4).

Observation of the patient

To confirm the presence of any abnormalities in the process of urination noted by the owner, the patient is observed. In some cases it may be difficult to be sure that an animal is actually passing urine. Placing the animal in a clean box with a dry concrete floor for 2 hours will often confirm evidence of urination. Time may not always be available for this procedure.

Dampness around the ventral commissure of the vulva in the female or on the preputial hairs of the male may indicate recent urination. Urination or attempted urination should be closely observed and a mid-stream sample of urine collected into a sterile container. Renal pain, prolonged attempts to urinate or straining after urination may cause the animal to stand with its back arched. The animal may also show signs of abdominal pain. Kicking at the ab-

Examination of the urinary system in cattle

Any abnormalities detected during observation of the patient should be followed up during the detailed clinical examination. The vulva or prepuce is examined to see if blood or pus is present which might have arisen from the urinary system. Any abdominal distension and ventral swelling observed, possibly caused by leakage of urine, should be investigated by palpation and if necessary by ultrasonographic examination. The skin covering areas of subcutaneous urine leakage may become cold and necrotic. The preputial hairs of male animals should be examined. Numbers of small uroliths attached

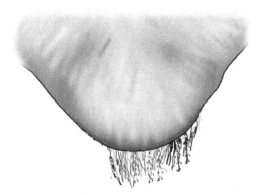

Figure 9.5 Prepuce of calf suffering from urolithiasis (or at risk of urolithiasis). Note uroliths on preputial hairs.

to the dry looking hairs are often seen in animals which have or are at risk of developing urolithiasis (Fig. 9.5).

Rectal examination

This is an important and essential part of the assessment of the urinary system in cattle. The caudal pole of the left kidney should be palpated (Fig. 9.1). Pain, enlargement or loss of the lobulated pattern of the kidney may all indicate renal disease. In pyelonephritis the left kidney may be painful to the touch. In renal amyloidosis the kidney is enlarged and its lobulated pattern is indistinct. The ureters are normally only palpable if diseased. Pain on palpation of the bladder may be seen in cases of cystitis or acute urinary retention. In the cow or heifer the bladder may, if empty, be partially obscured by the uterus which lies above it. The uterus in the female and the accessory sexual glands in the male should also be palpated to check that they are not also involved in any disease process. Large quantities of free fluid in the abdomen can be palpated *per rectum* and also be detected by external ballottement or paracentesis.

Ultrasonographic examination of the structures palpated and ballotted provides useful additional information, and should be carried out whenever possible. The scan should be carried out *per rectum* and a transabdominal scan can provide further useful additional information.

Examination of the genitalia

Vagina
Vaginal examination in the female, preferably by speculum, should also be performed. This will allow a visual examination of the vagina and the external urethral orifice to be completed and the presence of discharges of uterine origin or urovagina (Fig. 10.9) to be detected.

Penis
In the male, the external course of the penis should be followed by palpation. Details of this examination are given in Chapter 11.

Congenital defects

Hypospadia

This is failure of closure of the male urethra. The mucosal surface of the urethra is exposed from the perineum to the tip of the prepuce. Affected animals are often able to live a normal life and urine emerges from just beneath the anus (Fig. 9.6).

Patent urachus

This is less common in cattle than in the foal. Urine may leak from the umbilicus or there may be a closed cyst-like structure filled with urine adjacent to the umbilicus (Fig. 9.7). *Urachal infection* may be a sequel to umbilical infection leading to abscess formation. The enlarged urachus can often be palpated running caudally from the umbilicus towards the bladder. Ultrasonographic confirmation of diagnosis and the extent of tissue involvement is very helpful.

Kidney aplasia and ectopic ureters

These are very rare in cattle.

Hydronephrosis

This may occasionally be seen in calves. It has also been seen in older cattle recovering from enzootic haematuria (see below). Hydronephrosis may be

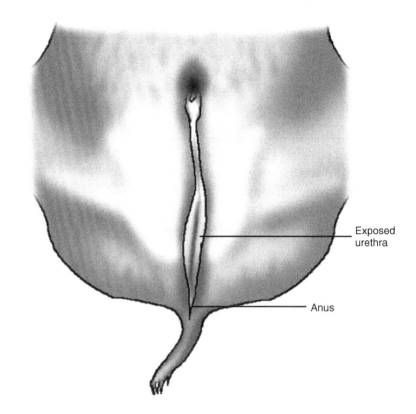

Figure 9.6 Male calf with congenital hypospadia.

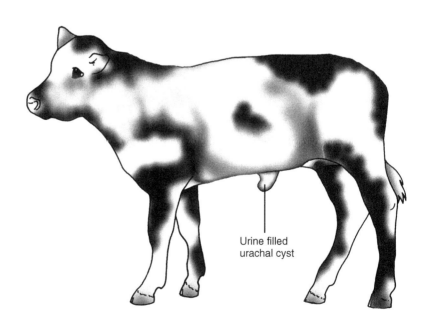

Figure 9.7 Heifer calf with congenital urachal cyst.

symptomless unless severe. Grossly enlarged kidneys may be (unusually) palpable in the sublumbar fossae beneath the lateral processes of the lumbar vertebrae. They can also be detected and evaluated by an ultrasonographic scan through the right dorsal flank.

Notes on specific clinical signs associated with some common bovine urinary system diseases

Diseases of the kidney

Pyelonephritis

Usually sporadic, often in fat, middle aged cows; can also affect calves.

Clinical signs   Insidious onset, pyrexia 39.5 to 41°C, loss in condition, frequent painful urination, may stand with back arched and may show colicky signs. The urine contains pus, blood, protein and bacteria. Uraemia in terminal cases. One or both kidneys are affected. The left kidney may be enlarged and painful on rectal examination and one or both ureters may be enlarged and thickened. *Chronic pyelonephritis* – few external signs and detectable only on rectal examination or through urine analysis is occasionally seen. In *calves* pyrexia and frequent passage of bloody urine may be seen.

Renal amyloidosis

Seen mostly, although rarely, in older postparturient dairy cows.

Clinical signs   Non-pyrexic, severe diarrhoea, generalised subcutaneous oedema, depression, anorexia. Left kidney is enlarged and rounded on rectal examination. May see polyuria and/or polydypsia if animal lives long enough. Severe proteinuria; severe hypoproteinaemia. Rapid deterioration and terminal uraemia.

Glomerulonephritis, interstitial nephritis and nephrosis

Specific physical clinical findings may not be present.

Renal neoplasia

Rare, but gross and irregular renal enlargement may be found on rectal examination aided by an ultrasonographic scan.

Diseases of the bladder and urethra

Cystitis

Mostly sporadic and may involve the bladder only or be part of the pyelonephritis complex (see above). Cystitis is more common in females than in males and often occurs shortly after parturition, especially when dystocia has occurred. It may also follow careless use of a urinary catheter.

Clinical signs   Mild pyrexia, seldom inappetant, frequent passage of small quantities of urine often with much straining and posturing. Discoloured urine contains numerous red and white blood cells, cells, pus and bacteria. Blood clots are sometimes seen in the urine or protruding from the external urethral orifice. The bladder wall may feel thickened, hard to the touch and painful on rectal examination.

Urolithiasis

May be sporadic but outbreaks may occur on some units. It can be difficult to diagnose and treat, and may be accompanied by heavy losses. In cattle the uroliths are usually calcium magnesium ammonium phosphate ($CaMgNH_4PO_4$).

The case history may include a number of factors which predispose to precipitation of solutes in the urinary tract. These are as follows:

- water deprivation – no water or some animals unable to reach the trough
- abnormal urinary pH
- high concentrate diet
- abnormal Ca : P ratio in diet; high phosphorus and low calcium levels are particularly dangerous
- gender – urolithiasis is more common in the male (especially the castrated male) than the female
- urinary infection – may provide foci of pus or debris which predispose to solute precipitation.

Clinical signs   Usually a progression of obstruction to urethral rupture, then bladder rupture; signs vary with the progress of the problem and the tissue damage.

Urethral obstruction – animal often uncomfortable and restless; grinds teeth; kicks at abdomen. Farmer often thinks the animal is constipated. May strain to urinate. Preputial hairs dry and impregnated with numerous small uroliths. Box floor dry – no urination. Pulsation of urethra on rectal examination. This also occurs during urination or on palpation, and may cease after rupture of the bladder has occurred.

Urethral rupture ('water belly') – subcutaneous swelling above and around prepuce as trapped urine accumulates. Initial decrease in prerupture pain. Skin becomes necrotic and discoloured (Fig. 9.4).

Rupture of bladder – animal is initially brighter as pain decreases. Urine builds up in abdomen causing distension. Gradual development of uraemia causes the patient's health to deteriorate. Death may follow in 7 days.

Urethral dilatation – occasionally seen in bulls. Affected animals have a perineal swelling; aspiration may reveal urine, blood and debris.

An *ultrasonographic scan of the abdomen and preputial area* may be helpful diagnostic aids. The scan may show free fluid in the ventral abdomen and no evidence of a distended bladder. *Abdominal paracentesis* – aspirated fluid smells of urine and has very high levels of urea and creatinine (several times higher than in the patient's plasma).

Diseases causing haematuria in cattle

Enzootic haematuria

A chronic non-infectious disease of cattle aged over 1 year characterised by the formation of haemangiomata in the bladder which may lead to severe bleeding and possibly death. Seen in certain areas where animals are exposed to bracken fern.

Clinical signs Haematuria and large clots of blood may be seen in the urine (and occasionally coming from the nostrils). This may lead to severe anaemia, recumbency and death in severe cases. In milder cases there may be gradual development of anaemia, thickening of bladder wall (and occasionally masses in the bladder) palpable *per rectum*, and the establishment of infection in the compromised bladder.

Diseases causing haemoglobinuria in cattle

Bacillary haemoglobinuria

An uncommon condition seen in animals over 1 year of age. The disease is caused by exposure to spores of *Clostridium haemolyticum* and liver fluke.

Clinical signs The animal may be found dead. There may be sudden acute illness with pyrexia (39.5 to 42°C), pain, abdominal stasis and brisket oedema. The urine is red, the faeces dark and watery. Later if the patient survives, jaundice and anaemia may be seen. Abortion may occur in pregnant animals. Dyspnoea is seen in severely ill cases.

Babesiosis

Seen in tick infested areas and chiefly in the spring, summer and autumn months in non-immune animals.

Clinical signs *Acute form* – pyrexia (to 43°C), depression, anorexia, red urine, pipe-stem diarrhoea, abortion in pregnant animals, anaemia, death in untreated cases. Occasionally see CNS signs as *Babesia* infested erythrocytes accumulate in the brain. *Subacute form* – transient dullness may be seen in immune animals. *Babesia divergens* or *Babesia major* are found in red blood cells.

Postparturient haemoglobinuria

An uncommon condition seen chiefly in Scotland in harsh weather conditions. High yielding dairy cows are affected, especially during lactations 3 to 5. Sporadic cases are seen in the first 4 weeks after calving. Animals are on a low phosphorus diet and often feeding on rape, cabbage, turnips and kale.

Clinical signs Sudden onset, reddish brown urine, weak, staggering, dyspnoeic, milk yield and appetite fall. Pallor of membranes, jaundice, collapse and death.

CLINICIAN'S CHECKLIST – THE URINARY SYSTEM

Abnormal urination
Urine inspection and analysis
Patient observation
External examination of urinary system

Rectal examination
Vaginal examination
Signs of specific urinary system
    disease

PHYSICAL SIGNS OF DISEASE ASSOCIATED WITH THE URINARY SYSTEM

N.B. Some of these physical signs are associated with diseases of other body systems and regions and are not unique to the urinary system.

Abnormal behaviour
  Bruxism
  Bellowing

Demeanour
  Lethargy
  Depression

Appetite
  Decreased

Drinking
  Increased
  Decreased

Hydration status
  Dehydrated

Urination
  Tenesmus
  Increase frequency
  Dysuria
  Painful

Volume of urine produced
  Anuria
  Oliguria
  Polyuria

Abnormal urine
  Discolouration
    Red
      Haematuria
      Haemoglobinuria
    Brown
    Yellow
  Abnormal contents
    Blood
    Pus
  Smell
    Ketones

Abdomen
  Pain
  Kicking abdomen
  Swelling of skin around
    prepuce
  Skin around prepuce cold and
    necrotic
  Preputial hairs have uroliths
    attached
  Bilateral ventral distension

Mucous membranes
  Pale

Faecal quality
  Diarrhoea

Umbilicus
  Closed cyst
  Urine
  Pus

Rectal examination
  Pole of left kidney
    Painful
    Enlarged
    Loss of lobulated pattern
  Bladder
    Thickened
    Painful
  Urethra
    Pulsation
  Bladder
    Enlarged and tense
    No bladder palpated

Vaginal examination
  Urovagina

Clinical Examination of the Female Genital System

Introduction

Examination and assessment of the genital system is an important part of the veterinary management of dairy cows. The target on many dairy farms is for cows to achieve a calving to calving interval of 365 days. To achieve this target the reproductive performance of the cow has to be closely managed. Some consider this calving interval to be an unattainable and possibly undesirable goal in high yielding cows. On many farms it is only achieved by close monitoring of the cows' reproductive performance and intervention with strategic hormone therapy. An assessment of herd fertility should involve examination of animals, including any problem animals, as they are presented for routine fertility checks. It should also involve consideration of the farm husbandry and management. Information required should include the overall disease profile of the farm, milk yields and both past and present fertility records.

The cow has an average gestation length of 283 days. To achieve a calving interval of 365 days she must conceive again within 82 days ($365 - 283 = 82$) of her previous calving. Uterine involution is normally complete and resumption of overt ovarian activity has normally commenced by 40 days after calving. Conception should ideally occur in the period of 40 to 82 days after calving.

Beef cows are subject to less intense pressures because their milk production has to be sufficient only for their own calf. None the less, a calving interval of 365 days is very important to enable the herd to calve at approximately the same time and over a short period each year. A short calving period enables the herd and their calves to be fed and managed as a group. Monitoring of the reproductive performance is also important in beef cattle.

Much routine fertility work consists of specific and often limited examinations of the cow's genital system. A more detailed and comprehensive examination may be requested and is necessary when a particularly valuable cow fails to conceive. In every case it must be remembered that the genital system is just one part of the patient. Unless the patient is in good health and her genital system is functioning normally, conception may not occur. Whenever the genital system is examined the veterinarian should also assess the general health of the patient and be alert to the possibility that disease involving other body systems may also be present.

Applied anatomy

The anatomy of the female genital system is illustrated in Fig. 10.1. Details of the anatomy of the individual genital organs are given under clinical examination below.

Signalment of the case

The age of the patient is very important. Maiden heifers have never bred and a small proportion may prove unable to do so. Some may be freemartins being the twin to a male calf and having the genital tract of an intersex. Other congenital defects resulting in infertility are rare but none the less must be considered in such a group of animals. Fertility problems tend to increase with the cow's parity because the risk of acquired abnormalities increases with the birth of each calf. Maiden heifers have not yet sustained injuries at calving or experienced problems associated with a retained placenta. These problems are more frequent in older cows. Such animals are

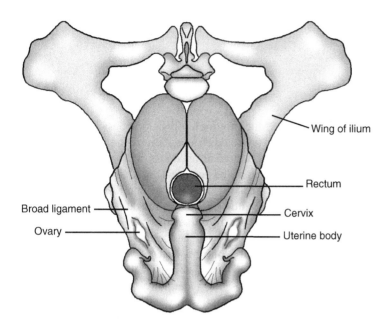

Figure 10.1 The bovine genital tract in a non-pregnant animal.

more likely to be exposed to dietary deficiencies which can have an adverse effect on fertility.

History of the case

Details of both herd and individual patient history are of great importance in the recognition and diagnosis of problems in the female genital system.

History of the herd

The clinician should seek answers to the following questions:

(1) What is the herd size? Has it increased recently?
(2) Are fertility records for the herd available? On many dairy farms retrospective computerised records are kept. A number of indices of fertility may be available and consideration of them all is beyond the scope of this book. Among important indices is the *herd submission rate* which assesses the vital oestrus detection rate of the herd. The *conception rate* and its seasonal change monitored by *cumulative sum* (Q sum) are also very important. Poor fertility indices may in-

dicate overall poor performance. They may also indicate that one section of the herd, for example first calf heifers, is performing badly. It should also be possible to identify how the herd is performing in the current year compared with previous years.

(3) Herd management – what staff are employed? Have there been recent changes of staff? What method(s) of oestrus detection are used? Is a fertility control scheme in place? Does it include a postnatal check, prebreeding examination and pregnancy diagnosis? What is the herd policy on cows not achieving herd targets such as being in calf by 82 days?
(4) Feeding and production – what feeding regime is used? Has the diet changed recently? Are trace element deficiencies known in the area? Are metabolic profiles taken from cows to assess feeding and identify deficiencies? Does the farm have a seasonal policy for milk production?
(5) What is the incidence of herd lameness, metabolic disease and mastitis? Have these problems increased recently?
(6) How many cases of abortion occurred during the last year? Was the cause of abortion diagnosed? Is a vaccination policy in place?

(7) Is the herd self contained? What was the health profile of any recently purchased animals?

(8) Is artificial insemination (AI) used? Is DIY AI used? Are the staff skilled in using AI? Do any staff members have poor cow AI conception rates? Is on-farm semen storage satisfactory? If natural service is used, is the bull known to be fertile?

History of the cow or heifer

Further questions should be asked or records inspected to ascertain the following details of the patient's history:

(1) The age and parity of the cow.
(2) Has the cow had any previous breeding problems? What were these? Was treatment successful?
(3) Details of last calving – date, parturient problems including dystocia, retention of fetal membranes.
(4) Dates of observed oestrus since calving – has the cow cycled regularly? Is she cycling now? Have her cycles been excessively short or prolonged?
(5) Service details – dates and method of service, operator, bull or semen used.
(6) Production records of this cow.
(7) Health record of this cow – details of lameness, metabolic disease, mastitis, abortion.

Observation of the patient

Cows presented for fertility investigation may be confined to a stall or in the parlour. Wherever possible the cow should be viewed from all sides without restriction, so that her general health and condition can be assessed. Certain specific changes may be seen which relate to the patient's reproductive state. Many of these are normal physiological changes, but the clinician should look carefully for obvious signs of abnormality which can be investigated further at a later stage.

The *condition score* of the cow should be estimated and confirmed by palpation of the lumbar and sacral regions when the cow is handled. The score (range 1

= very thin to 5 = obese) has an important influence on fertility. Cows should have a condition score of 3 at calving, 2.5 when served and 2.5 to 3 when dried off.

The *cow in oestrus* may appear slightly excitable. A vaginal discharge of clear tacky mucus (the 'bulling string') may be present. Scuff marks may be seen on her hindquarters and in front of her tuber coxae caused by the feet of other animals mounting her. Dried saliva from other cows may be seen in similar places. Approximately 48 hours after oestrus the cow may pass a dark red watery vaginal discharge.

Animals suffering from *long term cystic ovarian disease* may show abnormalities of body shape. *Virilism*, in which bull-like changes are seen, may occur in animals chronically affected by luteal cysts secreting progesterone. Increased development of the neck muscles may occur and the animal may become aggressive. Chronic exposure to oestrogens produced by follicular cysts may produce signs of *nymphomania*. In addition to displaying frequent signs of oestrus, affected animals may show slackening of the pelvic ligaments with apparent prominence of the tail head.

A degree of *abdominal distension* is anticipated during pregnancy, especially in the last trimester. Animals carrying twins may show greater than normal abdominal distension. *Pathological abdominal enlargement* may be seen in cases of hydrops allantois or hydrops amnion in which the uterus contains excessive amounts of fluid. The clinical signs of these two conditions are discussed below. Other causes of abdominal enlargement such as ascites must always be borne in mind and should be detected during the general examination.

In the *last few days of pregnancy* the sacrosciatic ligaments become relaxed. The vulva lengthens and appears slightly oedematous. Tail tone appears to be reduced. The udder continues to enlarge and may become oedematous. In some animals the teats leak colostrum. Mucus from the cervical plug may appear at the vulva. Body temperature may fall.

Immediately after calving the vulva is still enlarged and a scant bloodstained vaginal discharge is normal for 7 to 10 days. The pelvic ligaments begin to tighten up again and the perineum returns to its preparturient state. A foul *brown or red vaginal discharge* may indicate the presence of a potentially serious septic metritis. *Retained fetal membranes* occur quite frequently in cattle. They are usually clearly visible as strands of necrotic chorioallantois and amnion hanging from the vulva. In some animals there is no external sign of retained fetal membranes and these are only detected later during vaginal examination. *Prolapse or eversion of the vagina* may be seen in the periparturient period. *Uterine prolapse* with exposure of the endometrium and caruncles may be a complication of the postparturient period.

In the normal breeding period, 40 to 82 days after calving, the clinician should look for any signs of abnormal vaginal discharge. At this stage a creamy white discharge, either scant or profuse, may indicate the presence of *endometritis*.

CLINICIAN'S CHECKLIST – REPRODUCTIVE HISTORY AND OBSERVATION OF THE COW

Reproductive history of herd
Reproductive history of cow
Observation of cow
    General condition (condition score) and signs of health
    Signs of oestrus
    Evidence of abnormal vaginal discharge
    Changes in body shape

Examination of the female genital system

This has the following components:

(1) external examination of the female genital system,
(2) rectal examination of the genital system including ultrasonographic appraisal,
(3) vaginal examination,
(4) special diagnostic tests if required.

When possible and appropriate all components of the examination should be carried out. At the *postnatal check* 21 days after calving, specific checks are made for uterine involution, evidence of uterine infection and ovarian activity. When the cow is pre-

sented for pregnancy diagnosis and is found to be pregnant further examination is not performed. If not pregnant at pregnancy diagnosis a full gynaecological examination is carried to detect any reasons for failure of conception.

For reasons of hygiene, vaginal examination should precede rectal examination. Vaginal examination – especially if a speculum is used – may, however, result in aspiration of air into the vagina which can make subsequent rectal examination more difficult as the vagina feels grossly enlarged. Any air in the vagina can be expelled by gently pressing downwards and backwards on the vagina with the hand in the rectum. If the rectal examination is performed first, care must be taken to ensure that faecal material is not carried into the genital tract.

(1) External examination of the female genital system

Any abnormalities already observed should now be followed up by visual and manual examination with the cow restrained in a crush or AI stall. This examination is chiefly confined to the vulva and caudal vagina. Evidence of a vulval or vaginal discharge may be seen at this stage and will require further investigation. In the last trimester of pregnancy the fetus may be ballotted through the lower part of the right abdominal wall. Fetal presence and sometimes its viability can be detected. Detailed fetal appraisal by ultrasonography will be discussed later.

Vulva
The vulval lips should form a seal which, with the cervix, prevents the entry of potentially dangerous organisms into the uterus. The vulva should be positioned vertically below the anus. The lips of the vulva should normally be of approximately similar size and should have no visible space between them.

Sinking of the anus
Sinking of the anus in an anterior direction is seen in many older cows. It is also seen in younger animals in certain breeds, for example the Charolais. As a result of anal displacement the upper commisure of the vulva is dragged forwards, causing a variable degree of distortion of the vulva; thus the vulval seal may be

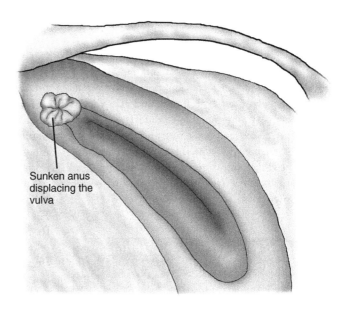

Figure 10.2 Poor perineal conformation in a cow with sinking of the anus and displacement of the vulva.

compromised and the risk of faecal contamination is increased (Fig. 10.2). At the mucocutaneous junction or just within the vulva, areas of *necrotic vaginitis* may be present caused by fetal or human pressure at calving. Early lesions appear dark and congested; later lesions are green and necrotic.

In the immediate postparturient period, the vulval lips may be oedematous and bruising may be present. *Scar formation* in the tissues of the vulval lips may follow injuries sustained during calving. This can also reduce the efficiency of the vulval seal and lessen the likelihood of successful conception.

Vulval and/or vaginal discharge

The colour, quantity and consistency of this should be observed. Its origin will probably require further investigation. The clear bulling string, the red metoestrus bloodstained discharge and the appearance of retained fetal membranes have been mentioned above. Although some bloodstained or purulent material may originate from the bladder or renal pelvis, most bovine vulval and/or vaginal discharges emanate from the reproductive system. A white or yellowish discharge may indicate the presence of *endometritis* or *pyometra*. A foul-smelling bloody and purulent discharge may be associated with *acute septic metritis* or with a *macerated fetus*. It

may also occur in cases of *abortion* or threatened abortion. This type of discharge can also be seen in cases of *necrotic vaginitis* and in association with infected wounds in the vaginal wall. A black-brown foul-smelling discharge in a very sick animal may be an indication of a *clostridial infection in the uterus*. The clinician must always check, through a full clinical examination, that any unpleasant odour at the hind end of the patient is actually emanating from the vagina. *Granular vulvovaginitis* may be caused by mycoplasma infection. *Infectious vulvovaginitis*, a venereal disease caused by bovine herpesvirus 1, causes painful inflammation of the external genitalia of the cow and the bull.

Ballottement

Ballottement of the *right side of the abdomen* in the last trimester of pregnancy will often make contact with the fetus and sometimes cause it to move. Signs of movement confirm the presence of fetal life. Absence of movement, either spontaneous or by ballottement, does not necessarily mean that the fetus is dead. Further evaluation of fetal well-being can be made by rectal examination and by ultrasonography. All or part of the fetus can be scanned *per rectum* in the first trimester of pregnancy. After this time the fetus slips down into the abdomen beyond reach and may not be palpable *per rectum* until the last month of pregnancy. Transabdominal ultrasonography through the clipped flank in late pregnancy usually confirms the presence of fetal fluids and placentomes. Parts of the fetus can sometimes be seen, depending on its exact location within the abdomen and also within the uterus. It may be possible to detect fetal heart movements, check fetal pulse rate and the expected absence of echogenicity in the normal clear fetal fluids. The use of ultrasonography in examination of the female genital system is discussed in greater detail below.

> ## CLINICIAN'S CHECKLIST – INSPECTION OF THE VULVA
>
> Position and conformation of the vulva
> Efficiency of the vulval seal
> Vulval and/or vaginal discharge – colour, quantity and consistency

(2) Rectal examination of the female genital system

This must be carried out methodically and with great care and sensitivity. The examination should provide useful information about all palpable parts of the female genital tract. It should reveal the whereabouts, size and condition of the cervix, the uterine body and horns, and the right and left ovaries. It may prove possible to identify and assess the ovarian bursae and the oviducts. These structures may be more readily detected when they are diseased than when they are normal.

As a result of rectal examination it should be possible to determine whether the animal is more than 6 weeks pregnant, whether she is cycling and the stage of her oestrous cycle. The reproductive information and history available for each animal will to some extent direct the rectal and other examinations, to provide the detailed assessment required at that time. Thus in the recently calved cow rectal examination will reveal how well the uterus has involuted. At 40 to 82 days postcalving, palpation of the ovaries should indicate whether the ovaries are active and in

many cases the approximate stage of the patient's current oestrous cycle. The accuracy of such findings can be enhanced in many cases by the use of ultrasonography *per rectum* and also by an appraisal of the progesterone profile of the cow.

The clinician must always be aware that the reproductive history of a cow may be inaccurate. The findings reported must always be those actually identified and where possible confirmed. In some cases a further rectal examination after a finite period of time may be necessary to confirm a tentative clinical observation and diagnosis made at the first visit. *Findings should be accurately recorded* and preserved at the time of each rectal examination.

Preparing for rectal examination

The animal must be restrained to ensure animal and operator safety. Confinement in an AI stall or crush is preferable to the milking parlour. Fingernails should be short and all hand jewellery removed before commencing rectal examination. Waterproof protective clothing is required. Both arms should be covered with long plastic sleeves, and ideally these should be changed between cows. Either the right or left hand may be used. Some clinicians prefer to use both hands sequentially during a rectal examination.

The fingers and thumb are formed into a cone and the gloved hand is covered with obstetrical lubricant. A further small amount of lubricant may be placed against the anal ring of the patient. The hand is gently but firmly advanced through the anus into the rectum. The anus normally relaxes after a few moments allowing the hand and wrist to enter the rectum. Any faeces are gently removed by enclosing them in the hand and carrying them out through the anal ring.

Care must be taken to avoid large quantities of air entering the caudal rectum. The risk of this occurring can be reduced by the clinician easing faecal material through the anal ring without fully withdrawing the hand on each occasion. If distended with air, the rectal wall becomes so tense that palpation of structures such as the uterus becomes quite impossible. The cow can usually be encouraged to expel rectal air. The clinician's hand is advanced into the anterior rectum where normal peristaltic tension in the walls is still present. By making gentle stroking movements with the fingers on the rectal wall muscular tension is restored and flatus is expelled.

Position of the female genital tract

In heifers and young cows the whole genital tract may be palpable lying on the pelvic floor. In older animals part or all of the uterus may hang over the pelvic brim. In these animals it is necessary to attempt to *retract the uterus into the pelvis* so that its component parts can be more readily examined. This may be done by hooking a finger over the inter-cornual ligament or by using the hand to scoop the anterior parts of the genital tract back into the pelvis (Fig. 10.3). Once retracted, the uterus is held in place by gentle manual pressure before being examined and then released to slip back over the pelvic brim.

The genital tract of the cow is supported by the *broad ligament* of the uterus which is attached to the sides of the pelvis (Fig. 10.4). A small fold of the broad ligament – the *ovarian bursa* – loosely surrounds each ovary. The ovarian bursa may become adherent to the ovary in cases of *ovarian bursitis*.

Middle uterine artery   This is the main source of blood for the uterus. The artery arises from the internal iliac artery shortly after this vessel leaves the aorta. In non-pregnant animals it passes caudally through the broad ligament, over the wing of the ilium into the pelvic cavity. It then enters the concave ventral surface of the uterus. As pregnancy progresses the artery is pulled forwards by the enlarging uterus. By the second half of pregnancy it may be palpated 5 to 10 cm anterior to the wing of the ilium. The blood flow through the middle uterine artery increases greatly as pregnancy progresses. It can be readily recognised when the clinician's hand is passed laterally and upwards from the uterus and cervix. The internal iliac artery is relatively immobile and is found just anterior to the wing of the ilium. The pudendal artery is palpable in the wall of the pelvic canal 10 cm anterior to the anus. The middle uterine artery is quite mobile and somewhat tortuous within the broad ligament. At 5 months of pregnancy a *turbulent flow* ('*fremitus*') is usually palpable within the artery on the pregnant side of the uterus. Towards the

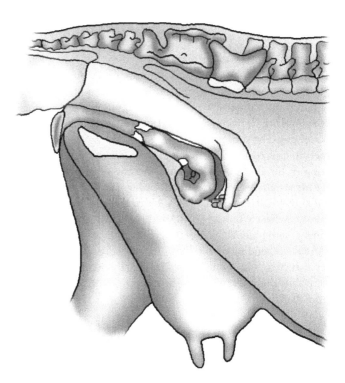

Figure 10.3 Retraction of the non-pregnant uterus of a mature cow. See text for details.

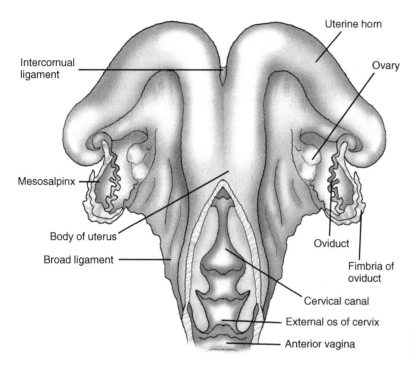

Intercornual ligament

Uterine horn

Ovary

Mesosalpinx

Body of uterus

Broad ligament

Oviduct

Fimbria of oviduct

Cervical canal

External os of cervix

Anterior vagina

Figure 10.4 Anatomical details of the bovine genital tract.

end of pregnancy fremitus is palpable in both middle uterine arteries.

Findings on rectal examination

The clinician's hand enclosed within its protective plastic sleeve and the rectum can be moved quite widely within the cow's pelvis. The bony limits of the pelvis can be readily identified as firm immobile structures. The roof of the pelvis is formed by the sacrum and coccygeal vertebrae, the walls by the wing of the ilium on either side and the floor by the fused pubic bones. The caudal border of the lobed left kidney can be palpated just anterior to the pelvic inlet: it lies just to the right of the midline beneath the lumbar vertebrae. The size of the genital tract is very variable depending on the age of the animal and its reproductive state. The cervix is usually readily found and the other parts of the tract can be identified from that point.

Cervix This is found close to the midline of the pelvic floor. It is located by initially exerting gentle manual pressure on the pelvic floor and resting the fingers on the pubic bones. The fingers are then moved laterally from one side to the other but maintaining downward pressure until contact is made with the firm, smooth cylindrical cervix. In heifers the cervix is about 2 cm in width and 4 cm in length. In these animals, where the entire genital tract is within the pelvis, the cervix is found on the pelvic floor approximately half way between the caudal border of the pubis and the pelvic brim cranially. The cervix is much firmer than adjacent soft tissues and can be moved laterally to a limited extent.

In older multiparous cows the cervix is 4 to 5 cm in width and 8 cm in length. Just before and after calving the cervix feels softer to the touch and may be 10 cm or more in width. It may lie just behind, on or over the pelvic brim. In pregnant animals lateral movement of the cervix is very limited as it is pulled tightly forwards by the weight of the pregnant uterus.

Uterus This is located by moving the hand forwards from the cervix. In heifers the body and horns of the uterus, which normally lies entirely in the pelvis, can be readily enclosed in the clinician's hand.

In older animals only part of the uterus can be enclosed in the hand in this way. The body and horns may lie on the abdominal floor anterior to the pelvic brim. Palpation may be aided by gently retracting the uterus (see above). Retraction may be impossible in pregnant animals or in those in which uterine adhesions are present. The uterine horns are coiled and their anterior extremities are not directly palpable.

The uterus feels turgid and very tightly coiled in animals in oestrus, but such turgidity can also be induced in some cattle by manual palpation of the genital tract. In early pregnancy the uterine walls are lacking in muscular tone. Later on as fetal size and uterine fluid content increase the tone of the uterine wall also increases The short *uterine body* is palpable as a cylindrical structure just in front of but much softer and slightly wider than the cervix. In heifers the uterine body is approximately 3 cm in length. In non-pregnant animals the two *uterine horns* should normally be approximately the same size (2 to 3 cm wide). In older animals the horns are larger and there may be a disparity of size caused by an earlier pregnancy. The uterus undergoes great enlargement during pregnancy.

Uterine involution commences immediately after calving. Initial involution is rapid in healthy animals but may be delayed by dystocia, uterine inertia and retained fetal membranes. The anterior poles of the uterus should be palpable by 14 days postpartum. Uterine involution should be complete by 25 to 50 days. Postpartum uterine fluid normally disappears within 7 to 10 days of calving. After that time the uterus should contain little fluid. In some animals a low grade infection – *endometritis* – is present in the uterus and is accompanied by the accumulation of varying amounts of purulent fluid. A visible vaginal discharge may be present and the uterus may be found to be enlarged and fluid filled on rectal examination. The presence of purulent material can be confirmed by ultrasonography.

Large amounts of purulent material are present in the uterus in cases of *pyometra* but the animal rarely shows signs of systemic illness. In the serious disease *acute septic metritis* the uterine wall may be hard and occasionally emphysematous on rectal examination. Very occasionally, and possibly following injury at parturition, a *uterine wall abscess* may be

detected. An irregular area on the uterine wall may be palpated *per rectum* and can be further evaluated by ultrasonography.

Pregnancy diagnosis by rectal palpation Details are beyond the scope of this book. The main findings may be summarised as follows:

35 days – unilateral enlargement of the pregnant horn; presence of corpus luteum on the ipsilateral ovary

42 days – palpation of *amniotic vesicle* (2 to 3 cm in diameter) in the pregnant horn

42–70 days – palpation of *membrane slip*. The uterine wall is lifted and allowed to slip between the clinician's finger and thumb. The additional chorioallantoic membrane slipping independently of the uterine wall is palpable at this stage. Disparity between pregnant and non-pregnant horns is more distinct (Fig. 10.5)

>120 days – *cotyledons palpable* in the dorsal wall of the uterus. At this stage they are 3 to 4 cm in diameter, increasing to 6 to 8 cm towards the end of pregnancy. Cotyledons have been described as being like 'corks floating on water'. They are initially quite close together but later, as allantoic fluid volume increases, they move further apart. Cotyledons are readily detected by advancing the hand as far forward as possible *per rectum* and then moving the palm backwards and downwards stroking the dorsal wall of the uterus. The cotyledons are palpated as elevations in the uterine wall

150 days – *fremitus palpable* in the middle uterine artery on the pregnant side

240 days – *bilateral fremitus palpable*; the exact timing is variable

The fetus, which is very small, is not palpable within the tense amniotic vesicle in the first 10 weeks of pregnancy. After this, fetal extremities may be palpable through the uterine wall. By 14 weeks the fetus has often passed beyond reach. Fetal extremities may be palpable again from 26 weeks of pregnancy. In the last 4 weeks of pregnancy the calf is usually readily palpable as it increases in size. Touching the fetal head or gently squeezing its feet may cause it to move, thus confirming its viability

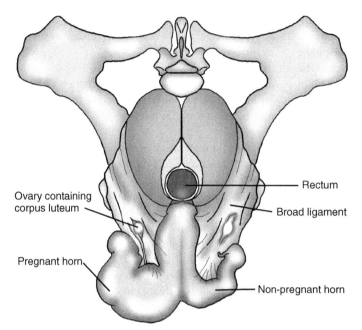

Ovary containing corpus luteum

Pregnant horn

Rectum

Broad ligament

Non-pregnant horn

Figure 10.5 The bovine uterus at approximately 10 weeks of pregnancy.

(Fig. 10.6). In the last few days of pregnancy the feet of the calf often enter the pelvis in preparation for birth. Occasionally, if the calf is very large and heavy, in late pregnancy it may slip under the caudal parts of the rumen and cannot be palpated *per rectum.*

Ovaries In non-pregnant animals these are located on the pelvic floor approximately level with and quite close to the junction of the body and horns of the uterus (Fig. 10.7). In searching for them *per rectum* the clinician should remain in manual contact with the uterus to which they are attached. Maintaining contact with the uterus enables the clinician to limit the area in which the ovaries may be sought. Occasionally one ovary, often the left, is not immediately palpable and may have slipped under the anterior border of the broad ligament. Digital pressure exerted in a downward and anterior direction on the broad ligament will usually cause the ovary to move back into a palpable position. Very occasionally animals are found in which only a single ovary is present.

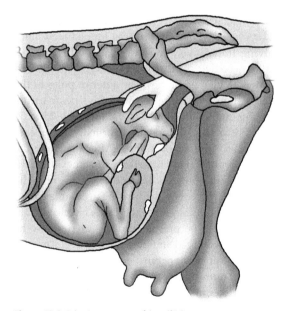

Figure 10.6 Palpation *per rectum* of the calf in late pregnancy.

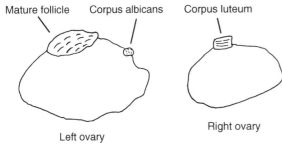

Figure 10.7 Diagrammatic representation of a cycling cow. The cow has a mature follicle on her left ovary and the regressing corpus luteum from the previous cycle on her right ovary. A corpus albicans from an earlier pregnancy is still palpable on the left ovary.

The ovaries are firmer than adjacent tissues and one, currently the more active ovary, is larger than the other. Inactive ovaries in postpubertal cattle are 1 to 1.5 cm at their largest diameter. Active ovaries are usually 2.5 to 3.0 cm in diameter, but are occasionally larger. Ovarian shape is very variable and is influenced by the ovary's physiological activity and the presence of follicles and corpora lutea. Cystic ovaries may be considerably enlarged and are discussed below.

Once located, the ovaries should be palpated in detail. They can be picked up by the clinician using the thumb and second finger. The surface of the ovary is palpated with the first finger (Fig. 10.7). As much of the ovarian surface as possible is explored, testing for shape and consistency. *Ovarian follicles* are fluid filled and readily compressible, with a smooth surface often rising just above the ovarian surface. More than one follicle may be present, but as oestrus approaches a single follicle may become dominant and grow faster than the others. Mature ovarian follicles are up to 2 cm in diameter. Just before ovulation the ripening follicle may soften. Immediately after ovulation a small depression may be palpated at the site of ovulation. This is later palpable as the spongy *corpus rubrum* which later becomes luteinised as the corpus luteum. *Corpora lutea* project from the ovarian surface and are firm and non-compressible to the touch (Fig. 10.7). The young corpus luteum is slightly compressible. It hardens with age and sinks back into the ovarian stroma but may still be palpable as a small

corpus albicans after it ceases to be active. During pregnancy the ovaries are palpable until about 90 days after conception. After that they are pulled forward beyond reach by the enlarging uterus.

Both ovaries must be examined before the clinician can evaluate their activity and identify the stage of the patient's oestrous cycle. Evidence of previous cyclical activity is often present. Ovulation may occur sequentially on the same ovary or alternate between the two ovaries. The absence of follicles or corpora lutea may suggest that the patient is in anoestrus. A further rectal examination should be made 10 to 14 days later to confirm or refute the absence of cyclical ovarian activity. Further evaluation of the ovaries by ultrasonography and a plasma or milk progesterone profile of the patient are extremely useful in confirming the physiological state of the ovaries. These techniques are discussed in greater detail below.

Cystic ovarian disease   Ovarian cysts are very common in dairy cattle and can be readily diagnosed on rectal examination. In most cases a single ovary is involved, but occasionally bilateral cysts are seen. Cysts are defined as being fluid filled structures greater than 2.5 cm in diameter. Ovaries containing cysts may be grossly enlarged and their overall diameter may occasionally exceed 5 to 6 cm. Ovarian cysts are broadly classified into two main groups whose clinical and diagnostic features are summarised below.

Follicular cysts – may be associated with short oestrous cycles, irregular oestrus and nymphomania. Cysts are normally thin walled (<3 mm) and may be multiple. They do not secrete progesterone.
Luteal cysts – often associated with anoestrus, may show signs of virilism, and are usually single and thick walled (>3 mm); progesterone is secreted.

Granulosa cell tumours   These large irregular tumours are uncommon in cattle. They usually involve one ovary which is grossly enlarged, has a variable hormone secretion and may hang over the pelvic brim.

Ovarian bursae These may not always be readily palpable *per rectum*. It may be possible to pass the fingers into the shallow bursa as it lies adjacent to the ovary. Small physiological adhesions may form between the ovary and the ovarian bursa. In cases of *ovarian bursitis* the bursa become tightly adherent to the ovary and may completely enclose it in a thick outer covering. This may physically prevent both the release of ova and also detailed palpation of the ovary by the clinician.

Oviducts These firm tortuous tubes 1 to 2 mm in diameter may sometimes be palpable in the specialised part of the broad ligament – the mesosalpinx – which carries them. If they become inflamed and obstructed, for example in *salpingitis*, they may become enlarged, thickened and sometimes more readily palpable.

Ultrasonographic examination of the genital tract

This technique has become an increasingly important part of the gynaecological examination of cattle. It provides additional information and also confirmation of the findings at manual examination. A linear array or sector scanner with a probe in the 3.5 to 7.5 MHz frequency range is used. The probe, coated with a couplant, is covered with a plastic sleeve before use. Ideally, a separate sleeve or outer sleeve should be used for each animal. The probe is easily damaged and the clinician should be constantly aware of its vulnerability when using it on the farm.

The brightness mode (B mode) scanner produces an image compounded from the reflection of ultrasonic waves directed by the probe into the tissue to be investigated. Water does not reflect ultrasound (it is said to be non-echogenic) and is seen as a black image on the screen. Dense tissue such as bone is impenetrable to ultrasound; it is said to be echogenic and produces a pale grey or white image. Other bodily tissues reflect ultrasound to an extent between the extremes of water and bone.

The bovine genital tract is very suitable for ultrasonographic evaluation. The technique enables *details of ovarian structure* to be demonstrated or confirmed. It is possible to recognise ovarian follicles as non-echogenic structures less than 2 cm in diameter. The *waves of follicles* that develop during the oestrous cycle can be seen and counted at serial examinations. Corpora lutea appear as echodense structures protruding through the ovarian wall. Ultrasound is also very useful in the *evaluation of ovarian cysts*. The wall thickness of ovarian cysts can be seen and measured. An echogenic band around an ovary may confirm the presence of *ovarian bursitis*.

Pregnancy diagnosis Ultrasonographic scanning of the uterus and its contents enables pregnancy to be easily and reliably diagnosed at 30 days; this is 12 days before the earliest time that pregnancy can be diagnosed by manual palpation of the uterus *per rectum*. Twins may also be identified and sexing of fetuses is possible by a skilled operator using a high quality scanner. It is possible that a percentage of very early pregnancies will not survive until term. It is advisable to check by palpation and scan that the animal has maintained pregnancy at 6 to 10 weeks.

Confirmation of fetal life can be demonstrated ultrasonographically from 30 days. It may be possible to see fetal heartbeats and at a slightly later stage fetal movement. Clear non-echogenic amniotic fluid with evidence of fetal viability suggests a healthy pregnancy. Cloudy amniotic fluid with fetal tachycardia or severe bradycardia suggests that fetal life is at risk.

In *later pregnancy* the fetus or its fluids are clearly demonstrable using ultrasound. The presence of cotyledons involving the uterine wall and the chorioallantois can also be clearly demonstrated from 90 days onwards.

The ultrasonographic probe can also be used per vaginam. Very detailed information concerning ovarian morphology can be obtained in this way. The probe is held against the vaginal wall. The ovary is secured *per rectum* and is carefully brought to the probe for evaluation.

Ultrasound is also used in the diagnosis of a number of pathological conditions of the female genital tract which are discussed below.

(3) Vaginal examination

This may be carried out manually or using a speculum. Many cows and most heifers find a manual vaginal examination uncomfortable but tolerate a speculum well. In the absence of a speculum much useful information can be obtained from a careful manual vaginal examination. Two main types of speculum are available. Plastic or polished cardboard tubular speculae with a light source at their distal end allow close and well illuminated examination of the vagina and the cervix. Their tubular parts are interchangeable and sometimes disposable, and a separate tube can be used for each animal. Metal, hinged 'duck-billed' specula can also be used. Light can be provided by a pen torch.

Before the examination, the perineum and vulva must be carefully washed with warm water and a small amount of dilute antiseptic. The distal end of the speculum is lightly smeared with obstetrical lubricant before being carefully introduced into the vagina. At this point the patient may aspirate air into her vagina, allowing a panoramic view of the vagina and cervix. This is particularly likely to happen with the duck-billed speculum. The tension on the vaginal walls and cervix may reveal lesions which are not visible in the non-dilated vagina.

Vaginal walls

The vaginal walls should be carefully inspected for signs of laceration or superficial damage. *Perivaginal haematomata* caused by calving injuries may cause distortion of the vaginal wall and reduce the size of the vaginal lumen. Their presence can be readily confirmed by rectal or vaginal ultrasonography when the typical segmented appearance of a haematoma can be confirmed. The *external urethral orifice* can be seen in the vaginal floor over the pubic bones.

Vaginal contents

The small *clitoris* may be seen on the ventral floor of the caudal vagina. In *freemartins* the clitoris may be prominent, occasionally surrounded by a small number of long hairs. The vagina is usually severely shortened (<5 cm) in freemartins and there is no cervix.

Hymenal remnants are quite rare in cattle. In some cases they occur, often just anterior to the external urethral orifice, as part of the *white heifer disease syndrome* where there may also be deficiencies in other parts of the tubular structures of the uterus and oviduct. Leiomyoma and squamous cell sarcoma are among *tumours* occasionally found near the vulval lips or within the vagina. *Vertical pillars* covered with mucous membrane are occasionally seen in the anterior vagina and are thought to be embryological remnants. Their presence should be noted, however, as they may cause problems at calving. A double cervix may be seen in some animals.

Cervix

The cervix is closely examined. When fully dilated at or immediately after calving the cervix is indistinguishable from the vaginal or uterine walls. It normally closes within a few days of calving, complete closure being delayed by the presence of infection or retained fetal membranes. The external os of the cervix is visible surrounded by a prominent rosebud-like protrusion into the anterior vagina (Fig. 10.8). In older cows a partial prolapse of the caudal part of the cervical canal into the vagina may be seen. In such cases one or more of the *annular rings* may be visible. Although noteworthy, this is thought to have no adverse effect on subsequent fertility. *Segmental laceration of the cervix* may occur at calving and resultant scar tissue may prevent closure of the cervical seal.

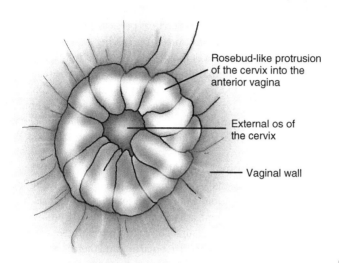

Rosebud-like protrusion
of the cervix into the
anterior vagina

External os of
the cervix

Vaginal wall

Figure 10.8 The bovine cervix as viewed through a vaginal speculum.

Such laceration may only be visible when the vagina is distended with aspirated air. In the non-pregnant cow the cervix is closed but opens slightly when the animal is in oestrus.

The vaginal lumen should normally be empty and any contents may be pathological. In cases of *urovagina* urine runs forward from the external urethral orifice pooling in the anterior vagina where it partially or completely covers the cervix preventing successful conception (Fig. 10.9). The clear thick mucus of the bulling string may be seen through the speculum in animals examined during oestrus. It is much thicker than obstetrical lubricant from which it is easily distinguished. A red watery metoestral discharge may be seen 48 hours after oestrus. A white or creamy white discharge coming through the cervix and pooling on the vaginal floor is seen in cases of *endometritis* and *pyometra*.

CLINICIAN'S CHECKLIST – VAGINAL EXAMINATION

Vaginal walls
Vaginal contents
Cervix

---

(4) Special diagnostic tests

These are only necessary in a few cases of diseases involving the female genital system. They are described in summary form below, together with some of their uses.

Milk (or plasma) progesterone assay

This can be used to confirm the presence of an active corpus luteum in one of the ovaries. Elevated progesterone is also seen in luteal ovarian cysts, in cases of a mummified fetus (see below) and in pregnant animals 19 to 23 days after service. Falling progesterone levels may be seen in failing pregnancies. Cows correctly diagnosed as being in oestrus have very low progesterone levels. Progesterone can be detected qualitatively or quantitatively in either milk or plasma using an ELISA test. A progesterone level of more than 5 ng per millilitre is regarded as being positive.

Oestrone sulphate test

This can be used to confirm the presence of a pregnancy of more than 105 days in cattle. The test is useful in cows in which the pregnant uterus is not accessible to palpation *per rectum* because of adhesions, or if transabdominal ultrasonography is not available.

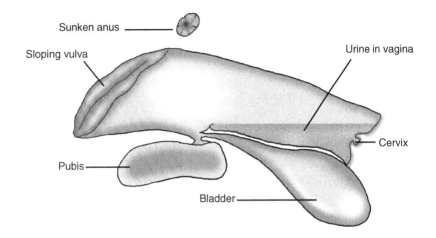

Figure 10.9 Urovagina in a cow.

Bovine trophoblast protein
This can be detected in the blood by an ELISA test in early pregnancy.

Oviduct patency test
Phenol red dye is placed in the uterus or one of its horns using a Foley catheter. If the oviducts are patent the dye will pass through them into the peritoneum. It passes into the circulation and is excreted through the kidneys. The bladder is catheterised and urine collected at 5 minute intervals. If dye is not seen in the urine within 40 minutes, the oviducts are not patent.

An alternative test is the *starch grain test* in which 1 g of sterile granular starch is placed over one ovary using a long needle via the sacrosciatic ligament. The cervical region of the vagina is flushed daily with 5 ml of sterile saline which is then stained with iodine. If the oviduct on that side is patent, starch can be identified in the saline within 48 hours.

Uterine biopsy
A sample of endometrium is taken by inserting a long pair of biopsy forceps through the cervix. Histological appraisal may indicate the presence of low grade inflammatory changes within the mucosa.

Clinical signs and diagnosis of some other conditions affecting the female genital system in cattle

Some of these conditions have been mentioned briefly above and additional information is given here.

Freemartin

A twin to a male calf. It may have a prominent clitoris, always has a shortened vagina (<5 cm) and no cervix. A vestigial uterus-like structure with no cervix is palpable *per rectum*. The gonads are placed very laterally in the pelvis (they are only palpable *per rectum* in older animals). The karyotype (XX/XY) can be demonstrated in a heparinised blood sample.

Hydrops allantois

Seen in late pregnancy. The cow is in poor condition with severe abdominal distension. Numerous small accessory cotyledons are palpable *per rectum* and demonstrable ultrasonographically. The distended uterus is pushed up into the pelvis. The calf is small and often not palpable. Paracentesis for uterine fluid – sodium, 50 mmol/l; chloride, 20 mmol/l.

Hydrops amnion

Seen from 6 months of pregnancy. The cow is in good condition, with normal cotyledons. The calf is palpable but often has a cleft palate. Paracentesis for uterine fluid – sodium, 120 mmol/l; chloride, 90 mmol/l.

Macerated fetus

The calf dies during pregnancy, the corpus luteum regresses and the cervix opens. A foul vaginal discharge is present. Fetal bones are palpable through the partially opened cervix. Uterine debris can be confirmed ultrasonographically.

Mummified fetus

The calf dies during pregnancy but the corpus luteum persists. Normal abdominal enlargement is not seen. The uterus is contracted around the fetus. The absence of fetal life or fluids is confirmed by ultrasonography. The cervix is closed. There is no vaginal discharge.

PHYSICAL SIGNS OF DISEASE ASSOCIATED WITH THE FEMALE GENITAL SYSTEM

Condition score
  High
  Low

Conformation
  Overdeveloped neck muscles
  Virilism
  Prominence of tail head
  Relaxed pelvic ligaments
  Bilateral ventral abdominal
    enlargement

Behaviour
  Increased aggression
  Nymphomania

Oestrus
  Not observed
  Interoestrus interval >24 days
  Interoestrus interval <18 days
  Interoestrus intervals irregular
  Oestrus >18 hours

Vulva
  Sloping conformation
  Swollen
  Lacerated
  Discharge
    Blood
    Creamy

Haemorrhagic and foul
  smelling
  Black-brown and foul smelling
  Placental debris >24 hours post-
    calving

Vagina
  Enlarged clitoris
  Vaginal prolapse
  Vaginal discharge
    Blood
    Creamy
    Haemorrhagic
    Urine in anterior vagina
  Vaginal mucosa
    Erosions
    Granular lesions
    Pustules
    Necrosis
    Perivaginal swelling
  Vaginal length
    Short

Cervix
  Open
  Lacerated
  Purulent discharge
  Double
  Absent

Uterus
  Distended
    Unilateral
    Bilateral
  Contents
    Fluid
    Emphysematous
    Bones (macerated fetus)
    Amorphous mass (mummified
      fetus)
  Uterine prolapse
  Mural swelling
  Abnormal size and shape

Ovaries
  Absent
  Abnormal position
  Cystic (>2.5 cm)
  Mass
  Ovarian bursa adherent to ovary

Oviducts
  Enlarged and palpable
  Thickened

Placenta
  Retained placenta

Pregnancy
  Abortion
  Stillbirth

Clinical Examination of the Male Genital System

Introduction

The majority of male cattle are castrated, and in these animals the genital system acts chiefly as a conduit for the passage of urine. Breeding bulls are an important part of the herd. To be effective sires, bulls must be in good health, have a satisfactory conformation and be free, as far as known, from genetic defects. They should also have a good libido, be able to mount and achieve intromission of the erect penis into the cow's vagina. They must be able to ejaculate semen of sufficient quality to fertilise the ova of healthy cows. In order to establish that a bull has these qualities a comprehensive and methodical examination is necessary.

Applied anatomy

The anatomy of the male genital system is illustrated in (Fig. 11.1). Details of the anatomy of individual genital organs are described below under 'Clinical examination'.

Signalment of the case

Details of this can be useful in the diagnosis of male breeding problems. Although puberty may be reached at 9 months, bulls are generally not used as sires until they are 18 months of age or over. Younger animals may have a poorly developed libido and poor semen quality. Excessive use of very young animals may also compromise sperm production. Libido may fall off in older bulls, and heavy bulls may have physical difficulty in mounting to serve. Some strains of Hereford bulls have a poorly developed libido.

History of the case

The general history of the case will have been discussed earlier in the diagnostic process. The owner should be questioned to determine the nature of any current fertility problem, the origin of the bull and his past performance. The following questions should be asked:

(1) Has the bull been recently purchased? If so are details available of his past performance? Has he ever sired a calf? When was he last known to have sired a calf?
(2) Has the bull been in good general health? Has he lost condition recently? Have there been any signs of lameness or other orthopaedic abnormality?
(3) Did his herd of origin have any past fertility problems? What was its health status? Was the herd known to be free from bovine virus diarrhoea infection and other diseases which may affect fertility? What is the disease status of his present herd?
(4) Has the bull served cows presented to him individually (in hand) or has he been running with the herd?
(5) If serving cows individually, has he been frightened in any way? Are the staff handling him experienced in their work?
(6) How many female animals was he running with? Is he still with them and if not when was he removed from their group? Has normal oestrus behaviour been observed in the group? Have they been bred from successfully before?
(7) What is the condition of the female animals? If in poor condition for how long has this been a problem? Has the cause of their poor condition been investigated?

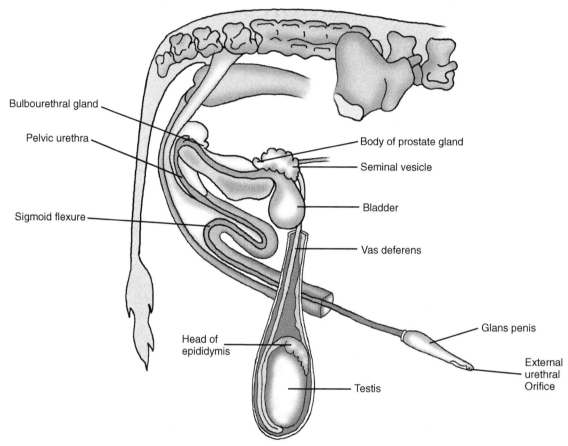

Figure 11.1 The genital organs of the bull.

(8) Has the bull been seen to serve? Was his service behaviour normal? Were any specific abnormalities during service noticed? In many cases close observation of service may not have been undertaken and the owner may be unaware of important details of service behaviour.

(9) Has pregnancy diagnosis been undertaken on the animals with which the bull has been running? What method of pregnancy diagnosis was used and was it capable of diagnosing early pregnancy (at 30 days)?

(10) Have the female animals been exposed subsequently to another bull? Has the other bull bred with them successfully?

Observation of the patient

The bull should be quietly observed to see if any obvious abnormalities which might affect his breeding ability are visible. Few reproductive problems in the male are visible externally. Obvious lameness could affect his ability to serve. Gross abnormalities in scrotal size or a disparity in testicular size may be visible, but must be confirmed and investigated during the full clinical examination.

Clinical examination of the male genital system

This has the following five component parts:

(1) full clinical examination including a rectal examination,
(2) assessment of libido,
(3) observation and assessment of service behaviour,
(4) semen collection and evaluation,
(5) further diagnostic tests if required.

Logically the clinician might wish to start with the full clinical examination to establish the health status of the patient and to diagnose any visible and palpable reproductive problems. Most bulls are infrequently handled and may be aggressive, requiring confinement for clinical examination. Young bulls may be nervous when handled and their libido may be suppressed. In practice, therefore, it may be best to observe libido and service behaviour, collect semen and complete the clinical examination after this.

The examination will be described in the order listed above.

(1) Full clinical examination including rectal examination

Physical examination of the bull – observation and inspection of the male genital system

The bull is initially observed from a distance. Orthopaedic abnormalities such as lameness, which could affect the bull's ability to mount or thrust, are noted at this stage. The prepuce, part of the penis and the scrotum are the only parts of the male genital system which are visible. Temporary *prolapse of the preputial mucosa* is seen in some bulls during periods of rest. In other animals, preputial prolapse is pathological and the exposed mucosa becomes oedematous and infected. In severe cases it may become impossible for the bull to extrude his penis (*phimosis*) or to retract his penis (*paraphimosis*).

Gross *enlargement of the scrotum* or disparity between its two sides may be noticed and will be further investigated by palpation at a later stage. The penis is normally fully enclosed within the prepuce, but a swelling may be seen anterior to the scrotum in cases of *rupture of the tunica albuginea* of the penis ('fractured penis'). This condition is discussed under penis below.

Detailed examination of the bull

Great care must be taken during all stages of the clinical examination of bulls. They are potentially dangerous animals and, although mostly distracted by the presence of a female animal, they should be watched carefully for signs of aggression.

The bull should be examined in a crush large enough to accommodate him comfortably and safely. His *identity* should be checked and his *ear number* recorded for inclusion in any report on his potential fertility. The *condition score* of the bull is assessed, since both very poor and excessive bodily condition may have an adverse effect on fertility. Temperature, pulse and respiratory rate should be checked. The chest and abdomen should be auscultated to ensure that the heart, lungs and gastrointestinal organs are functioning normally. Any problems with the bull's general health can also have an adverse effect on fertility. The bull's legs and feet are examined closely for signs of orthopaedic disease. The genital organs are then examined methodically. Much of the examination must take place behind or beside the bull and in range of his hind legs. The clinician must take care to avoid being kicked. In difficult animals it may be helpful to raise one of the patient's hind limbs whilst the prepuce and penis are being examined.

Scrotum This should be examined visually and then carefully palpated. The skin of the scrotum is mobile and covered with a coat of fine short hair. It should be free of any evidence of skin disease which, if inflammatory, may have an adverse influence on spermatogenesis. An increase in scrotal skin temperature may indicate inflammation of either the skin or the contents of the scrotum. Conversley, a decrease in temperature may indicate a loss of blood circulation within the skin or deeper tissues. The right and left sides of the scrotum should be symmetrical. Contraction of the cremaster muscles or of the subcutaneous tunica dartos may cause one or both testes to move dorsally, causing crinkling of the scrotal skin. There should be no free fluid within the scrotum. In cases of urethral rupture occurring near the scrotal neck, urine may leak into the scrotum. As a result, damage to scrotal tissues, especially the skin, may occur. In animals which have been vasectomised, vertical scars are seen on the skin of the scrotal neck, usually on its anterior surface.

Testes These should be mobile within the scrotum. Enclosed by the tunica vaginalis, their movement is aided by the lubricating action of small amounts of peritoneal fluid. The greatest testicular movement is within the dorsoventral plane. Lateral movements are restricted by the scrotal septum formed by layers of the tunica dartos. The testes are most effectively examined by gently moving them ventrally in the scrotum using pressure from the clinician's fingers and thumbs (Fig. 11.2). The surface of the testes should be smooth and firm, and their consistency that of a ripe tomato. Occasionally, defects in the tunica albuginea which covers each testis may be palpated. The testicular contents may bulge through such defects in the form of a *spermatocoele* or *sperm granuloma*. Such lesions may develop as a result of obstruction of semen outflow following vasectomy or injury.

The two testes should be approximately the same size and consistency. In the uncommon condition of *testicular hypoplasia* both testes are much smaller and softer than usual. In this hereditary condition sperm output is absent or severely decreased. *Testicular*

degeneration can also result in a reduction of testicular size and is often caused by an earlier infection. Sperm output is again reduced and large numbers of abnormal sperm may also be seen. *Cryptorchid* animals have only one scrotal testis and should not be used for breeding. The other organ may be retained within the abdomen, be partially descended or palpable near the external inguinal ring.

Disparity in testicular size may be seen in cases of *orchitis* affecting one testis. The affected organ may be enlarged, giving the scrotum an asymmetrical appearance. The affected testis may be painful to the touch, firmer than the normal testis and also less mobile within the scrotum.

Overall testicular size and volume are approximate measures of sperm output and can be equated with the scrotal circumference measured with a tape-measure at its largest point (Fig. 11.3). Scrotal circumference increases with age and is normally within the range 28 to 35 cm.

The testes can be evaluated by ultrasound either directly or using a stand-off technique. Both testes normally have a similar echodensity and have a number of horizontal bands of greater echodensity. In cases of chronic inflammatory disease the affected testis may have scattered areas of increased echodensity.

A testicular biopsy may be collected by direct removal of a small portion of testis or using a needle biopsy technique. The biopsy can provide useful his-

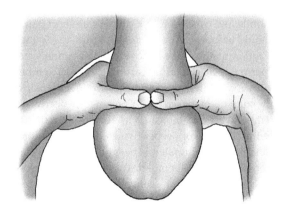

Figure 11.2 Palpation of the testes – see text for details.

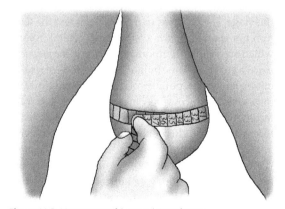

Figure 11.3 Measurement of the scrotal circumference.

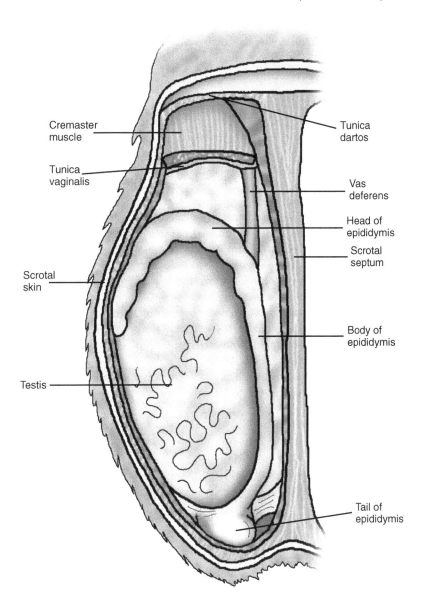

Figure 11.4 The structures within the scrotum.

tological information, but may result in temporary suppression of spermatogensis.

Epididymes Each epididymis has a head, body and tail (Fig. 11.4) which are quite closely attached to their adjacent testis. The two epididymes are normally of the same size and consistency. Very occasionally, part of the epididymis becomes detached from the testis. The organ may become enlarged and painful to the touch in the presence of infection. Each epididymis should be methodically palpated commencing with its head, which is usually slightly firmer to the touch than the tail. The body of the epididymis runs down the medial side of the adjacent testis, becoming quite narrow and difficult to palpate in places. The tail of the epididymis contains the fluid-filled ductus epididymis which is quite compressible. The epididymes can be readily assessed ultrasonographically. The efferent ducts of the head and the ductus epididymis of the tail are readily demonstrable as fluid filled channels which are less echodense than the surrounding tissues.

Spermatic cords   These are readily palpable as they run dorsally from each testis towards the inguinal canal. The cords should be approximately equal in size, consistency and compressibility. The cords may become thickened, less mobile and painful to the touch when inflamed. They contain the spermatic artery, veins (including the pampiniform plexus), lymphatics, nerves and the vas deferens. The contents of the cord can be gently compressed, allowing them to be identified and compared. The vas deferens is readily identified as it runs dorsally in the medial part of the spermatic cord. It is approximately 3 mm in diameter and less compressible than surrounding tissues. In fat animals, deposits of adipose tissue may surround the lower part of the cord within the tunica vaginalis. Inguinal hernia is a rare condition in cattle. If present, a loop of bowel or mesentery may be palpable and in many cases is readily pushed back up into the peritoneal cavity.

Penis   This runs from the caudal part of the pelvic urethra to the glans penis, which in its non-erect, fully retracted state lies within the caudal part of the prepuce. The pointed anterior tip of the penis can be palpated through the preputial skin 10 cm or more caudal to the preputial orifice. The penis is covered by the thick, smooth and flexible tunica albuginea which encloses the two main erectile channels – the corpora cavernosae penis. A smaller erectile channel – the corpus cavernosum urethrae – surrounds the urethra . Penile erection is a reflex act which is induced by neurohormonal stimulation. The arterial blood supply to the penis is increased whilst venous drainage is decreased. Relaxation of the retractor penis muscle allows the sigmoid flexure to straighten and the penis to be extruded from the prepuce. Occasionally *abnormal vessels or anastomoses* between the arterial and venous circulations prevent penile erection from occurring. Affected animals are described as being impotent and unable to serve.

Glans penis   This can only be inspected after it is exposed by passing through the preputial orifice. Abnormalities such as a *persistent frenulum* deviating the penis downwards when erect and *spiral deviation of the penis* ('corkscrew penis') may be observed at this stage (Fig. 11.5). In prepubertal calves the glans penis is adherent to the prepuce and cannot be extruded. A brief inspection of the glans penis can be carried out at the time of service or when the bull is sexually aroused. A more detailed examination requires either a general anaesthetic or a pudendal nerve block to allow relaxation of the retractor penis muscle. Massage of the accessory glands *per rectum* may result in penile extrusion, but is unreliable. The glans

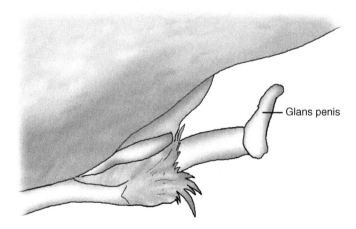
— Glans penis

Figure 11.5 Spiral deviation of the penis.

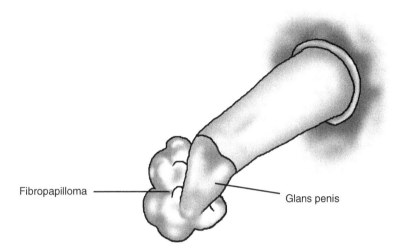

Figure 11.6 Fibropapilloma attached to the glans penis.

penis is pointed and covered with moist, pink mucous membrane. The urethra can be identified towards the tip of the glans on the right side. The external urethral orifice is a few millimetres caudal to the tip of the glans penis. *Penile warts* (viral fibropapillomata) may be seen on the glans penis (Fig. 11.6). They often have a narrow neck attached to the glans penis close to the external urethral orifice. These and other tumours such as *squamous cell carcinoma* should be identified histologically. Tumours may become so large that the penis cannot be moved through the preputial orifice. *Ulceration of the penile mucosa* is seen in cases of infection, including balanoposthitis (see under prepuce below).

Bleeding at the time of service may occur from the penile tumours mentioned above. Bleeding may also occur from small pinpoint lesions in the erect penis or arising in the urethra. Their position can seldom be identified in the non-erect penis.

Penis caudal to the prepuce　This can be identified by palpation through the covering skin and subcutaneous tissues. It can be readily identified back to the scrotal neck, and it is in this area that damage to the tunica albuginea with haematoma formation ('*fractured penis*') can occur (Fig. 11.7). This type of injury is more common in younger bulls, especially those serving young and inexperienced heifers. The dam-

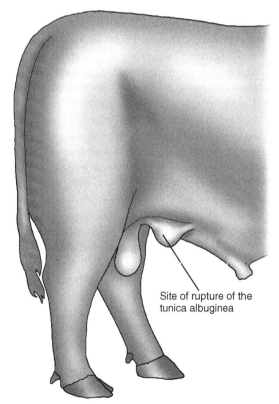

Figure 11.7 Rupture of the tunica albuginea of the penis ('fractured penis').

age to the tunica albuginea may occur if the bull or heifer moves suddenly during service. Caudal to the scrotum, parts of the sigmoid flexure may be palpable in younger bulls and older bulls who are not overweight. Very occasionally, damage to the tunica albuginea may also occur in this area. The penis is seldom palpable as it leaves the pelvis and runs down the perineum towards the sigmoid flexure.

Prepuce   This is situated on the ventral surface of the body running forward from the neck of the scrotum to a point near the umbilicus. It is covered in a loose layer of skin and lined by a mucous membrane which is reflected onto the surface of the penis. When the penis is fully retracted, the prepuce forms a sac 25 to 40 cm in length. During penile erection the sac is everted and the mucous membrane extended and exposed.

The *preputial orifice*, which has a sphincter, is found on the anterior end of the prepuce. It is surrounded by long hairs which are usually damp. If the animal is suffering from *urolithiasis* the hairs may be dry with adherent uroliths. This condition is discussed under the renal system (Chapter 9). A purulent preputial discharge may indicate infection of the prepuce.

In cases of *balanoposthitis*, some of which are associated with infectious bovine rhinotracheitis/infectious pustular vulvovaginitis/infectious pustular balanoposthitis (IBR/IPV/IPB) infection, the prepuce and penile surface may become severely inflamed and ulcerated. The area is painful to the touch, and the bull may become unwilling or unable to extrude or retract his penis. In some bulls, especially those at AI stations, the preputial mucosa may be periodically everted but retracts fully if the bull is disturbed. If the preputial mucous membrane is exposed to the air for long periods or is damaged, it readily becomes dry and infected. Withdrawal then become difficult or impossible.

The prepuce should be examined and palpated from its origin near the scrotum to its orifice. Soft, fluctuant and sometimes painful swellings at its anterior end may be caused by *subcutaneous abscesses*. Firm caudal swellings caused by local enlargement of the underlying penis just anterior to the scrotum may be caused by rupture of the tunica albuginea of the penis ('fractured penis'). This is also discussed above under 'Penis'. These swellings can be more fully investigated with the help of ultrasound, and in some cases by needle aspiration and identification of contents.

Rectal examination

This is an important and essential part of the examination of the genital system of the bull. It enables the accessory sexual organs which are situated mainly on the pelvic floor to be examined and appraised (Fig. 11.8). These structures are rarely involved in disease, but may individually or together become infected with serious consequences for semen quality and fertility. They should be methodically examined in the bull, commencing with the pelvic urethra to which the other structures may be readily related.

Pelvic urethra   This is readily palpable in the midline of the pelvic floor as it runs backwards from the neck of the bladder to the perineum. It is firm and non-compressible. Pulsations can be felt when the animal is passing urine or attempting to pass urine, and may be induced by palpation.

Ampullae of the vas deferens   These are palpable as firm tubes 4 to 8 mm in width as they pass round the anterior border of the pubis and enter the dorsal wall of the urethra adjacent to the seminal vesicles. They can be moved slightly in a lateral direction and are normally non-painful to the touch.

Bovine prostate gland   The prostate gland has two parts. The *body* is a firm, smooth, elastic structure approximately 1 cm long (anteroposterior size) and 2 cm in width. It is a saddle-like structure which is readily palpable as a protuberance on the cranial part of the pelvic urethra. The *disseminated part* of the prostate surrounds the pelvic urethra and is not normally identifiable. The bovine prostate is rarely involved in disease, but if inflamed the body may be painful to the touch.

Bulbourethral glands   These are small, paired and situated at the caudal end of the pelvic urethra just before it turns ventrally to run down the perineal area. The glands are usually covered by the bulbospongiosus muscle and are rarely palpable.

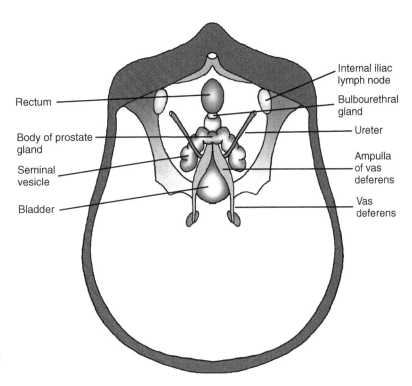

Rectum

Body of prostate gland

Seminal vesicle

Bladder

Internal iliac lymph node

Bulbourethral gland

Ureter

Ampulla of vas deferens

Vas deferens

Figure 11.8 Diagram of the accessory sex glands palpable *per rectum*.

Seminal vesicles These flattened, leaf-shaped structures with irregular surfaces lie on either side of the anterior part of the pelvic urethra. They are approximately 10 to 15 cm long and 3 to 6 cm wide in adult bulls, and are readily located by moving the hand laterally from the pelvic urethra. They are normally the same size, but one or both may be enlarged and painful to the touch if they are inflamed or infected. Problems with the seminal vesicles are relatively uncommon, but may lead to quantities of inflammatory cells and other debris in the semen.

Semen In most cases it is essential that clinical examination of a bull should include semen collection and evaluation. Semen is normally collected using an artificial vagina, and the act of collection may influence both libido and service behaviour. If service behaviour is known to be normal and the bull is thought to have a poor libido, it may be advisable to attempt to collect semen as he mounts the cow for the first time. If libido is good but details of service behaviour are unknown, service should be closely

observed first and semen collected later. Once all parts of the examination are complete the bull's overall health and fertility can be reported.

The bull's environment
This should be observed. In beef herds the bull usually runs with the cows and heifers he is serving. In dairy herds he may be confined to a bull pen into which animals for service are introduced. Details of the pen, including its height and floor surface, should be carefully observed to ensure that no adverse factors might compromise the bull's ability to serve. Details of the quality and quantity of his food and water supply should also be obtained at this stage.

Presence of a female animal in standing oestrus
This is essential for all the stages of the bull's examination except the detailed clinical examination. The clinician should arrange for such an animal to be available. In many cases oestrus is induced by prostaglandin injection to coincide with the pro-

posed time of examination of the bull. A mature cow is usually a better teaser animal for a bull than a young inexperienced heifer. If the bull or the cow's behaviour suggests that she is not in standing oestrus she should be examined to determine if the changes associated with oestrus are present. A mature ripening ovarian follicle is normally palpable on rectal examination, and a quantity of clear mucus (the bulling string) is usually found in the vagina.

The teaser cow should be restrained in service stocks or allowed to be free in a large box with a high roof where the bull can be readily and closely observed. If attempts are to be made to collect semen, restraint of the cow is advisable but may put the bull off in some cases.

(2) Assessment of libido

The bull is observed as he approaches the cow in oestrus. Normal bulls should show an immediate sexual interest. Libido may be quantified by libido score or reaction time.

Libido score
Scores are given in Table 11.1.

Reaction time
This is the time from time of introduction of the bull to the teaser cow to the first attempt at mounting. This should be less than 10 minutes for the bull to

Table 11.1 Libido score for bulls

Score	Behaviour
0	Bull shows no sexual interest in presence of cow in oestrus
1	Passing interest only, sniffs perineum, no attempt to mount
2	Interest in cow shown on more than one occasion
3	Active pursuit of cow with persistent sexual interest, no mounting
4	Single mount/mounting attempt but no service
5	Two mounts/mounting attempts but no service
6	More than two mounts/mounting attempts but no service
7	Single service, no further sexual interest
8	Single service with continued sexual interest including mounting
9	Two services, no further sexual interest
10	Two services followed by persistent sexual interest including mounting

have an adequate libido. It is less than 0.5 minute in an animal with an excellent libido and 10 to 30 minutes for an animal with a weak libido.

(3) Observation and assessment of service behaviour

Normal mating behaviour is the result of the stimulation and completion of a number of reflexes. Mating in the bull is normally completed in less than 15 seconds, and observation must therefore be made quickly and carefully. In a bull with good libido several matings can be observed in a short period of time.

Normal mating in the bull – sequence of events

(1) *Sexual excitation* The bull makes contact with the cow, smells and touches her with his muzzle and tongue. He may rest his head on the cow's gluteal and sacral regions. The bull licks her perineum, udder and flanks. The cow may pass urine at this point. The bull may taste the urine, champ his jaws, lift his head and show flehmen (retraction of lips and elevation of muzzle). Reflex penile erection commences. The penis protrudes freely from the prepuce and erection may be partial or complete. Small quantities of clear seminal fluid may be passed. In normal adult bulls at least 10 cm of the erect penis protrudes from the prepuce. When the penis is fully erect, up to 40 cm of the penis protrudes. Full penile erection may not be seen in some animals until the bull mounts the cow.

(2) *Mounting* Taking his weight on his hind limbs, the bull rears up to place his sternum on the cow's lumbosacral region. The penis should be fully erect at this stage. The bull clasps the cow with his forelegs, each leg being anterior to the cow's tuber coxae. Correct positioning by the bull is important, and failure to mount effectively may inhibit completion of coitus.

(3) *Intromission* Once mounted the bull makes seeking movements with his penis until he finds the vulval entrance and makes contact with the vaginal mucosa.

(4) *Thrusting and ejaculation* Once within the vagina

the bull makes thrusting movements with his penis and back. These may be progressively more intense until the final thrust. At this point the bull usually jumps. His hind legs briefly leave the floor, allowing the penis to reach the anterior fornix of the cow and triggering the ejaculation reflex.

(5) *Dismounting* The bull usually dismounts immediately after ejaculating, sliding backwards and sideways off the cow to take his weight on his four legs.

(6) *Penile retraction* Contraction of the retractor penis muscle should normally result in rapid retraction of the penis back into the prepuce.

Observation of mating should reveal any abnormalities in service behaviour and ability. If libido is good, a further service may be observed to see if the abnormality noted is a feature of each service. If equipment is available, service can be recorded on video for further viewing and analysis.

Specific abnormalities
Specific abnormalities which may be confirmed and elucidated by observation and enquiry are described below with the most important causes of each problem.

Deficient libido Immaturity, old age, systemic disease, fear and other psychological factors.

Inability to mount Orthopaedic abnormalities of the feet, legs and back. Neurological injuries or deficits. Unsuitable floor or ground surfaces.

Inability to achieve intromission Disparity in body size between male and female. Inability to extrude the penis (phimosis), persistent frenulum, spiral deviation of the penis. Inability to fully erect the penis (anastomoses between arterial and venous blood vessels interfering with the normal erectile mechanism). Adhesions between the penis and prepuce, for example in rupture of the tunica albuginea of the penis ('fractured penis'). Neoplasia, for example very large fibropapillomata arising from the glans penis. Smaller fibropapillomata may not prevent penile movements but may cause exposure of the

spermatozoa to blood arising from minor trauma and adversely affect fertility. Failure of the retractor penis muscle to relax may also prevent extrusion of the penis.

Inability to fertilise This may occur if sperm production is reduced or absent through injury to or infection of the testes and other organs of reproduction. Genetic and immunological factors can also reduce sperm production. Transmission of venereal diseases, such as campylobacteriosis and trichomoniasis, may also have an adverse effect on fertility of the bull or the cows he serves.

(4) Collection of semen from the bull

Semen is normally collected using an artificial vagina in the presence of a cow in oestrus. Semen can also be collected by electroejaculation and in some cases by massage of the intrapelvic urethra and accessory sex glands.

Collection of semen using an artificial vagina
The construction of the artificial vagina (AV) is shown in (Fig. 11.9). The AV is carefully prepared before use and the cow is secured ready for collection. The AV is filled with warm water at a temperature of 40°C. The caudal part of the AV is lubricated with an inert jelly. The clinician, who should wear a hard helmet, stands close to the bull ready to place the AV in position as he mounts the cow. If the clinician is too close there is a possibility that a nervous bull may be inhibited from serving. If too far away the clinician cannot reach the bull before he achieves intromission and serves the cow before the AV can be correctly positioned.

As the bull mounts the cow, the clinician grasps the prepuce to deviate the penis laterally towards the AV. The AV is placed over the tip of the glans penis and moved back towards the prepuce. This movement normally stimulates the final thrust and ejaculation, and the bull dismounts. As the bull dismounts the caudal part of the AV is raised to allow the semen to pass into the collecting vessel at the cranial end of the AV.

Most bulls serve quite readily into the AV. If the bull is reluctant to serve, the temperature and

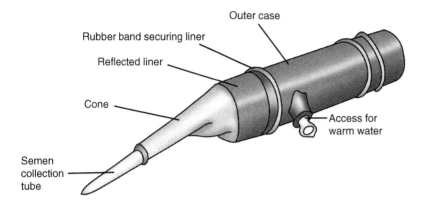

Figure 11.9 Artificial vagina for semen collection from the bull.

amount of water in the AV should be checked and adjusted as necessary. A very brief visual inspection of the penis can be made as it is extruded from the prepuce and before it enters the AV. Gross abnormalities, such as severe injury or blood loss, may be observed but will require more careful examination.

The semen sample must be kept warm and examined as soon as possible. Semen volume, density and motility are determined immediately. A drop of semen is placed into eight drops of nigrosin–eosin stain, and smears are made to enable the percentage of live, normal, and live and normal sperm to be determined. The smears are examined microscopically using an oil immersion lens. Dead sperm take up the nigrosin–eosin stain; living sperm do not. Sperm defects, such as detached heads and coiled tails, are identified and counted by direct observation.

Normal semen parameters in the bull

These are given in Table 11.2; slight variation from the reported parameters is acceptable, and some bulls of proven fertility may have, for example, low sperm density. Wherever possible, high standards of semen quality are desirable.

(5) Further diagnostic tests

Blood sample

A blood sample may be taken to check whether the bull has been exposed to infection by such organisms as IBR/IPV/IBP virus. Antibody and antigen tests are taken for diagnosis of bovine virus diarrhoea (BVD) infection.

Table 11.2 Normal semen parameters in the bull

Parameter	Value
Volume (ml)	5–10
Density (sperm/mm^3)	0.5–1.5×10^6
Live sperm (%)	75
Normal sperm (%)	80
Live and normal sperm (%)	75
pH	7
Motility	>3 (range 0–5)
Progressive motility (%)	>80
Methylene blue reduction time (min)	<15

Preputial washings

These may be used to diagnose the presence of *Trichomonas fetus* or *Campylobacter fetus* infection. Fluorescent antibody techniques can be used to detect the presence of viruses. The bull, who should have had no sexual contact with cows for 4 days, is restrained in a crush. The outer surface of the preputial orifice is washed with warm water and soap, disinfected and dried. Hair is clipped carefully away and 200 ml of sterile normal saline is carefully introduced via a plastic catheter into the prepuce from a collapsible plastic bag. The clinician encloses the preputial orifice by pressure from finger and thumb. The catheter is left in place and the distended prepuce manipulated to allow the fluid to reach all parts. After 5 minutes, samples are withdrawn for laboratory investigation.

Final report

Having completed the examination of the male genital system, the clinician may be asked to prepare a report on his or her findings. This will be based on the clinical examination of the patient, observation of mating and semen evaluation. Current, past and future fertility can never be guaranteed. A description of current potential fertility can be made.

PHYSICAL SIGNS OF DISEASE ASSOCIATED WITH THE MALE GENITAL SYSTEM

Libido
  Poor

Scrotum
  Skin abnormally hot
  Skin abnormally cold
  Asymmetrical
  Enlarged
  Vasectomy scars on proximal anterior skin
  Reduced mobility of testes
  Circumference small/large
  Fluid present in scrotal sac

Prepuce
  Prolapse of mucosa
  Skin/prepuce anterior to neck of scrotum
    Swollen
    Hot
    Painful
    Cold
    Necrotic
  Prepucial orifice constricted
  Crystals on prepucial hairs around orifice

Penis
  Cannot be extruded (phimosis)
  Cannot be retracted (paraphimosis)
  Spiral deviation
  Ventral deviation
  Non-erectile penis
  Bleeding
  Mass on penis

Adhesions
  Inflamed
  Ulcerated
  Painful on palpation

Testes
  Cryptorchid (only one testicle in scrotal sac)
  One or both testes
    Small
    Enlarged
    Painful
    Hard
    Soft
    Bulge in surface of testicle
    Surface uneven and nodular

Epididymes
  Enlarged
  Painful on palapation

Spermatic cord
  Thickened
  Loss of mobility
  Painful

Pelvic urethra
  Fremitus-like pulsation

Prostate
  Painful on palpation

Seminal vesicles
  One or both may be enlarged
  Painful on palpation

Clinical Examination of the Udder

Introduction

The udder is responsible for milk production and delivery of milk. Milk is the main source of income in dairy herds, and conditions that reduce the quality or quantity of milk will adversely affect the profit margin. In addition, conditions that affect the milking process will increase the milking time and may predispose the udder to mastitis. It is estimated that mastitis costs £100 per cow per year in the UK. This chapter will describe the clinical examination of the ligaments and the skin of the udder, the teats, the mammary gland and the milk. A clinical appraisal of suspected cases of mastitis will be described.

Applied anatomy

The udder is composed of four mammary glands, each with its own teat. The weight of the udder is supported by the medial and superficial and deep lateral ligaments (Fig. 12.1). These ligaments are attached to the pelvis and/or the abdominal muscles. Each gland is composed of milk producing alveolar cells, a reservoir for the milk produced called the gland cistern and a teat (Fig. 12.2). The teat has an annular fold at the base which partially separates the gland cistern from the teat cistern. The teat cistern is intermittently filled with milk from the gland cistern during milking. At the apex of the teat is the streak (teat canal) and the teat orifice through which milk passes during milking. The teat canal has a muscular sphincter which opens during milking but which is sealed during the dry period. There is a specialised area at the proximal end of the streak canal called the rosette of Furstenberg which is concerned with defence against infection. The skin covering the teat is hairless and strongly adherent to the underlying tis-

sues. The supramammary lymph nodes are palpable from the rear as described in Chapter 3.

Restraint

Examination of the udder of a fractious suckler cow or a painful udder can be difficult. Restraint in a crush is advisable unless the patient is a docile trustworthy dairy cow. Additional restraint may be necessary to prevent kicking. This may include an antikick bar, an udder kinch placed around the abdomen just anterior to the udder, raising of the tail or lifting the contralateral leg to the side of the udder being inspected.

Rupture of the ligaments

Observations of the contour and the anatomical position of the udder from the lateral aspects and the rear are required to detect the changes caused by rupture of the supporting ligaments of the udder.

Rupture of the medial ligaments

This is the most common type of rupture and results in a lateral displacement of the right and left halves of the distal udder. When viewed from the rear this is recognised by the teats splaying outwards. The teats are no longer perpendicular to the ground or parallel with each other. Care is needed to differentiate this from poor conformation. The farmer may notice a sudden change in the udder confirmation, and there is a loss of the dividing curvature between the two halves of the udder.

Rupture of the lateral ligaments

This is most easily recognised and results in a dramatic lowering of the udder below the hocks.

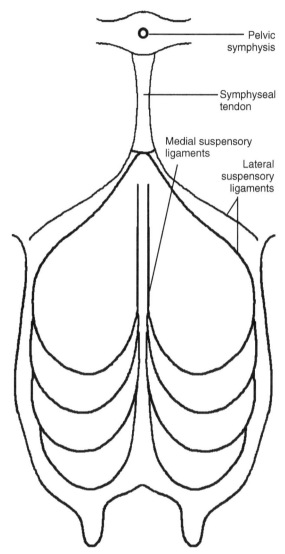

Figure 12.1 Suspensory ligaments of the udder.

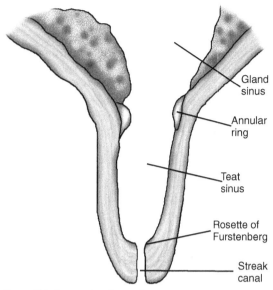

Figure 12.2 Cross-section of a normal teat.

Conditions of the skin of the udder

The skin of the udder is examined in detail by visual and olfactory inspection, and palpation. Good lighting is essential and a helmet with a light attachment leaves the clinician's hands free for the examination. The general examination should precede the examination of the udder to identify clinical signs which may be present and related to the udder lesions. The lesions associated with photosensitisation are examples.

Staphylococcal impetigo

This condition of the udder skin may present as numerous erythematous papules.

Mange

Chorioptic and, occasionally, sarcoptic mange may infest the skin of the udder causing papules, abrasions, alopecia and thickening of the skin. Lesions are likely to be present on the perineum or around the tail head.

Rupture of the anterior sections of the ligaments

Sometimes this occurs and presents as a gross enlargement in front of the udder. Haematomas and rupture of the abdominal wall may have similar presentations.

Intertrigo

In cows with pendulous udders or heifers with udder oedema, intertrigo may develop in the skin between the two halves of the udder or between the leg and the udder. The condition may be first suspected by an unpleasant smell emanating from the ventral surface of the udder. The affected area is inflamed, painful and suppurative.

Photosensitisation

The skin of the udder is usually unpigmented and is often affected when an animal is photosensitised. In the early stages, the skin of the udder is painful and erythematous. The skin then becomes dry, cracks and peels, often forming scrolls of parchment. Lesions will be present on other areas of unpigmented skin.

Udder oedema

This condition is most common in first calf heifers. The udder is sometimes painful, but not always. The condition may begin 2 to 4 weeks before calving. Excessive sodium intake during the dry period is associated with this condition, the severity of which increases as the lactation begins. The udder and the subcutis of the adjacent anterior ventral abdomen may become grossly swollen with pitting oedema. The condition may ameliorate over 2 to 4 weeks or, less commonly, persist throughout the lactation. Cows may also be affected and on occasion localised udder oedema has begun during mid-lactation. Necrotic dermatitis and milking difficulties may result.

Conditions of the skin of the teats

The surface of the skin is examined visually and by palpation. Good lighting is essential.

Supernumerary teats

Supernumerary teats are a common congenital abnormality. A diagnosis of supernumerary teats is made when more than four teats are present. Upending a calf facilitates this inspection. The supernumerary teat may be attached to the main teat, but is usually entirely separate. The identification of which of the teats is (are) the supernumerary teat(s) may be more difficult. Accurate identification is important because surgical amputation is the preferred treatment. If a teat is not in the correct anatomical position, is smaller and thicker, and the teat cistern is absent on palpation, then it is likely to be a supernumerary teat. If in doubt, delaying the decision until the animal is older may assist in identifying the supernumerary teat.

Hyperkeratosis (HK)

This presents as a smooth or roughened raised ring of tissue around the teat orifice, comprising fronds of teat duct keratin. The degree of hyperkeratosis may be assessed and scored from normal (0) to severe (5) (Figs 12.3 and 12.4). Milk machine faults are responsible, and the severe forms can predispose to mastitis and/or the development of blackspot.

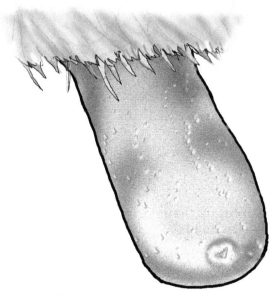

Figure 12.3 Mild hyperkeratosis.

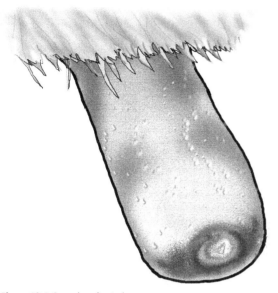

Figure 12.4 Severe hyperkeratosis.

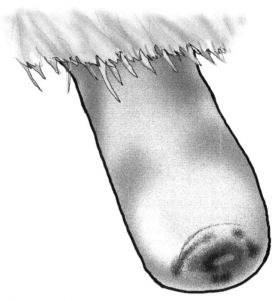

Figure 12.5 Blackspot.

Blackspot (BS)

This is a secondary bacterial infection around the teat orifice by *Fusobacterium necrophorus* alone or in association with *Staphyloccocus aureus*. Blackspot may be superimposed on either moderate or severe hyperkeratosis. The teat end appears ulcerated and blackened with granulation tissue present (Fig. 12.5).

Congestion, oedema and wedging

These are temporary phenomena caused by the milking machine, and are observed immediately the cluster is removed. They are of no clinical significance. *Congestion and oedema* usually occurs at the distal end of the teat. The teat appears hyperaemic and feels turgid. *Wedging* is a flattening of the teat, so that a white line appears across the teat end following the plane of teat cup liner closure. Occasionally this condition develops further to show roughened skin along the line of wedging.

Pseudocowpox (PCP)

Pseudocowpox is caused by a parapoxvirus. Small vesicles appear which later form characteristic horseshoe-shaped or circular scabs on teats and occasionally on the udder (Fig. 12.6). Diagnosis is usually based on the clinical signs. Confirmation is by virus isolation or detection by electron microscopy.

Bovine herpes mammillitis (BHM)

This condition is caused by bovine herpesvirus 2. Initial vesicles on the teat rupture to produce raw ulcerated areas (Fig. 12.7) which become covered in thick brown scabs (Fig. 12.8). It is a painful condition.

Warts

Teat lesions may be caused by papovavirus types 1, 5 and 6. The morphology of the warts can vary in different outbreaks. The warts may be multiple and fulminating in appearance or singular (Figs 12.9 and 12.10). Two common types are feathery and nodular teat warts. Morbidity can be high, particularly in heifers or in naïve introduced cows joining an infected milking herd or following the introduction of infected animals to a naïve herd.

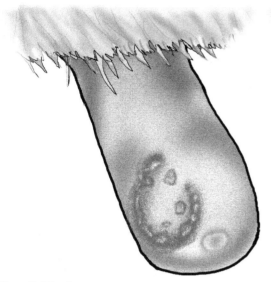

Figure 12.6 Pseudocowpox.

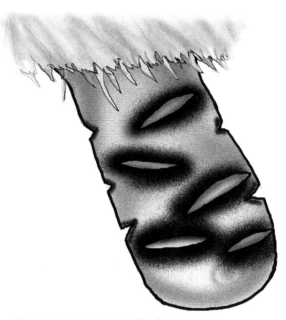

Figure 12.8 Bovine herpes mammillitis (late stages).

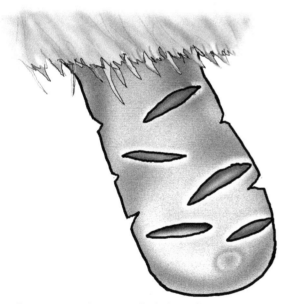

Figure 12.7 Bovine herpes mammillitis (early stages).

Foot-and-mouth disease

The teat lesions caused by foot-and-mouth disease may resemble those of bovine herpes mammillitis, but are invariably seen in association with the char-acteristic vesicles, bullae and ulcerated areas on the muzzle, tongue and coronary bands. Secondary mastitis is a feature. Affected animals are anorexic, pyrexic, salivate profusely and are lame.

Cowpox

Is not now thought to occur as a clinical entity in cattle in the UK.

Chaps

Chaps are superficial cuts and abrasions on the teat skin (Fig. 12.11). These lesions are seen on the teats of suckler cows with older calves. They are the result of trauma caused by the sharp edged incisor teeth of the calf. Similar lesions are seen in dairy cows and are associated with ill-fitting teat cups exacerbated by a cold wet environment.

Cut teats

Cut teats will be obvious on visual inspection, but it is important to establish the severity of the lesion and

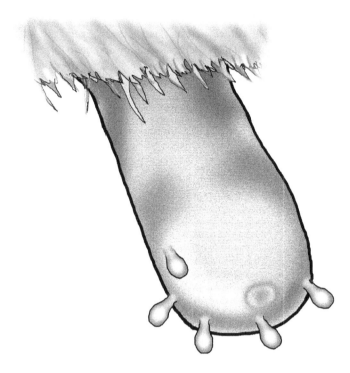

Figure 12.9 Warts: widely dispersed.

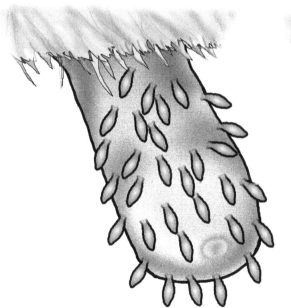

Figure 12.10 Warts: densely packed together.

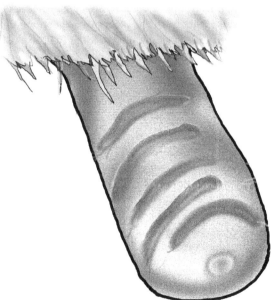

Figure 12.11 Chaps.

whether the teat cistern has been penetrated. The wounds can be categorised as flap wounds, deep lacerations without teat cistern penetration and deep lacerations with teat cistern penetration. Leakage of milk following let down is diagnostic of teat cistern penetration. Secondary mastitis is common.

Fly irritation

During summer months, persistent fly worry may cause self-mutilation by licking and produce abrasions on the teats.

Bruising

Trauma of the udder can result in bruising. The udder presents with a bluish discolouration of the skin. Differentiation from gangrenous mastitis is important.

Teat obstructions (Fig. 12.12)

Patients with teat obstructions present as hard milkers or with a total absence of milk delivery at milking. Careful palpation to assess the presence of milk in the teat cistern and other internal abnormalities is required. Good lighting to identify fibrosis of the teat orifice is essential.

Basal obstruction (spider teat)

Milk and/or colostrum cannot pass from gland sinus to teat sinus following calving and the teat cistern is empty. This condition is usually caused by adhesions across the annular fold following chronic inflammation due to infection during the dry period. In first calf heifers non-patency of the annular fold may indicate a congenital condition. A Hudson's probe and spiral can be used to clear the obstruction and confirm the diagnosis.

Mid-teat obstructions

Total, partial or intermittent obstruction of the teat cistern may result from neoplasia (papilloma),

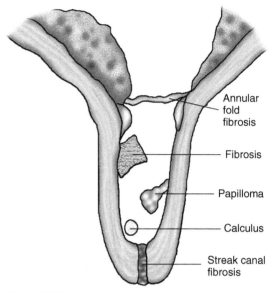

Annular fold fibrosis

Fibrosis

Papilloma

Calculus

Streak canal fibrosis

Figure 12.12 Teat obstructions.

chronic inflammation or mineral calculi. Calculi are sometimes known as teat peas because of their shape and size. These lesions can be palpated externally by rolling the teat between finger and thumb.

Apical obstructions

Fibrosis and stenosis of the streak canal may cause it to be totally or partially blocked. Palpation of the teat indicates the cistern is full of milk but that no internal lesions are present. The condition can usually be diagnosed from visual inspection of the end of the teat. Obstruction can be confirmed by the use of a probe. Further confirmation is achieved by the flow of milk if the probe is used to penetrate a complete obstruction.

Further investigations

Open teat surgery may be needed to confirm a basal or a mid-teat lesion. Contrast radiography, endoscopy and ultrasonography have been used to characterise internal teat lesions.

Mastitis

Introduction

An investigation into a mastitis problem and the predisposing factors at a herd level is beyond the scope of this book. This section will describe the examination of a cow suspected to have mastitis.

Inflammation of the glandular tissue of the quarter of the udder is called mastitis. Mastitis can be divided into subclinical mastitis and clinical mastitis. *Clinical mastitis* causes abnormalities in udder or milk and these can be detected during physical examination. There may also be systemic signs present. *Subclinical mastitis* cannot be detected by physical examination.

Mastitis may be part of a generalised infection with systemic haematogenous spread to the udder: leptospirosis is an example. More usually, pathogens gain entry to the mammary gland through the teat orifice. Most of these infections remain localised in the mammary glands; however, some of these pathogens may cause an endotoxaemia with systemic effects.

The causal agents are usually classified according to the predominant reservoir of infection. If the udder is the reservoir of infection, the pathogens are classified as contagious. If the environment is the source of infection, the pathogens are called environmental. Common pathogens and frequency of isolation are as follows:

- Contagious
  Staphylococcus aureus (coagulase positive) (18%)
  Streptococcus agalactiae and *Streptococcus dysgalactiae* (7%)
  (*Streptococcus uberis*)
- Environmental
  Escherichia coli (30%)
  Streptococcus uberis (26%)

History of the farm

Records on the farm may indicate the incidence of mastitis, the range of important pathogens present on the farm (bulk milk analysis), the common aetiological pathogens (bacteriology of clinical cases), the seasonality of cases, the antibiotic tube usage, vaccination programmes for leptospirosis and *Escherichia coli*, the age of the cows affected and their stage of lactation, the mastitis recurrence rate, the herd somatic cell counts, the dry cow tube usage and the number of cows culled because of mastitis. This information may focus the investigation.

History of the patient

The individual mastitis records should indicate the dates of previous episodes of mastitis, which quarters were affected, if bacterial culture was attempted and the results, and which treatments were used. Somatic cell counts from composite samples of all quarters from the patient may be available from previous monthly recordings. These will indicate the chronicity and the severity of the problem regarding the contribution of the patient towards the bulk tank milk quality. The clinical signs that have been observed, results of any Californian milk tests (CMT), and if and when milk samples for bacteriology have been taken should be established. The stage of lactation and the duration and type of treatments that have been administered should be obtained.

General examination of the cow

It is important to perform a general clinical examination whenever mastitis is suspected to ensure that systemic signs are not missed and the severity of the condition is recognised. Toxic mastitis can easily be confused with hypocalcaemia and the clinical examination should be performed with great care.

Observations at a distance

The conformation and symmetry of the udder should be examined from both lateral aspects and from the rear to identify absolute and relative enlargement of the affected quarters. Pain caused by mastitis may result in apparent lameness with abduction of the limb adjacent to the painful quarter.

Clinical classification of mastitis

A classification system for mastitis based upon the changes in the milk, quarter and the presence and absence of systemic clinical signs has been devised and is presented in Table 12.1.

Examination of the mammary gland

All four quarters of the cow should be visually inspected at close range and palpated. The supramammary lymph nodes should be palpated to assess their size. In addition, milk samples from all the quarters should be obtained for gross visual inspection and additional tests.

The clinical presentations of subclinical mastitis, clinical mastitis of the udder, toxic mastitis and summer mastitis are described below.

Subclinical mastitis

This is very common but cannot be detected by physical examination of either the cow or udder or milk. However, there can be large numbers of somatic cells produced by the inflammation in the affected gland. This results in milk with a high somatic cell count (SCC) which is expressed as cells/ml. Cows with

subclinical mastitis can contribute a significant proportion of bulk tank SCC. This may reduce the payment received for the milk. In addition, subclinical mastitis results in a reduction in the volume of milk produced of 2.5% for each 100 000 cells/ml above 200 000 cells/ml. Detection of the cow and the quarter affected with subclinical mastitis is important.

In some herds, individual cow composite samples composed of milk from all four quarters are taken at monthly intervals and the SCC measured. Cows with an SCC of over 200 000 cells/ml are likely to be infected and have subclinical mastitis. The CMT test can be used to identify the quarters of these cows with high SCC. Samples can then be taken for bacteriology if desired. In herds without SCC records, CMT tests can be performed on all the lactating cows.

Clinical mastitis

In cows with clinical mastitis the affected quarter(s) may be enlarged relative to the uninfected quarters, although on occasion all four quarters may be affected equally. On palpation the affected quarter(s) may be hard, hot and painful. In mild cases the affected quarter is normal. *Staphylococcus aureus* can produce a gangrenous mastitis in association with severe systemic illness. Gangrenous mastitis is caused by the alpha toxin that damages blood vessels, resulting in ischaemic coagulative necrosis of the adjacent tissue. The affected quarter becomes purple and cold. There is often a clear demarcation of dead and surviving tissue. The necrotic gland will eventually slough if the animal survives.

Chronic mastitis

In chronic mastitis, which is often caused by *Staphylococcus aureus*, there is a gradual replacement of secretory tissue by fibrous tissue with a loss of milk production. Abscesses may also be present. A fibrotic quarter is indurate and is shrunken in size compared with the normal quarters. On deep palpation the fibrotic regions are painless and hard with an uneven surface. Abscesses vary in size. They are most commonly located in the stroma of the gland on the caudal aspect of the udder. They present as hemispheres, often the size of squash balls, bulging out from the surface of the udder. They are usually well circumscribed, thick walled and spherical. Confirmation is

Table 12.1 Classification of normal and mastitic quarters

Normal	Milk normal appearance, has no pathogens, few neutrophils, udder feels normal on palpation, cow normal
Subclinical	Milk normal appearance, milk has pathogens, many neutrophils, udder feels normal on palpation, cow normal
Clinical	
Grade 1 (mild)	Quarter normal, cow normal but milk clots, many neutrophils, milk has pathogens
Grade 2 (moderate)	Quarter abnormal, cow normal, milk abnormal
Grade 2A (acute)	Quarter is swollen, hot, painful and sometimes discoloured
Grade 2C (chronic)	Quarter may be hard, lumpy, fibrosed, reduced in size
Grade 3 (severe)	Cow systemically ill, quarter usually abnormal, milk usually abnormal

by needle aspiration and gross examination of the sample. Ultrasonographic scanning can also be used to characterise suspicious superficial focal lesions.

Toxic mastitis

This may occur at any time including the dry period (usually following the application of contaminated dry cow antibiotic tubes), but it is more common in early lactation. The udder may or may not show signs of inflammation. The milk may be more watery than normal but without discolouration, although sometimes it is haemorrhagic. *Escherichia coli* is most commonly isolated, although *Staphyloccocus* and other pathogens may cause the condition. In a recent study, 60% of cases occurred within 1 month of calving and 29% within 4 days of calving. During this study the following sign frequencies were recorded: lethargy (92%), pyrexia (18%), dehydration (44%), diarrhoea (23%), tachypnoea (23%), recumbency (18%), staggering (18%), discoloured milk (90%). Other clinical signs include tachycardia and ruminal stasis. Biochemical parameters included a high urea (31%) and a high blood creatinine (42%). Haematology revealed severe leucopenia (56%).

Summer mastitis

This is a severe suppurative mastitis, usually of dry cows and heifers, but occasionally of newly calved and lactating cows. Supernumary teats may also be infected. Occasionally vestigial mammary tissue of bulls and steers can be affected. The disease produces extensive permanent damage to the udder tissue and sometimes toxic effects systemically. It usually occurs in the summer months. The frequency of occurrence of bacteria associated with the condition is *Arcanobacterium pyogenes* (85%), *Peptostreptococcus indolicus* (62%) and *Streptococcus dysgalactiae* (24%). Surveys indicate that 20 to 60% of dairy farms are affected and between 1.0 and 1.5% of all cows will have the condition.

In the early stages in the dry cow there is lethargy, pyrexia, loss of appetite and reduced rumination. The animal may separate itself from the herd at grass. The udder is swollen, hot and painful. In the later stages there is a purulent, foul smelling teat secretion which is sometimes inspissated. With increasing severity there may be hind leg lameness, swelling of the hock joints, toxaemia, abortion, weak full term

calves and permanent loss of a productive quarter. In rare cases the cow may die. Mild cases may be missed and it is only after calving that a blind quarter is detected with a thickened teat and a fibrotic core replacing the teat cistern.

Summer mastitis is transmitted by *Hydrotaea irritans*. A small number of cases are diagnosed at other times of year and in areas which do not have *Hydrotaea irritans*. This fly prefers woods, copses and damp ground which are sheltered from the wind. Larvae overwinter in light, sandy soils and usually emerge as adults in July. Adult flies are active during (June) July, August and September (October), which are the most common months for summer mastitis. Legs, abdomen and udder are preferred sites for blood sucking. The flies are attracted to teat sores. *Hydrotaea irritans* is active only during the daytime.

Examination of the milk

Milk samples from all four quarters of mastitic cases should be examined for signs of mastitis. Visual appraisal is facilitated by placing the milk sample onto a black surface. Strip cups are very useful for this purpose as they minimise environmental contamination. Alternatively, black tiles on the floor of the parlour may be available. As a last resort a wellington boot can be used, but judicious washing and disinfecting should follow. In clinical mastitis, clots caused by cellular debris derived from gland inflammation are often present. The clots may have been detected by the herdsman in the parlour by inline filters which are designed for this purpose. Other gross changes include milk which is more watery and discoloured.

The discolouration may be yellow, port wine or red. Red indicates blood in the milk and/or colostrum. This is seen in a proportion of newly calved cows. One, several or all quarters may be affected. This condition is of no pathological significance, although it must be differentiated from acute mastitis (e.g. *Bacillus cereus*) that can sometimes present with a haemorrhagic milk sample which has a darker port wine appearance.

Identification of the infected quarter is further assisted by using a CMT to identify which quarter(s) have a high somatic cell count indicating mastitis. This is described below.

Further tests on milk

Californian milk test (CMT)   The CMT measures the quantity of DNA in a milk sample and gives an indirect measure of the number of somatic cells present. This test is quick, cheap, easy to perform and is often used routinely by herdsmen. A milk sample is placed from each quarter into each of the four wells of a plastic paddle supplied in the test kit (Fig. 12.13). The volume of the sample is adjusted by pouring off the excess using a marker in the paddle. An equal volume of a supplied detergent is applied to each well and the paddle swirled gently. The more viscous the mixture becomes, the greater is the somatic cell count. Interpretation is provided in Table 12.2. Counts of over 200 000 cells/ml indicate the presence of mastitis. There is also a pH indicator present which turns from purple to yellow with an acidic pH. However, although a decrease in pH is associated with some types of mastitis, lack of colour change does not rule out mastitis and often the colour remains purple in the presence of mastitis.

Conductivity   Early in the course of the mastitis some 24 to 36 hours before there is a rise in the SCC, there is an increase in the sodium chloride concentrations of the milk and an increase in the electrical conductivity. Hand-held conductivity meters are available, and conductivity meters can also be fitted inline in the parlour. Conductivity is usually measured relative to the other quarters in the affected cow, although high absolute values often indicate an early mastitis.

Collection of mastitic milk samples for bacteriology

Contamination of the sample is common following poor sampling technique, and the results of the culture are often misleading or meaningless. The following protocol is suggested.

The teat to be sampled should only be washed if obviously dirty, and should be dried immediately. Hands should be washed and dried thoroughly. The end of the teat should be cleaned with cotton wool swabs dampened with surgical spirits. The end of the teat is cleaned until the end of the swab is no longer discoloured by cleaning. A pair of new disposable latex gloves should be worn. Two draws of foremilk are discarded. The top is removed from a wide necked universal sample bottle. The lid should be kept clean, preferably by holding it in the crook of the little finger. The sample bottle is held away from the udder, to avoid contamination from debris falling from the udder skin, with the opening pointing to-

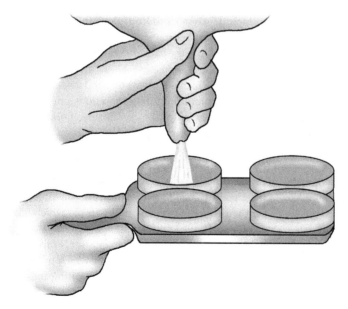

Figure 12.13 Milk sampling for the Californian milk test.

Table 12.2 Interpretation of the Californian milk test

CMT score	Interpretation	Visible reaction	Total cell count/ml
0	Negative	No reaction	0–200 000 0–25% neutrophils
T	Trace	Slight precipitation	150 000–500 000 30–40% neutrophils
1	Weak positive	Distinct precipitation but no gel formation	400 000–1 500 000 40–60% neutrophils
2	Distinct positive	Mixture thickens with gel formation	800 000–5 000 000 60–70% neutrophils
3	Strong positive	Viscosity greatly increased. Strong gel that is cohesive with a convex surface	>5 000 000 70–80% neutrophils

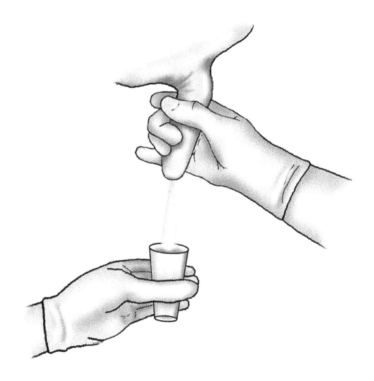

Figure 12.14 Taking a milk sample for bacteriological culture.

wards the teat to be sampled. The teat is held angled towards the sample bottle; milk is withdrawn and directed towards the open mouth of the sample bottle (Fig. 12.14). The bottle is filled with milk and the lid replaced. The bottle is labelled with the cow number, the date and the quarter.

Freezing milk samples

Milk samples for bacteriological culture can be frozen and batched for later culture to reduce the cost. Storage for up to 3 months results in only a small reduction in the number of successful cultures achieved.

CLINICIAN'S CHECKLIST

Examination of the udder support ligaments

Examination of the skin of the udder

Examination of the skin of the teat

Examination of teat obstructions

Examination for mastitis
    General examination for systemic signs
    Supramammary lymph nodes
    Mammary gland
    Gross examination of milk
        CMT
        Conductivity
    Milk sample for bacteriological culture

PHYSICAL SIGNS OF DISEASE ASSOCIATED WITH THE UDDER

Silhouette, conformation and position of udder
    Teats splayed outwards
    Loss of dividing fold (rear view)
    Dropping of the udder below the hocks
    Swelling of ventral abdomen anterior to udder
    Enlarged swollen udder with pitting oedema

Skin of the udder
    Erythematous papules
    Papules
    Alopecia
    Abrasions
    Skin thickening
    Suppurative
    Foul smell
    Dry, cracked, peeling, fissured
    Bruising
    Cold
    Gangrenous
    Necrotic
    Sloughing

Skin of the teat
    Supernumerary teats
    Raised tissue around teat orifice
    Focal black, granulated, ulcerated teat-end lesion

Swelling of teat
Teat flattened longitudinally
Horseshoe shaped small vesicles and scabs
Painful multiple raw ulcerated areas with thick brown scabs
Nodular lesions
Feathery lesions
Vesicles/erosions
Horizontal fissures
Lacerations
Abrasions
Sores
Cold
Blue
Thickened teat

Hard milkers (teat obstructions)
    Teat cistern empty of milk
    Teat cistern full of milk
    Mass present in cistern
    Teat orifice non-patent

Mammary gland
    Enlarged
    Painful
    Hard
    Abnormally warm
    Indurate
    Fibrotic
    Flaccid

Circumscribed swellings bulging from surface
Sloughing

Milk/discharge
    Clots
    Milk watery
    Purulent
    Discolouration
        Yellow
        Bloodstained
        Port wine (haemmorrhagic)

Systemic signs (N.B. These physical signs may be associated with diseases of other body systems and regions.)
    Lameness
    Abduction of hind limb
    Diarrhoea
    Lethargy
    Pyrexia
    Recumbency
    Staggering
    Tachycardia
    Ruminal stasis
    Reduced appetite
    Separation from herd
    Swelling of hock joints
    Abortion
    Weak calves

Clinical Examination of the Musculoskeletal System

Introduction

The musculoskeletal system is composed of the bones of the skeleton, joints, ligaments, muscles and tendons. In addition to the nervous system, the musculoskeletal system is important for the maintenance of posture and for locomotion.

Lameness is a common presentation and 25 to 35% of dairy cows are affected by lameness each year. *It is an important condition in terms of welfare and economic losses*. Severe conditions may result in recumbency. Foot lameness accounts for 88% of all lamenesses in cattle. Hind leg lesions account for 86% of all foot lamenesses. The lateral claw of the hind leg accounts for 85% of the hind leg lesions. Front foot lameness is divided equally between medial and lateral claw.

The aim of the clinical examination is to identify the site and the cause of the lameness. In most cases clinical examination precedes the identification of possible risk factors. This section will describe the examination of the foot, the limbs and the special case of the downer cow. Musculoskeletal conditions of the head and neck are described in Chapter 5.

History

Defining the problem

- *Date of onset, duration and signs observed* should be obtained.
- *Individual problem or herd problem?* Conditions such as digital dermatitis and foul are usually herd problems, whereas cases of septic arthritis are sporadic.
- *Acute or chronic?* Injuries such as fractures usually appear suddenly, whilst problems such as degenerative joint disease may have a more chronic history.
- *Mild or a severe condition?* Bruising may produce a mild lameness, whilst solar ulcers often produce severe lameness.
- *Static or progressive?* Animals with infections such as septic arthritis usually deteriorate rapidly. Traumatic injuries such as bruising may improve rapidly. Animals with chronic arthritis may show no change over time.

Management

- *Is there a routine health care programme?* Foot-baths and foot trimming protocols should be checked for compliance.
- *Vaccinations* Clostridial diseases are important in certain areas and vaccination is important for prevention.
- *Animal movement* Loading, mixing or moving cattle can result in lameness. A cow showing severe lameness with crossing over of the front feet that has recently been unloaded from transport may have sustained a fractured pedal bone.

Recent oestrus will have been accompanied by mounting and other physical activities during which injury may be sustained. A cow that has been in oestrus recently may have sustained a traumatic injury such as a sacroiliac subluxation.

Records

Farm records may indicate the range of recent and current problems diagnosed on the farm. The incidence of each condition may be obtained. Locomotion scores may be helpful in identifying herd and individual problems and their progression. Individual cow records indicating previous problems and their anatomical locations may highlight a recurrent problem. Seasonality of problems and the groups affected can be identified. The main reasons for culling may indicate that an abnormally high proportion of culls are due to lameness.

Signalment

New-born calves may present with contracted tendons, arthrogryphosis or congenital joint laxity and dwarfism. Older calves may present with spastic paresis. Growing cattle may present with physitis, and adult cattle may present with interdigital hyperplasia. First calving dairy heifers in early lactation may be adversely affected by solar ulceration and subacute laminitis. Older cows may have chronic recurrent problems. Conditions may be inherited and be breed or family related, such as hip dysplasia and corkscrew claw.

Environment

The type of housing (cubicles or straw yards) and the specifications and management of the system should be established. The number of cubicles and cubicle dimensions, including slurry management, may be significant. Flinty soils, muddy area around water troughs, stony gateways and unsuitable cow paths from pasture to the milking parlour may all be important risk factors.

Nutrition

Laminitis, solar ulceration and white line disease may be related to the composition of the diet, the method of feeding, and sudden changes in energy density and availability. The management of the first calving heifers prepartum and postpartum is particularly important in influencing the prevalence in first calving heifers. Congenital joint laxity and dwarfism in suckler calves is associated with feeding silage as the major winter feed. Inadequate diets may result in copper deficiencies or vitamin E and/or selenium deficiencies. Calcium and phosphorus mineral imbalance may result in osteodystrophies.

General clinical examination

This should precede the detailed examination, as the locomotory defects may be related to abnormalities in other body systems or be part of a generalised condition. A focal septic lesion in the foot may be related to a tricuspid valve murmur caused by a vegetative endocarditis. An infected umbilicus may be related to a septic polyarthritis in a calf. Locomotary abnormalities may not be related to the musculoskeletal and nervous systems but to reduce the pain caused by normal locomotion, such as in severe mastitis when the mammary gland is extremely painful.

Observations during recumbency, rising, standing and during locomotion

Identification of the affected limb, the site of the lesion within the limb and assessment of the severity of the lesion, are primary aims of the initial part of the examination. Localisation to a foot or an upper limb problem may be possible by observation. Abnormalities of posture and gait, weight bearing and gross swellings, wounds and deformities should be noted.

Recumbency

The normal posture of a recumbent animal is to lie with both carpi flexed with the sternum for support. The hind legs are slightly flexed and with one hind leg beneath the abdomen with the upper leg free of weight bearing. Lame animals will often spend prolonged periods in recumbency and adopt a posture which will minimise the pain. A painful hind limb will be kept uppermost, with the normal limb tucked under the abdomen. A forelimb with a painful foot condition may be held with the foot out to the front with the carpus in extension.

Rising

Severely lame animals are reluctant to rise. Normal cattle raise their hindquarters first, followed by their

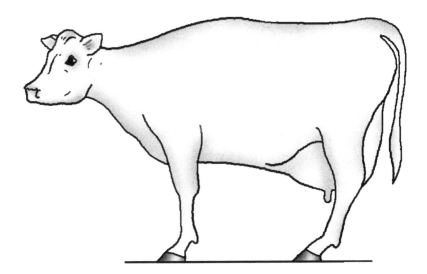

Figure 13.1 Camping forward.

forequarters. Pain may result in abnormal struggling movements with instability and obvious difficulty, with the animal sometimes failing to rise after repeated efforts to do so.

Standing

Once standing, the conformation, symmetry and posture of the animal can be assessed. These should be viewed from the cranial, caudal and lateral positions.

Conformation
Refers to the outline, shape or profile of the animal. An abnormal conformation may be symmetrical or asymmetrical. An example of the former is a bilateral sacroiliac subluxation and of the latter is localised muscle atrophy.

Symmetry
The body of the normal animal should be symmetrical around the median plane which divides the body into two equal parts. The sizes and shapes of the joints, bones, tendons and muscles of each limb and its contralateral limb should be similar. In addition, absolute changes, irrespective of symmetry, should be investigated thoroughly. For example, septic polyarthritis may be symmetrical but present with bilateral swollen joints.

Posture
To relieve pain, abnormal postures may be adopted with reduced weight bearing on affected limb(s). With conditions affecting the foot of a single limb, the weight bearing may be reduced by flexing the limb slightly with the weight being taken by the contralateral limb. In severe cases the limb may be held completely clear of the floor or just with the toe touching. In the latter case, hyperalgesia may result in a quick and repeated withdrawal of the limb if the toe does touch the floor. *Adduction* to allow the weight to be taken by the lateral claw of the limb usually indicates a painful medial claw. *Abduction* to allow weight to be taken by the medial claw usually indicated a painful lateral claw lesion. *Paddling of the hind legs* where the weight is shifted from one leg to the other may indicate painful lesions in both feet. In *camping forward*, the hind feet are placed further forward than normal under the body to take weight on the heels and reduce pain caused by lesions such as horizontal or vertical fissures in the toe region of the hind feet (Fig. 13.1). In *camping back*, the hind feet are placed further caudally than normal to take the weight on the toes and reduce pain caused by lesions in the heel region, such as solar ulceration (Fig. 13.2).

Examination of the gait

Identification of the affected limb(s) before restraint

169

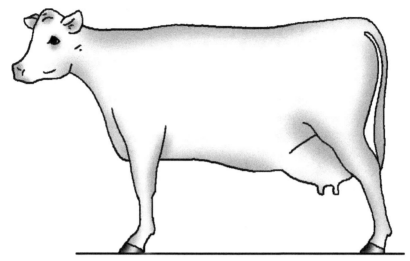

Figure 13.2 Camping back.

and detailed examination is a primary aim if this has not already been decided. Gait abnormalities, such as abduction, adduction and forward and camping back, should be noted as these may indicate the location of the lesion. Care is needed to distinguish incoordination caused by weakness or a neurological lesion and abnormal gait caused by painful musculoskeletal conditions. Care is also needed to distinguish abnormalities of the gait caused by overgrown and uneven claws, and pathological lesions.

The animal should be observed on a non-slippery concrete floor without straw to hinder detailed observation. Ideally, the animal should be observed during forward motion, backward motion, circling, and mounting and dismounting a kerb. The animal should be observed from the cranial, caudal and both lateral aspects. This is rarely possible unless the animal is halter trained. Opportunism is therefore required. Moving the group and observing the affected individual may indicate the degree of lameness and the limb affected without resorting to restraint. Driving the animal in a secure space or observing movement forwards or backwards in a race may provide useful information regarding the abnormality.

Identifying the affected leg is dependent upon the change in gait. The more severe the lameness, the more abnormal the gait. With foreleg lameness the head is raised when the affected limb is bearing weight. In hind limb lameness the pelvis is raised when the affected limb is weight bearing, but pelvic symmetry is maintained.

Localisation of the lesion to the foot or upper limb can sometimes be achieved by the character of the lameness: supporting limb lameness is associated with lesions of the foot and swinging leg lameness with lesions of the upper limb. Supporting limb lameness is characterised by a shortened weight bearing phase and a quick swing phase. This movement tends to limit the contact time of the painful part of the foot with the floor. In animals with upper limb lesions, flexion causes pain and so the limb is held in extension during the swing phase resulting in a *swinging leg lameness*.

The *degree of the lameness* should be assessed on a scale of zero to ten ranging from no injury (0) to the limb being totally non-weight bearing (10). *A locomotory score* can also be assigned where 1 indicates minimal adduction/abduction of limb, no uneven gait and no tenderness in the limb and 5 indicates difficulty in rising and unwillingness to walk.

Clinical examination of the foot

Functional anatomy (Fig. 13.3)

Corium

This structure forms the papillae of the coronary band and sole. It also forms the laminae suspensory system. It is responsible for the supply of blood to these structures which are involved with the production of horn and its physical attachment to the underlying structures. Damage to the corium can result in poor horn formation and the detachment of the hoof.

Periople

This covers the coronary band and produces a waxy coating which prevents water loss and keeps the horn of the wall supple; damage may result in a vertical fissure.

Wall of the claw

This is composed of horn produced by the corium of the coronary band. Horn is produced at a rate of 0.5 cm a month. The distance from the coronary band to the toe is 75 mm and takes it 15 months for horn produced there to come into wear.

Laminae

The hoof wall is firmly attached to the underlying structures by an interdigitating structure, the *laminae*, which forms part of the corium. The laminae support the wall but allow it to progress towards the toe.

Sole

The horn of the sole is formed from the papillae on the sole. There are no laminae on the sole. The horn of the wall meets the horn of the sole at the white line. It runs from the bulb of the heel to the toe and then back along the first one-third of the axial wall. Being a junction, this is a point of weakness and a common site of impaction of debris and entry of infection.

Heel

The heel or the bulb of the hoof is a rounded area covered by softer horn. The heel compresses during weight bearing and the stresses caused by this movement at the sole–heel junction of the abaxial wall may be responsible for the higher incidence of impaction

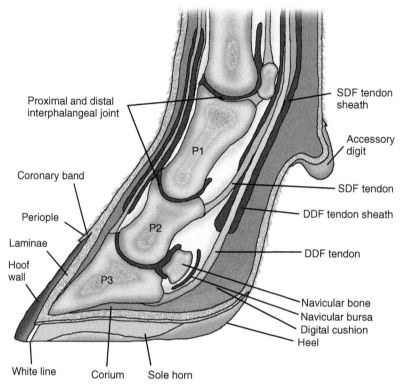

Figure 13.3 Functional anatomy of the bovine foot: SDF, superficial disital flexor; DDF, deep digital flexor.

and infection at this site in the white line. During movement the *digital cushion* acts as a pump to facilitate the circulation of blood in the foot. Lack of exercise may lead to corium anoxia.

Pedal bone (P3)

The pedal bone (P3) is attached to the horn via the suspensory corium laminae. The pedal bone posterior border is located three-quarters of the way along the sole. This is a prime site for solar ulceration which can be caused by the caudal border of the pedal bone pinching the corium at this site, resulting in poor horn formation.

Synovial structures

Purulent lesions affecting the anterior third of the sole or the heel can be painful, but are less likely to lead to serious complications than those involving the sole–heel junction. The middle third of the foot is anatomically close to three synovial structures: the

pedal joint capsule, the navicular bursa and the deep flexor tendon sheath. The navicular bursa is usually affected first. This may be followed by extensions to the other structures.

Restraint

Physical restraint that ensures the safety of the clinician and patient is essential for detailed examination of the foot. Ideally a Wopabox or a crush designed for foot work, or a foot trimming flip table should be used. However, basic crushes, AI stalls and swing gates can be used to good effect in combination with competent and judicious usage of roping techniques. Casting with ropes with the use of hobbles and/or chemical restraint using sedation can be helpful in extreme circumstances, but it is often difficult to control small forceful movements. Intravenous regional anaesthesia should be considered in patients with very painful conditions to enable thorough exploration and detailed examination, particularly where aggressive paring may be required. This technique is described on page 193 under 'Further investigations'.

Close inspection of the standing animal

Following restraint, the use of a hosepipe to remove gross contamination of the foot may be necessary. Gross lesions on the anterior aspect of the foot are easier to visualise before raising the leg.

Horizontal and vertical fissures of the hoof wall – may be seen (Fig. 13.4): a horizontal fissure that has progressed to the toe may cause a piece of the toe horn to snap off prematurely resulting in a 'broken toe' (Fig. 13.4).

Coronary band lesions – may be caused by digital dermatitis or trauma.

Severe swelling of the area proximal to the coronary band – may indicate a septic arthritis of the distal interphalangeal joint (Fig. 13.5), foul (Fig. 13.6) or ascending infection from white line disease.

Coronary band vesicles/erosions – if foot-and-mouth disease is suspected, a careful examination for vesicles or ruptured vesicles is required; if mucosal disease is suspected, erosions may be present.

Grossly overgrown and corkscrew claws – will be self evident.

Changes in claw conformation – may be seen in chronic laminitis and corkscrew claw. There may be horizontal ridges extending the length of the claw with a concavity of the wall giving the Turkish slipper appearance (Fig. 13.7). Corkscrew claw presents as a severe rotation of the hind-leg lateral claw.

Cleaning the raised foot

Once the leg is raised, the foot may need to be cleaned. *Cleaning the foot* with a hard bristled brush and copious quantities of water is usually necessary to remove mud and debris to facilitate examination. Sawdust is advocated once cleaning is complete to dry the hoof and make handling easier, but care must be taken to avoid blocking the drainage system. Following cleaning, the foot should be visually inspected in a systematic way.

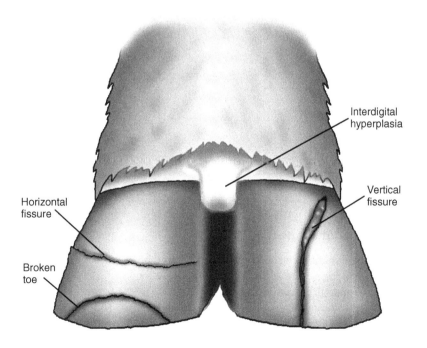

Interdigital hyperplasia

Vertical fissure

Horizontal fissure

Broken toe

Figure 13.4 Interdigital hyperplasia, broken toe and horizontal and vertical fissures.

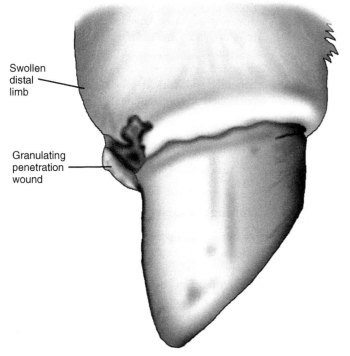

Figure 13.5 Septic arthritis of the distal interphalangeal joint.

Swollen distal limb

Granulating penetration wound

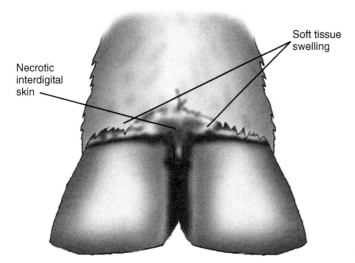

Soft tissue swelling

Necrotic interdigital skin

Figure 13.6 Foul in the foot.

Examination of the foot

The contralateral limb should always be examined to ensure a less severe lesion is not overlooked, for example solar ulcers can be bilateral.

The most common causes of lameness in cattle are: foul in the foot, white line disease, sole ulceration, penetration of the hoof by sharp objects, heel erosion, digital dermatitis and laminitis.

Interdigital space

The interdigital space can be examined by gently parting the claws. A pen torch can facilitate the search as the examination area is often poorly lit. Stones or other foreign bodies may be lodged here and can easily be missed (Fig. 13.8). Interdigital hyperplasia may be seen, particularly in the hind feet, and presents as a ridge of solid tissue which may force the claws apart (Fig. 13.4). The skin between the claws should be checked for integrity. Foul in the foot

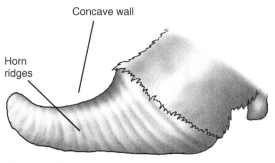

Figure 13.7 Chronic laminitis.

causes skin necrosis and a characteristic unpleasant odour (Figs 13.6 and 13.9). Puncture wounds caused by foreign objects may be seen in the interdigital skin, and if chronic the wound may be granulating. The wound may be associated with a septic distal interphalangeal joint (Fig. 13.5).

Bulbs of the heel

The bulbs of the heel should be carefully inspected for erosion of the heel horn which is often called slurry heel. This condition often produces a dark or tarry appearance with deep furrowing and fraying of the softer horn of the heel (Fig. 13.10). A painful swelling of the heel, with or without a sinus tract, is usually indicative of infection tracking from an entry point at the white line towards the back of the sole (Fig. 13.10). Haematoma of the heel may produce a discrete swelling of the bulbs of the heel. Lesions caused by digital dermatitis are commonly found on the skin between the bulbs of the heels and are recognised as a

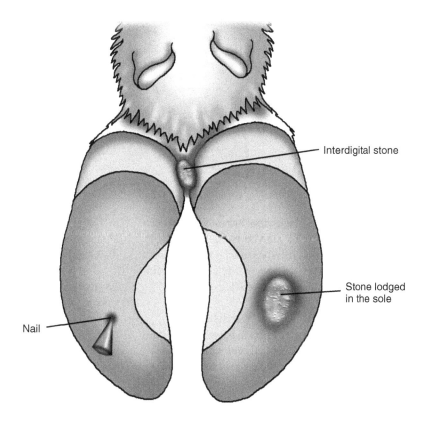

Figure 13.8 Foreign bodies.

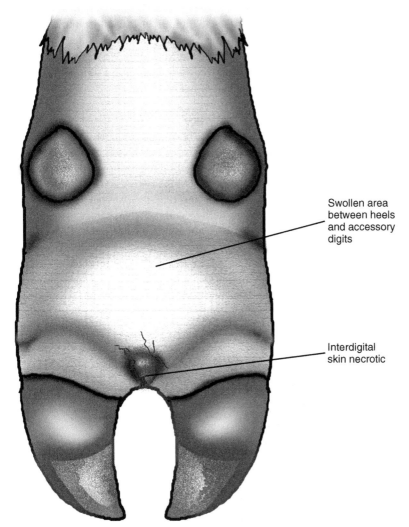

Swollen area
between heels
and accessory
digits

Interdigital
skin necrotic

Figure 13.9 Foul in the foot.

raw shiny area of skin with the shape and colour of a strawberry cut in half ('strawberry heel'; Fig. 13.11). The lesion is very painful when touched. In the chronic form known as verrucose dematitis, a plume of fulminating keratin 'threads' is seen (Fig. 13.12).

Swelling of the skin around the distal limb

Foul presents as a swelling of skin between heels and accessory digits caused by inflammation of the shin and subcutaneous tissue. The claws may be forced apart with necrotic interdigital skin (Fig. 13.9). Infection of the synovial structures of the distal limb,

including the distal and proximal interphalangeal joints, results in severe generalised swelling of the distal limb.

Examination of the sole

Corrective foot trimming using the Dutch five-step method is a useful starting point to examine conditions of the sole, as initial examination without corrective trimming can lead to a misdiagnosis and unjustified invasive paring. This method is described at the end of the chapter under 'Further investigations'.

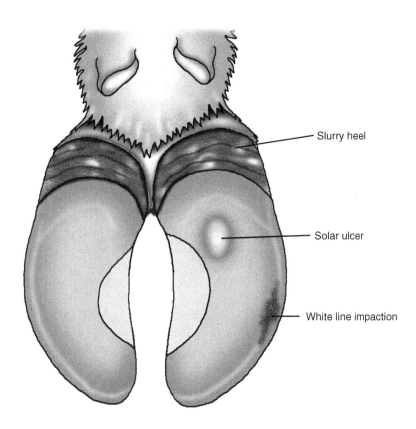

Figure 13.10 Slurry heel, white line impaction and solar ulcer.

In the correctly shaped foot, weight is taken on the heel and the wall with the exception of the middle one-third of the axial wall (no white line) (Fig. 13.13). Overgrowth of the toe leads to backward rotation of the pedal bone towards the heel. Erosion of the heel can exacerbate the degree of rotation. Rotation can cause corium pinching between the pedal bone and the hoof.

During corrective foot trimming when the sole has been reduced to the correct thickness, the condition of double sole may have been identified as a layer of poor quality dark flaky horn sandwiched between normal solar horn as the depth of sole was reduced. This reflects an historical period of poor horn production and may coincide with a bout of laminitis. Small flat stones and (particularly) shards of flint can sometimes be deeply embedded in the sole and will have been identified at this stage (Fig. 13.8).

Once the shape and thickness of the sole has been corrected, problem areas of the sole can be recognised and investigated. The sole of the hoof is often pigmented. These discrete pigmented areas should not be mistaken for abnormality.

Laminitis This causes pressure pain and loss of 'adhesion' of the horn to the underlying structures of the foot. The blood supply to the structures supporting and producing the horn of the hoof is compromised, and poor quality soft horn may result. Laminitis may predispose the foot to sole ulceration, white line disease, rotation and penetration of the sole by P3. A double sole may follow a bout of laminitis. Laminitis presents with a yellow exudative/haemorrhagic discolouration of the solar horn.

Bruised sole The sole may be worn thin from walking over hard rough surfaces and is easily bruised. Bleeding occurs beneath the sole. The condition is painful on compression of the sole. Differential diag-

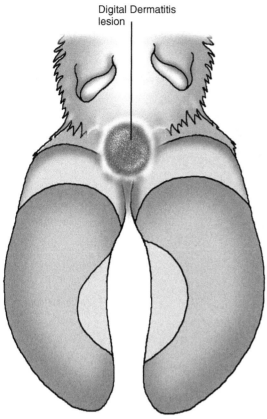

Digital Dermatitis
lesion

Figure 13.11 Digital dermatitis (strawberry heel).

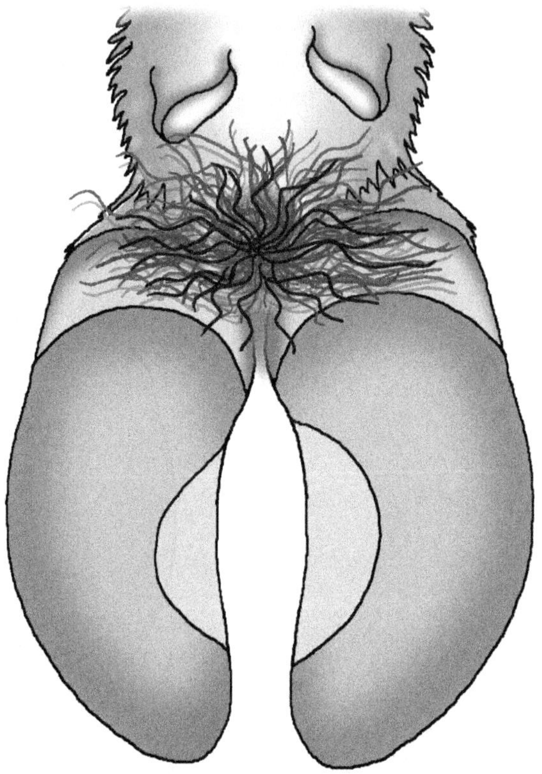

Figure 13.12 Digital dermatitis (verrucose dermatitis).

nosis is subclinical laminitis where the blood is in the horn of the sole not beneath it.

Classical solar ulcers These are recognised as circumscribed areas where horn is missing or the horn is of very poor quality. The corium is exposed or has been protected by the production of granulation tissue. The ulcers occur towards the back of the sole, two-thirds of the distance between the toe and the heel directly over the posterior border of the pedal bone. They are usually the size of a bottle top (Fig. 13.10). Less commonly *solar heel ulcers* may be present which are set further back on the sole. Ulcers are often bloody due to presence of granulation tissue, and very painful.

White line disease The white line is a point of weakness, and dirt may become impacted and provide a portal of entry for infection if the integrity of the join between the horn of the wall and the horn of the sole is compromised. Once the claw has been trimmed affected regions of the white line can be readily identified as distinct black thick zones (Fig. 13.10).

Solar abscess White line disease can result in ascending infections or lateral infections. The latter produce solar abcesses. These may be detected during corrective trimming by a sudden thinning of the sole followed by the appearance and drainage of pus. Alternatively, it may present as a painful pliable thin sole at the end of Stage 1b of the foot trimming process. Pain testers can be useful to localise the area of pain, and further thinning of the sole may puncture the abscess. Occasionally, on applying pressure, pus can be seen to exude from the original portal of entry in the white line.

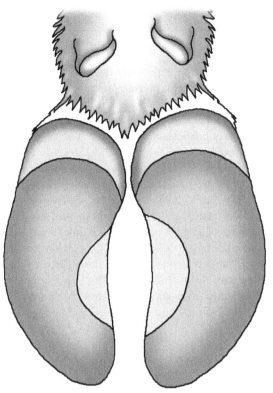

Figure 13.13 Weight distribution on a correctly shapes foot.

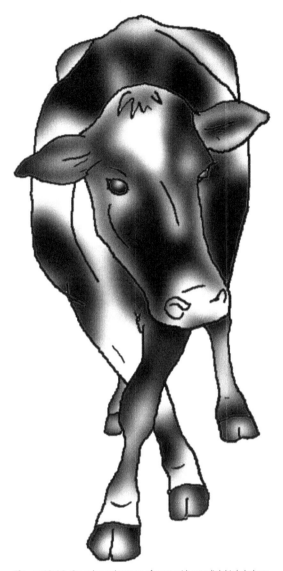

Figure 13.14 Cross-legged posture of a cow with a medial third phalanx fracture.

Deeper structures of the foot

Fractured pedal bone (P3) Fracture of the pedal bone is usually traumatic in origin, although sometimes pathological. Mounting activity or incorrect unloading from a transporter are usually responsible. The medial claw is usually affected and although most often unilateral, bilateral fractures can occur. There is acute pain, and lameness on moving is severe. When standing the animal adopts a characteristic cross-legged posture of the forelimbs to take the weight on the lateral claw and off the fractured medial claw (Fig. 13.14). Radiography will confirm the diagnosis.

Septic arthritis of the distal interphalangeal joint This produces lameness of rapidly increasing severity. There is swelling of the proximal soft tissue just above the coronary band which is hot and painful on palpation. A fistulus tract may be present just above the coronary band or at the point of penetration in the interdigital space (Fig. 13.5). Arthrocentesis of the dorsal pouch of the joint capsule is possible in a well restrained animal, preferably using intravenous regional anaesthesia. The site is located just proximal to the coronary band on the dorsal aspect. Radiography is less invasive. In an established infection the joint space will be increased when compared with the same uninfected joint on the opposite leg.

Tenosynovitis of the deep and superficial flexor tendons This is characterised by a moderate to severe lameness, and other structures may be involved concurrently. There is usually severe ascending diffuse swelling on the flexor aspect of the distal limb along the course of the infected tendon sheath. Rupture of the deep digital tendon results in an upward tilting of the affected claw. Ultrasonography will reveal the presence of abnormalities such as enlargement of the tendon sheath, abscessation and tendon rupture.

Osteomyelitis of the pedal joint This results in a chronic progressive lameness. Comparative radiography demonstrating lucency and sclerotic bone is diagnostically useful.

Further investigations

If the site of lameness in the foot cannot be identified, a block can be placed on one of the claws of the affected limb. If the lameness gets worse this suggests the lesion is located in the claw with the block. If the lameness improves this suggests the block has been placed on the limb without the lesion. If the cause of the foot lameness cannot be identified visually, then palpation, compression using hoof testers, percussion with a small hammer and manipulation, may be required to identify the seat of lameness. Further investigations, such as arthrocentesis, radiography, ultrasonography, regional anaesthesia, nerve blocks, scintigraphy and thermography, will provide more detailed information and are described under 'Further investigations' on page 192.

CLINICIAN'S CHECKLIST – EXAMINATION OF THE FOOT

Close inspection of the standing animal
Raise and clean the foot
Examination of the raised foot
   Skin of the distal limb
   Interdigital space
   Bulbs of the heel
   Sole
   Deeper structures of the foot
Further investigations

Limbs

Anatomy

The forelimb is composed of the scapula, humerus, radius, ulna, carpi, metacarpi and phalanges. The joints in the forelimb are the shoulder, elbow, antebrachiocarpal, intercarpal, carpometacarpal, metacarpophalangeal, proximal interphalangeal and distal interphalangeal (Fig. 13.15). The hind limb is composed of the femur, patella, tibia, fibula, tarsi, metatarsi and phalanges. The joints in the hind limb are hip, stifle, hock (tarsocrural, intertarsal, tarsometatarsal), metatarsophalangeal, proximal interphalangeal and distal interphalangeal (Fig. 13.16). The hind limb articulates with the pelvis at the hip joint. The pelvis consists of three bones on each side: the ilium, ischium and pubis. The pelvic bones are attached to the axial skeleton at the sacrum by the sacroiliac joints, one on each side (Fig. 13.17).

Clinical examination of the limbs

Most cases of bovine lameness involve the foot; none the less, upper limb lameness in cattle is quite common. A full clinical examination of the whole limb should be made in every case of lameness to ensure that no lesion is overlooked. More than one problem may be present.

Upper limb lameness may be caused by infection or injury to one or more of the following tissues: bones, joints, ligaments, tendons, muscles, skin, subcutis or nerves. It may be related to lower limb lameness, e.g. with ascending infection from the foot spreading up the upper limb, or it may be unconnected with the lower limb.

The examination of the proximal limb proceeds from the coronary band upwards. The bones, joints, ligaments, muscles and tendon sheaths are examined concurrently as the leg is ascended. The techniques used include visual inspection, palpation, manipulation, manipulation with auscultation, flexion and extension of the joint. The structures should be assessed for pain, swelling, heat, deformation, abnormal texture, atrophy, reduced movement, abnormal movement and crepitus. Particular atten-

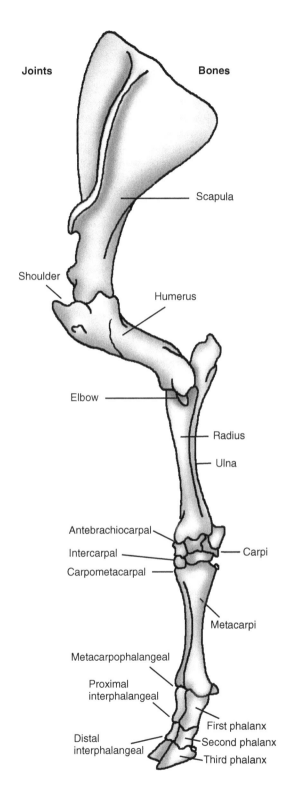

Joints

Bones

Scapula

Shoulder

Humerus

Elbow

Radius

Ulna

Antebrachiocarpal

Intercarpal

Carpi

Carpometacarpal

Metacarpi

Metacarpophalangeal

Proximal
interphalangeal

First phalanx

Distal
interphalangeal

Second phalanx

Third phalanx

tion and detail is given to localisation of the problem from earlier observations.

Joints

Lameness and altered stance are a features of conditions affecting the joints. There may be associated muscle atrophy as a result of disuse. Enlargement due to *joint capsule distention* or *apparent enlargements* of a joint due to bone abnormalities can be detected visually. Severe enlargement will be obvious, whereas mild enlargement may be more easily appreciated by comparison with the normal joint on the opposite limb. Palpation may reveal an enlarged joint capsule from the increase in synovial fluid within the affected joint, and heat and pain may be apparent. Manipulation may induce severe pain and crepitus due to abnormal periarticular bone or articular cartilage erosion. Rectal palpation is useful when trying to characterise abnormalities of the sacroiliac region and the hip joint.

Apparent joint enlargement   This may be caused by abnormalities of the growth plates (physitis), soft tissue (cellulitis) or tendon sheaths (tenosynovitis).

Physitis   This results in enlargement of the epiphyses. Juvenile physitis occurs in fast growing beef calves and usually affects the metacarpus and metatarsus. The condition may be accompanied by mild to moderate lameness, with mild resentment on palpation. Copper deficiency can also result in physitis and enlargement of the epiphyses, but with no accompanying pain. This is most apparent around the joints of the distal limb. Septic physitis is associated with *Salmonella dublin* infections and is accompanied by severe pain and systemic signs.

Septic arthritis   Pain is usually severe on palpation and joint movement in septic arthritis. The joint is hot on touching and the joint capsule distended on palpation. Weight bearing is reduced and lameness is usually severe and progressive. The animal may be recumbent and reluctant to rise. *Arthrocentesis* and

Figure 13.15 Bones and joints of the left forelimb skeleton.

Joints **Bones**

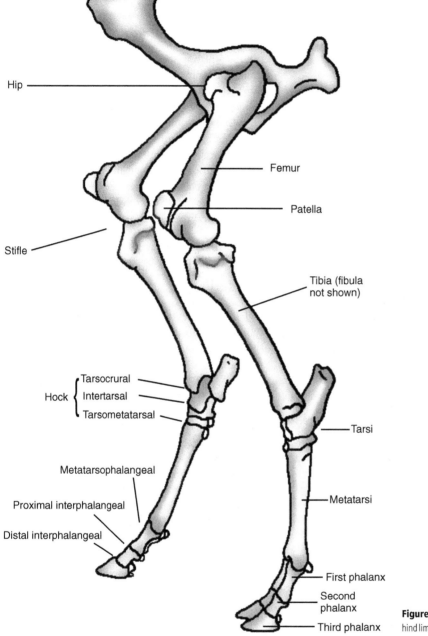

Hip

Femur

Patella

Stifle

Tibia (fibula
not shown)

Tarsocrural

Hock Intertarsal

Tarsometatarsal

Tarsi

Metatarsophalangeal

Metatarsi

Proximal interphalangeal

Distal interphalangeal

First phalanx

Second
phalanx

Third phalanx

Figure 13.16 The bones and joints of hind limbs.

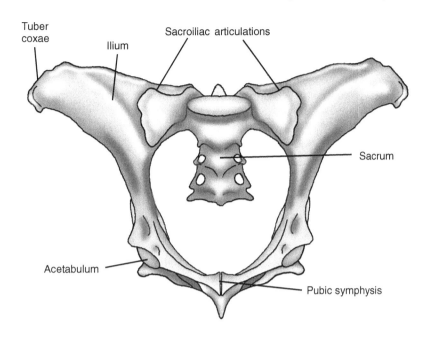

Figure 13.17 Pelvic girdle and sacrum.

synovial fluid analysis can be useful in diagnosing and differentiating septic and non-septic arthritis. This technique and the interpretive analysis are described at the end of the chapter under 'Further investigations'.

Septic arthritis or joint ill in calves is quite common and is a potentially crippling disease. Haematogenous spread of bacteria from a normal umbilicus acting as a portal of entry or an infected umbilicus acting as a source of infection is most common, but this is not always the case. One or more joints may be affected, with the carpus, hock and stifle being those most commonly involved (Fig. 13.18). The animal may have systemic signs of a septicaemia such as pyrexia, hypopyon and depression. Meningitis and encephalitis may also be present.

Septic arthritis occurs sporadically in adult cattle and is usually caused by trauma or local extension from adjacent infected structures. The presence of a skin wound over the joint may be evidence of a local penetration into the joint.

Differentiation of arthritis and physitis This can be achieved by palpation. Arthritis presents with enlargement of the joint with distended joint capsule(s), whereas physitis produces bony enlarge-ment some distance proximal to and/or distal from the joint over the growth plates.

Osteochondritis dissecans This is the splitting of the articular cartilage following ostechondrosis (abnormal growth plate development). Physitis and tibial and femoral subchondral bone cysts have also been recorded in cases of osteochondrosis. The condition is rare but may affect the stifle, hock and shoulder joints. Synovial effusion with joint capsule distention occurs and is usually associated with mild lameness. Radiography may be helpful, but the changes can sometimes be difficult to demonstrate. Arthroscopy is the most useful confirmatory diagnostic technique.

Degenerative joint disease This is most common in older cattle and may be primary or secondary to acute traumatic injuries or osteochondritis dissecans. The condition usually has a chronic course. The hip joint is most commonly affected, although any joint may be affected. This may be accompanied by crepitus on movement of the joint, the detection of which may be enhanced by placing the ear or stethoscope on the skin over the joint during movement if it is safe to do so. There is usually altered gait, some-

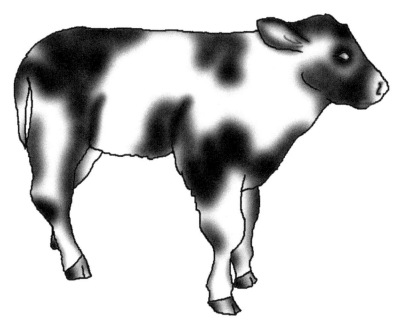

Figure 13.18 Septic arthritis of the hock and carpal joints of a calf.

times with chronic lameness and muscle atrophy. Further confirmation of the abnormal joint may be achieved by observing the improvement in gait following the intra-articular injection of local anaesthetic without adrenalin.

Hydrarthrosis   This is seen chiefly in the hock joints of young adults with a very upright hock conformation. The exact cause is unknown, but it may develop in response to repeated and chronic percussive injuries. The hock joint capsule becomes quite distended and obvious. These swellings may spoil the show potential of an affected animal as they are quite unsightly. No pain or lameness is present.

Hip dysplasia   Seen mostly in young fast growing beef bulls aged 3 to 12 months, it is an inherited condition and has been diagnosed in the Hereford, Aberdeen Angus, Galloway, Charolais and Beef Shorthorn breeds. The clinical abnormalities arise as a result of shallow acetabulae. This causes poor hip joint articulation and results in hip subluxation. Erosions of the articular cartilages develop, and joint instability and eventually degenerative joint disease may follow. A swaying gait in the hind limbs is seen

with the animal rolling from side to side as it walks. Some excessive hip joint movement and crepitus may be detected when the animal is walking or is rocked gently from side to side. Muscle wasting of the hindquarters develops, and the animal is reluctant to get up and finds it increasingly difficult to do so. The condition is usually bilateral and becomes progressively worse. Diagnosis is ideally by radiography with the animal anaesthetised or heavily sedated and lying in dorsal recumbency. A shallow acetabulum is seen with flattening of the femoral head.

Bone fractures

Fractures usually have a sudden onset with the affected limb becoming immediately non-weight bearing. Muscle tone in the affected limb is lost; the limb may hang limply. Unusual and abnormal movement of adjacent parts of the leg are possible. In general, the higher in the limb the site of fracture the more difficult the diagnosis. The large bulk of the upper limb muscles makes detailed palpation of the bones very difficult. Soft tissue swelling due to inflammation and haemtomata is usually severe in upper limb fractures. Crepitus may be palpable and audible when the limb is moved gently. Detection by auscultation will be increased with the use of a stethoscope placed on the affected limb close to the suspected fracture site. Superficial damage overlying the fracture may also have been sustained by the animal at the time of injury, which may assist identification of a possible fracture site.

Traumatic fractures of the tuber coxae   These are encountered and a sequestrum with a sinus tract may be formed. There is caudal asymmetry of the pelvis.

Fractures of the metacarpal and metatarsal bones These are the most common types of fracture encountered in cattle. This type of injury is seen in large calves delivered by traction. The new-born animal is lame with angular deformity and swelling of the affected distal limb. The condition is painful.

Epiphyseal displacements   These may occur when the bones of young animals are subjected to severe trauma. Displacement of the epiphysis (slipped capital femoral epiphysis) of one or both femoral heads can occur as a result of excessive traction being applied to a calf during delivery when foetopelvic disproportion is present. It may also occur as a result of other trauma. In such cases the calf may be unable to stand. Displacements of the distal epiphyses may occur in the extremities of all the long bones especially the metacarpals.

Osteomyelitis   This may arise through blood borne infection or may spread from (or to) sepsis in adjacent joint capsules. Entry by blood borne pathogens may be aided by trauma. Various organisms may be involved including *Actinomyces pyogenes* and *Salmonella* spp. Osteomyelitis should always be suspected when severe lameness is present without an obvious cause. In early cases of osteomyelitis in cattle few radiographic changes may be seen. Later radiographic changes include lysis of bone and irregular deposition of new bone. Sequestra may form and be associated with a discharging sinus tract.

Osteomalacia and rickets   These conditions are rare and occur in association with a severe imbalance of minerals (calcium and phosphorus) or gross deficiency of vitamin D. In calves, bending of the limbs and a rickety rosary on the costochondral junction of the ribs may be seen. In older animals pathological fractures of the long bones may occur.

Luxation/subluxations
May affect hip, stifle, shoulder and the lower joints of the fore- and hind limbs.

Luxation/subluxation of the hip   This may be the result of direct trauma and may also be a contributory factor to the 'downer cow' syndrome. Periparturient animals are predisposed to this condition by slackening of ligaments and muscles at calving time. Existing obturator paralysis is also a contributing factor. Hip luxation/subluxations may be craniodorsal, cranioventral or caudoventral. The craniodorsal luxation/subluxation is the most common, with the femoral head lying lateral to the ilial shaft. The condition is sudden in onset with no or greatly reduced weight bearing ability on the affected side. The stifle is rotated outwards, the hock inwards and attempts at movement are painful. The trochanter of the femur may appear more prominent, cranial and dorsal than normal when viewed from the rear. Attempts to move the joint may result in crepitus being felt or heard, and the movement is associated with pain. Confirmation in young animals may be possible by radiography. Rectal palpation of the obturator foramen may reveal a caudoventral luxated femoral head.

Upward fixation of the patella   This is rare except in draft animals abroad. It is a dorsal luxation/subluxation and is acute in onset; it is often recurrent. The patella is fixed in an abnormal dorsal position, preventing flexion of the stifle.

Medial or lateral luxation/subluxation of the patella This is described in fast growing young stock and results in a flexed stifle.

Femorotibial subluxations   These are more common in older animals. Ruptured collateral and/or cruciate ligaments are responsible. Often the onset is sudden and very painful, causing the affected limb to be almost non-weight bearing due to resultant instability. The onset may follow mounting activity. Excessive movement and crepitus are detectable in the stifle and there is pain on movement. In a heavily sedated animal, it may be possible to demonstrate the 'draw forward' movement.

Carpal luxation/subluxation and fetlock luxation/ subluxation These are associated with severe traumatic damage to the joint capsule and collateral ligaments. The condition is rare, occurring more frequently in calves.

Sacroiliac luxation/subluxation This may be the result of damage caused at calving or other trauma in the perinatal period, predisposed by relaxation of the pelvic muscles and ligaments. Obvious sinking of the sacrum may be seen externally, with crepitus and creaking on palpation and manipulation. The sacrum may appear displaced downwards on rectal examination, with a reduction of the dorsoventral diameter of the pelvic canal. There may be damage to the nerve supply of the hind limb.

Subluxation of the shoulder This is rare, but cases of forelimb lameness are seen in which some laxity of the shoulder joint is present with no evidence of loss of neurological function. Increased joint space is palpable between the lower extremity of the spine of the scapula and the proximal edge of the lateral humeral tuberosity. Some pain is experienced on extension and flexion of the shoulder joint.

Periostitis This may be caused by a variety of conditions, including osteomyelitis, trauma and fluorosis. The affected bone may have a raised hard area, sometimes with the shape of a 'volcano' if the problem is focal such as a sequestrum, or have a diffuse roughened surface if the condition is generalised as in fluorosis.

Congenital joint laxity and dwarfism (CJBD) The condition is encountered in spring- or summer-born suckler calves from cows fed predominantly on silage throughout the winter. The long bones are shortened, particularly the humerus and femur which have prominent epiphyses. There is joint laxity which results in fetlock joint overextension,

but this resolves soon after birth. The head is domed with a dished face and there is usually superior brachygnathia.

Arthrogryposis The term describes a permanent congenital joint contracture of the limbs.

Muscles and tendons
Muscle or tendon rupture This usually results from sudden excessive traumatic force. The *gastrocnemius* muscle may be ruptured or torn in heifers by unexpected mounting by the bull, or by a downer cow trying to rise. Affected animals are unable to extend the hock. The animal walks on its hocks if the rupture is total, or with flexion and dropping of the hock if the rupture is partial.

Adductor rupture This is seen in the downer cow. The recumbent cow may have a splay legged posture with localised swelling of the medial adductor group.

Peroneus tertius rupture This is caused by trauma and excessive flexing of the hock. Excessive restraint when elevating a foot during foot trimming, or damage during attempts to rise by downer cows are examples. At rest the animal may appear normal, but on moving the hock can be overextended whilst the stifle is flexed. The limb is dragged and the claw may scrape the ground. The limb may be manually extended caudally so that the tibia and metatarsus are in a straight line while the stifle remains flexed. Muscle swelling over the anterior surface of the tibia may be palpable.

Serratus ventralis rupture Rupture of this muscle may be unilateral or bilateral with the scapula blade protruding dorsally from the withers as a result of severe stretching of the normal sling mechanism. This change in conformation is sometimes called 'flying scapulae'. The condition may be accompanied by local haematomata. It is a condition seen in young fattening cattle and is probably related to vitamin E and/or selenium deficiency. Rupture of other skeletal muscles also occurs in calves with this deficiency. Rupture of this muscle has also be reported in the

Channel Island breeds. Ultrasonography is useful in the diagnosis of muscle ruptures. Muscle damage may result in the elevation of the muscle enzymes creatine phosphokinase (CPK) and aspartate aminotransferase (AST).

Clostridial diseases of muscle
Tetanus – proceeds rapidly from mild stiffness to opisthotonus with hypertonia.
Botulism – results in a flaccid muscle paralysis.
Blackleg – usually occurs in the hind legs in the gluteal region, although may it may occur in the brisket or shoulder muscles. The animal deteriorates rapidly. Lameness and swelling of the affected muscles are a feature. The animal is depressed and systemically ill. The affected area is crepitant but painless on palpation.
Malignant oedema – is associated with wound contamination. Stiffness is associated with castration wounds and lameness with hind-leg wounds caused by contaminated or inappropriate injections. The animal is severely ill with systemic signs.

Abscess formation in muscles   This condition may arise from a puncture wound or spread from adjacent or distant septic focus. It may occur in any muscle mass, but is more common on the caudal aspect of the hind limb with gross enlargement of the popliteal lymph node. Large amounts of pus accumulate within muscle tissues and extend along fascial planes. Needle aspiration will confirm the diagnosis.

Tendon strains   Strains of the deep and superficial flexor tendons are occasionally encountered, with some distension of the adjacent digital sheath. Ultrasonography is useful to characterise these lesions.

Contracted flexor tendons   This is a relatively common problem in neonatal calves, and several animals within a group may be affected. It can be associated with other abnormalities such as a cleft palate. Genetics, nutrition and *in utero* position have all been suggested as factors in this condition. The condition is usually bilateral and more commonly affects the forelegs. Mildly affected animals are able to stand, but weight is taken on the tips of the toes due to

flexion of the interdigital joints and the carpus (Fig. 13.19). More severely affected animal are unable to stand unaided.

Infections of the skin and subcutis associated with lameness
Tarsal and carpal bursitis   Hygromata are caused by chronic low grade trauma on pressure points of the hock, carpus and occasionally the elbow. Predisposing factors include poor cubicle design and construction. Uninfected hygromata contain golden viscous fluid which looks like synovial fluid. They are unsightly but do not usually cause pain and lameness unless infected. They may be associated with other painful lesions caused by the same predisposing factors.

Subcutaneous abscessation and cellulitis   Infection can spread upwards from sepsis involving the feet and produce a generalised cellulitis of the distal limb. This is characterised by a hard swollen distal limb. The back is another common site for subcutaneous infection, often caused by cows lying sideways in their cubicles and traumatising their backs on the bars when they attempt to rise. In severe cases, infection may spread along the entire dorsum of the back, breaking through the skin to the surface at intervals. Lesions may also extend down between the fascial planes of the limb musculature. They are very painful and, if involving the limb, cause lameness.

Decubital lesions   These may be present on the pressure points of the tarsal and carpal bones, and appear as ulcerated raw areas, sometimes with sepsis. They are often sensitive to the touch. They are commonly associated with prolonged recumbency or inappropriate housing.

Spastic paresis   This condition is characterised by a unilateral or bilateral spastic contracture of the gastrocnemius muscle in calves from 2 weeks to 12 months old. The hock is periodically forcibly extended so that the 'angle' is 180°. The limb may jerk without touching the ground when at rest. The gastrocnemius tendon has increased tension, but the hock can be flexed without difficulty. One or

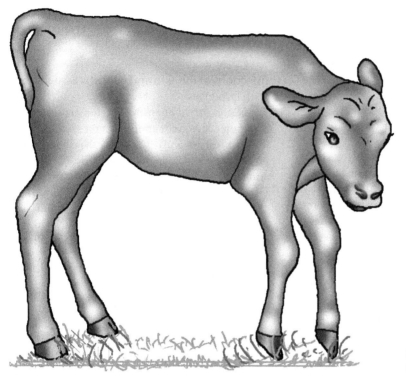

Figure 13.19 Contracted flexor tendons of the thoracic limbs of a calf.

both limbs may be affected, but not necessarily at the same time.

Ankylosing spondylitis This condition is caused by the fusion of the ventral parts of the caudal thoracic and the lumbar vertebrae, leading to reduced spinal flexibility. It is a condition of older animals, particularly breeding bulls, and may interfere with the ability to mount cows and serve successfully. This condition may lead to ataxia if there is compression of spinal nerves.

CLINICIAN'S CHECKLIST – CLINICAL EXAMINATION OF THE LIMBS

Examination of the proximal limb proceeds from the coronary band upwards

The skin, bones, joints, ligaments, muscles, tendons and tendon sheaths are examined concurrently as the leg is ascended

Techniques used include visual inspection, palpation, manipulation, manipulation with auscultation, flexion and extension of the joint

The structures should be assessed for pain, swelling, heat, deformation, abnormal texture, atrophy, reduced movement, abnormal movement and crepitus

Clinical examination of the downer cow

Downer cows are animals that have been recumbent for more than 24 hours (Fig. 13.20). The downer cow presents some physical difficulties to the clinician due to the anatomical position and weight of the animal, but in spite of these limitations useful diagnostic and prognostic information can be obtained. This scenario is most commonly found in adult dairy cattle from 2 days prepartum to 4 days postpartum. In one study of 433 periparturient recumbent cows 39% recovered, 30% died and 31% were euthanased. This section will focus on the periparturient dairy cow.

Common initial or primary causes of recumbency are milk fever and injuries sustained during dytocia. The most common injury sustained during parturition is pressure neuropathy of the obturator and sciatic nerves during passage of the calf through the birth canal. Other primary causes include toxaemia as a result of peracute mastitis or peracute metritis. Less common causes include fractured bones (e.g. fractured femur) and dislocated joints (e.g. dislocated hip), peritonitis (ruptured uterus and traumatic reticulitis), anaemia caused by a ruptured uterine artery, hypomagnesaemia, hypophosphataemia, fat cow syndrome and, rarely, bovine spongiform encephalopathy.

However, *secondary damage caused by the initial period of recumbency or by attempts to rise may result in continued recumbency.* An important and common cause of continued recumbency is *ischaemic muscle necrosis*, particularly of the hind-leg hamstrings and adductor muscles. Damage begins during the initial phase of the recumbency and is caused by the weight of the animal overlying the lower hind leg beneath the abdomen. This may result in continued recumbency and further muscle damage. *Pressure neuropathy of the peripheral nerves* (peroneal and tibial nerves) may also be caused by recumbency which will debilitate the animal and may result in uncoordinated attempts to rise with the danger of traumatic injury.

Injuries encountered when animals attempt to rise include ruptured muscles (gastrocnemius, adductors), luxation of joints (particularly the hip, but stifle and hocks have been reported), rupture of tendons (particularly of the hock) and occasionally fractured long bones (femur).

The chief aims of the clinical examination are to identify any remaining primary and current secondary causes of recumbency and to identify and quantify prognostic indicators. The welfare of the animal should be carefully considered.

History

The length of time the animal has been recumbent and whether recumbency was associated with dystocia or milk fever is important information. About 50% of downer cows will rise within 4 days. The prognosis is poor for those cows that are still recumbent after 10 days. Animals that are active and change their position regularly and demonstrate

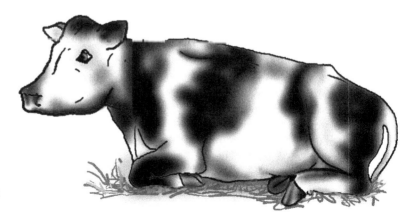

Figure 13.20 A downer cow in the correct sitting position.

good coordinated limb support following lifting have the best prognosis. Cows that show no attempt to rise, do not change position and are inactive when raised generally have poorer prognoses. The clinical signs of the animal before treatment and the response to treatment may rule in or rule out milk fever as a primary cause. Calcium can be cardiotoxic if administered incorrectly, and the dosage used and method of administration should be checked. The feeding regime of the dry cows and the incidence of milk fever in the herd should be established.

The quality of care following recumbency, including the provision of bedding and the frequency of turning, may also indicate the degree of secondary problems that may have developed. Observations by the owner regarding traumatic episodes, lameness and incoordination before going down may provide pointers to the original cause. Animals with systemic conditions may be depressed and inappetent, while other recubent animals are often bright and alert with normal appetites. The condition score of the dry cow group may be relevant to the current problem. Dry cows with high condition scores have an increased risk of developing postparturient fat cow syndrome.

Signalment

Multiparous high yielding dairy cows with previous episodes of milk fever are prime candidates for milk fever.

Observations

The position and posture of the animal should be carefully noted as this may suggest an underlying cause or prognosis.

Creeper or crawler cows – are animals that make repeated attempts to rise, move around the box and shift position frequently, often removing bedding underlying the hindquarters in the process. These cows often adopt a *frog legged posture* with the hind limbs partially flexed and extended caudally. The prognosis for recovery is usually good.

Non-creeper cows with the legs extended caudally in the frog legged position – those which make no attempt to move or use their hind legs usually have severe nerve or muscle damage and their prognosis is usually poor.

Cows with one or both hind limbs extended cranially reaching to the elbow joint – usually have upper limb problems such as a hip luxation/subluxation, severe muscle or nerve damage and have a very poor prognosis. These cows replace their legs back into the abnormal position even when repositioned to the normal position as this is more comfortable. Ischaemic muscle necrosis of the adductors is common in these cows.

Recumbent cows in the 'splits' position with both hind legs extended laterally – have a poor prognosis. These cows usually have severe injuries to the upper limbs as a result of complete abduction. The primary cause in these cows is usually obturator paralysis. Inability to abduct the hind limbs to support the body in the standing position can result in complete abduction and recumbency. Injuries sustained during this process include fractured femurs, luxated hips and ruptured adductor muscles.

Cows that consistently adopt lateral recumbency following repositioning in sternal recumbency – usually have a poor prognosis, provided that metabolic diseases have been ruled out as a cause. Brain damaged animals may lie in lateral recumbency with their heads drawn backwards.

Cows adopting a dog-sitting position with flaccid or spastic hind limbs – have vertebral lesions in the thoracolumbar region and a poor prognosis.

Clinical examination

Involvement of other organ systems and signs of systemic illness including anaemia, toxaemia, hyperaesthesia and flaccid paralysis should be detected during the general clinical examination which precedes the specific examination of the downer cow. Lifting the animal facilitates the clinical examination. Lifting equipment that provides good support and distributes the forces evenly, such as a webbing sling, are particularly useful, safe and comfortable for the cow. During the examination the animal should be closely observed for signs of pain, particularly during manipulation and palpation.

Rectal examination

This may indicate constipation and a full bladder which are associated with milk fever. Palpation of the obturator foramen may reveal the femoral head following a caudoventral luxation. Sacroiliac luxation may be palpable. Manipulation of the hind leg during rectal palpation may produce crepitus or creaking, which may indicate pelvic damage or a hip luxation.

Manipulation of the pelvis

This may reveal increased and abnormal mobility.

Examination of the mammmary gland

The detection of acute mastitis or developing mastitis as a result of recumbency is important. To examine the mammary gland in a cow that is in sternal recumbency, the cow must be pushed over into lateral recumbency so that upper quarters and teats can be examined. It is sometimes possible to examine all four quarters in this position, but placing the cow back into sternal recumbency and then pushing the cow over into lateral recumbency on the opposite side provides better access to the other quarters. Alternatively, the cow can be placed in dorsal recumbency to examine the mammary gland if there is sufficient manpower. Hoisting the cow will enable a thorough examination.

The quarters should be visually inspected and palpated for signs of mastitis. A milk sample should be taken and examined from each quarter. Gross changes in acute mastitis due to *Escherichia coli* may not be obvious and careful detailed clinical assessment of the animal is required to avoid a misdiagnosis. The clinician must proceed with caution whichever method is used, as some downer cows can sometimes kick out aggressively with their hind legs and butt aggressively with their heads.

Examination of the limbs

Abnormal contours and angularities may indicate torn muscles and/or tendons, fractures or luxation/subluxations. These are painful, and examination should proceed with care. With the animal in lateral recumbency it is possible to manipulate and palpate the joints of the limbs. Muscles should be palpated carefully, particularly the adductors, peroneal tertius and gastrocnemious for signs of rupture. Manipulation may reveal crepitus. Increased auditory sensitivity is achieved by using a stethoscope. Skin over the pressure points should be carefully examined for decubital lesions. Skin sensation can be tested by using a large gauge needle. Conscious awareness and limb movement are informative, but a poor response is noted in many downer cows due to their posture and apathy. It is often difficult to perform a detailed neurological examination of the limbs, and interpretation of abnormal responses may be unreliable.

Assessment of ischaemic muscle necrosis

Hard swollen rigid muscles indicate ischaemic muscle necrosis. The hamstrings and adductors are most often affected. There may be hyperkalaemia and associated cardiac dysrhythmias. Attempts should be made to obtain a urine sample either by perineal stimulation or by catheterisation. The urine may be rusty colour or brown due to myoglobinuria and have an increased protein concentration. The sample can be also tested for ketones. Myoglobin may cause renal damage and contribute to the raised urea levels due to muscle damage. AST and CPK levels are elevated.

Urea, AST and CPK levels have been used to predict the probability of the animal rising. In one study of 433 downer cows sampled on one occasion between days 2 and 7 of recumbency with urea levels above 25 U/l and/or AST levels above 890 mmol/l, the chance of recovery was only 5%. CPK has a shorter half-life than AST and is therefore a more sensitive indicator of ongoing muscle damage. The critical 5% recovery levels for CPK were 18 600 U/l on day 2, 10 600 U/l on day 4 and 3900 U/l on day 7. Testing CPK levels on more than one occasion is a useful way to monitor for increasing damage between days 2 and 7.

Examination per vaginam

A depressed toxaemic animal may have a severe metritis. A lubricated gloved hand should be introduced into the vagina and a careful examination made for retained fetus(es) and/or a putrid purulent haemorrhagic discharge indicative of acute metritis. More detail is provided in Chapter 10.

Biochemistry

A useful panel for downer cows is as follows: calcium, phosphorous, magnesium, creatinine, potassium, urea, ketones, AST and CPK.

CLINICIAN'S CHECKLIST – EXAMINATION OF THE DOWNER COW

Primary aims
  Identification of any remaining primary causes of
    recumbency
  Identification of current secondary causes of recumbency
  Quantification of prognostic indicators

History
  Length of time the animal has been recumbent
  Whether recumbency was associated with dystocia or milk
    fever
  Quality of care following recumbency

Observations
  Position and posture

Clinical examination
  Rectal examination
  Manipulation of the pelvis
  Examination of the mammmary gland
  Examination of the limbs
  Assessment of ischaemic muscle necrosis
  Examination *per vaginam*

Further investigations

Further investigations

Most cases of bovine lameness can be diagnosed without recourse to more complicated investigations. Such investigations include: radiography, ultrasonography, scintigraphy, thermography, arthroscopy, muscle biopsies and histopathology and the sampling of joint fluid and bone in certain cases.

Radiography

Radiographs of the lower limbs can be taken using portable sets available in practice but upper limb investigations may need more powerful machines in referral centres. In very heavily muscled animals diagnostic radiographs of the upper limb may be very difficult to achieve.

Ultrasonography

Ultrasonographic scans are useful for evaluation of soft tissue structures including abscesses, muscle and tendon injuries.

Scintigraphy

Scintigraphy uses radioactive technetium to detect focal areas of inflammation. It has a short half-life and is particularly useful for conditions of the hip joints in larger animals where radiography can be difficult. Availability is restricted to referral centres.

Thermography

Thermography uses a heat seeking camera to detect infrared rays. It can detect small temperature differences and is useful in identifying the presence of inflammation. Availability is restricted to referral centres.

Muscle biopsies and histopathology

These techniques are occasionally used and are diagnostically useful to identify white muscle disease and neurogenic disuse such a femoral nerve paralysis.

Arthroscopy

This entails the use of a fibreoptic scope to visualise the joint surfaces. Cruciate ruptures, degenerative joint disease and osteochondritis dissecans may be diagnosed in this way. General anaesthesia is required. Availability is restricted to referral centres.

Nerve blocks

These may be used diagnostically but are seldom used in practice due to the uncooperative nature of bovine patients.

Intra-articular anaesthesia and intravenous regional anaesthesia (IVRA)

These techniques are sometimes very useful to identify the site of lameness.

Arthrocentesis (joint tap)

Technique

Restraint and immobilisation of the patient are important to minimise the discomfort. The hair on the site over the selected joint is clipped and aseptically prepared. This requires great care to avoid introducing infection into the joint. A sterile 1.5 inch (3.8 cm) 19 BWG (1.10 mm) needle is commonly used, although a sterile 9 cm lumbar spinal needle of size 18 BWG (1.20 mm) with a stylet may avoid blockage of the lumen by soft tissue. The needle is introduced into the joint space and a sample of synovial fluid obtained by aspiration using a syringe (Fig. 13.21). One aliquot of the sample is then placed into an EDTA tube (for cytology and protein content) and another into a plain tube (for bacteriological culture).

Analysis and interpretation of synovial fluid

Gross examination   This is inexpensive and can quickly be accomplished at the cowside.

Normal synovial fluid – is clear, viscid, colourless or pale yellow, does not clot and does not form a stable froth when shaken.

Aseptic arthritis, hydrathrosis and degenerative joint disease synovial fluids – are grossly normal.

Septic arthritis synovial fluid – is turbid, sometimes with flocculent material present. There is a reduction in viscosity, producing a watery consistency. Inflammation causes the protein content to rise and a stable froth is formed when shaken. The fluid will clot on standing.

Bacteriology   The preparation of a smear on a glass slide followed by Gram staining may reveal bacteria in the sample and can be quickly accomplished in a practice laboratory. Culturing of synovial fluid samples from joints with septic arthritis frequently results in no growth. A negative sample does not rule out a septic arthritis or confirm an aseptic arthritis. The chances of identifying the causal organism in septic arthritis is enhanced by sampling before therapy and by sampling the synovial membrane using arthroscopy. The latter technique is expensive and confined to referral centres. In the event of a pathogen being cultured this further supports a

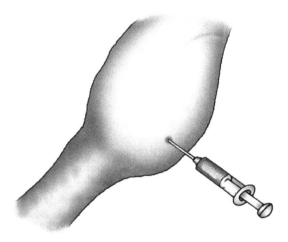

Figure 13.21 A joint tap of a septic carpal joint.

Table 13.1 Total and differential white blood cell count (WBC) and protein concentrations of synovial fluid from a normal joint, a joint with septic arthritis and a joint with degenerative osteoarthritis

Synovial fluid	Appearance	Clot	WBC × 10^9/l	Neutrophils (%)	Protein (g/l)
Normal joint	Clear	–	<0.25	<10	<18
Septic arthritis	Turbid	+	10.00	95	>40
Degenerative osteoarthritis	Clear or turbid	–	<0.25	<15	<20

diagnosis of septic arthritis, provided a competent sampling technique has been used.

Total and differential white blood cell count (WBC) and protein concentrations There is an elevated total WBC count with a neutrophilia in septic arthritis. The protein content is also elevated. The relative values are shown in Table 13.1.

Intravenous regional anaesthesia

Intravenous regional anesthesia provides analgesia which enables an otherwise painful invasive procedure, such as aggressive paring of the sole, to be accomplished. The technique involves injecting a local anaesthetic into a visible and superficial accessible vein of the distal limb following the application of a proximal tourniquet.

Depending on the procedure and the available restraint equipment, the animal may need to be sedated and cast. In the hind leg a tourniquet is applied above or below the hock. If the tourniquet is applied above the hock, padding in the form of a roll of dressing material is required to 'fill the gap' in the depression between the teres major tendon and the tibia on both medial and lateral aspects (Fig. 13.22). In the foreleg the tourniquet is applied above the carpus (Fig. 13.23). A disused long tube from the milking parlour makes an ideal tourniquet for this procedure. The position of suitable superficial veins for the hind leg are shown in Fig. 13.22 and for the foreleg in Fig. 13.23. In an adult dairy cow 30 ml of a 2% solution of lignocaine hydrochloride without adrenalin is injected rapidly into a superficial vein using a 1 inch (2.5 cm) 19 BWG (1.10 mm) needle. Smaller animals should be given proportionately lower doses. Following removal of the needle, topical pressure is applied to prevent the formation of a haematoma. Complete anaesthesia of the limb distal to the tourniquet occurs within 10 to 15 minutes. The interdigital skin is the last area to become desensitised, and pinching of the skin with forceps in this area is a use-

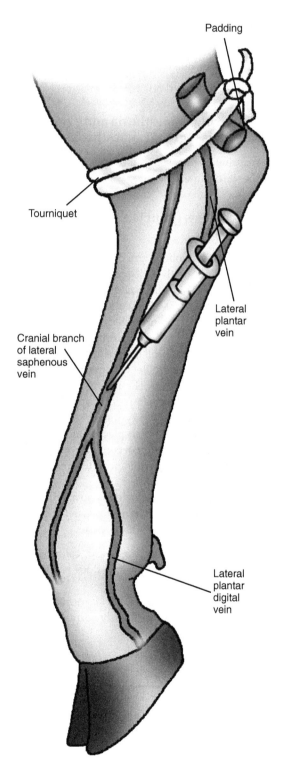

Figure 13.22 Intravenous regional anaesthesia of the pelvic limb foot (lateral view).

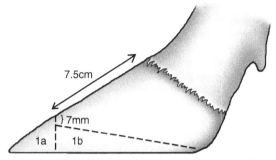

Figure 13.24 Dutch 'five step' method of foot trimming: steps 1a and 1b.

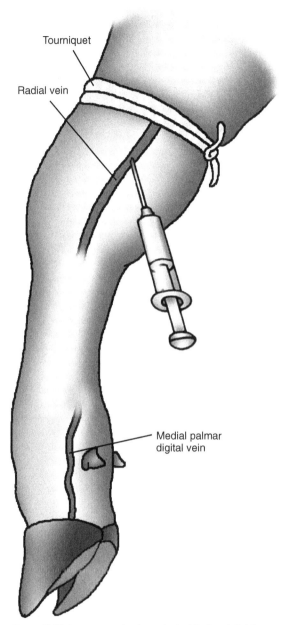

Figure 13.23 Intravenous regional anaesthesia of the thoracic limb foot (medial view).

ful test for anaesthesia. If the tourniquet needs to be removed soon after the administration, then it should be done slowly. The tourniquet should not stay in place for more than 60 minutes.

Dutch 'five step' method of foot trimming
(Fig. 13.24)

A wooden block 7.5 cm long and 7 mm deep is used as a guide to the measurements used in this method.

(1a) Cut the medial hoof wall to the correct length of 7.5 cm at the toe, ensuring the cut at the toe is perpendicular to the sole and is square across the toe.

(1b) Reduce the horn of the medial sole to the correct depth of approximately 7 mm:
   (i) the cut edge at the toe should be 7 mm;
   (ii) the white line will reappear as an ellipse around the toe when sole is correct depth;
   (iii) if the sole is pinking it is getting too thin.
   Using the handle of the knife check to ensure that the paring is producing a flat sole.

(2) Using the medial claw as a template, cut the toe of the lateral claw to the correct length and pare the sole to the correct depth.

(3) Hollow out the non-weight bearing axial surfaces between the white line and the heels of both claws (Fig. 13.13).

(4) Investigate any problems on the sole.

(5) Trim the heels if necessary. Be careful because the heels are sensitive. Do not be too aggressive:
   (i) remove any loose tags of horn;
   (ii) reshape the heel;
   (iii) reduce any deep furrows.
   Rasp the edges of the claws to prevent trauma.

Physical Signs of Disease Associated with the Musculoskeletal System

N.B. Some of these physical signs are also associated with diseases of other body systems and regions.

Posture
  Recumbent
    Posture
      Frog legged
      Frog legged with hind limbs extended caudally
      Hind leg(s) extended cranially
      Splits position
      Lateral recumbency
      Dog-sitting position
    Abnormal lying down position
    Foreleg extended in recumbency
  Standing
    Reduced weight bearing on limb
    No weight bearing on the limb
    Limb not touching ground at rest
    Immediate lifting of leg on contact with ground
    Adduction of limb
    Abduction of limb
    Camping back
    Camping forward
    Paddling of hind legs
    Crossing over of front legs
    Dangling leg (non-weight bearing)
    Stifle cannot be flexed
    Dropping of hock
    Hock touching the ground
    Scapulae elevated above axial skeleton
    Calf on tiptoes (forelegs)
    Unable to extend the digits

Actions
  Reluctant to rise
  Rising with difficulty
  Unstable during rising
  Repeated attempts to rise
  Fails to rise after repeated attempts
  Recumbent
    Creeper
    Non-creeper

Conformation
  Abnormal

Gait
  Lameness 0–10
  Locomotory score 0–5
  Ataxia
  Supporting limb lameness
  Swinging limb lameness
  Foreleg
    Bobbing head
    Head raised when painful forelimb bears weight
  Hind leg
    Pelvis raised (but symmetrical) when painful hind limb
      bears weight
    Swaying hind-leg gait
    Hyperextension of hock

Foot
  Claw
    Overgrown horn
    Corkscrew claw
  Wall of claw
    Horizontal fissure
    Vertical fissure
    Concave anterior wall
    Multiple ridges
    Broken horn at toe
  Coronary band
    Vesicles
    Erosions
    Erythematous
    Swollen
    Sinus tract
  Interdigital space
    Wedge of tissue occupying interdigital space
    Foreign body
    Necrosis of the interdigital skin
    Penetration wound
    Granulating penetration wound
  Bulbs of the heel
    Erosions
    Focal swelling
    Generalised swelling
    Midline superficial circular circumscribed
      erosion
    Fulmination keratin threads

(Continued on p. 197)

PHYSICAL SIGNS OF DISEASE ASSOCIATED WITH THE MUSCULOSKELETAL SYSTEM
CONTINUED

Sole
- False sole
- Foreign body
- Ulcer
- Abscess
- White line impaction and penetration
- Haemorrhage
- Yellow/heamorrhagic dicolouration of horn
- Painful
- Penetration by P3

Skin of distal limb
- Painful
- Hard
- Discharging sinus tract
- Swollen
  - Generalised
  - Focal
    - Heel
    - Coronary band
    - Flexor tendons

Limbs
- Joints
  - Single joint affected
  - Multiple joints affected
  - Swollen
  - Abnormally warm
  - Enlarged joint capsule
  - Crepitus
  - Pain on manipulation
  - Laxity of joint
  - Reduced mobility
  - Reduced range of movements
- Rectal palpation
  - Head of femur in obturator foramen
  - Sacrum displaced ventrally

Bones
- Epiphyses
  - Enlarged

Painful on palpation
Soft tissue swelling
Crepitus
Abnormal angularity
Fragments of bone visible
Costochondral junctions enlarged
Discharging sinus
Contour of bone abnormal
- Long bones bent
- Long bones short
- Surface irregular
- Local enlargement

Muscles and tendons
- Muscle
  - Atrophy
  - Swollen
  - Hard
  - Painful
  - Rupture
  - Emphysematous
  - Flaccid
  - Tetanic
  - Abscess
- Tendons
  - Contracted
    - Extension of carpal joint impossible
    - Tendon very tight on joint extension
  - Ruptured

Skin and subcutis
- Pressure points
  - Painless swollen area
  - Painful ulcers
- Distal limb hard, abnormally warm and painful
- Loss of skin sensation

Urine
- Brown colour

Clinical Examination of the Nervous System

Introduction

Conditions of the nervous system may result in abnormalities in mental status, behaviour, posture and balance, gait and muscle tone, and the special senses. The *brain* is responsible for consciousness, behaviour, voluntary and reflex movements of the head, initiation and refinement of voluntary movement, spatial awareness, modulation of muscle tone and appreciation of the senses: vision, hearing, taste, pain and touch. The *spinal cord* acts a conduit for information passing to and from the brain. In addition, in the ventral grey horns of the spinal chord are located lower motor neurons which are involved in involuntary spinal reflexes as well as voluntary actions. The *peripheral nerves* are composed of sensory nerves carrying information to the spinal cord and motor nerves carrying information to the muscle.

Neurological conditions of cattle are common and important. Milk fever and bovine spongiform encephalopathy are two examples. Examination of the nervous system can be difficult due to the lack of facilities for restraint, the size of the animal and the fractious nature of some infrequently handled patients. Testing of some of the reflexes cannot be readily accomplished. However, with care, a great deal can be achieved despite these limitations. In many cases a definitive diagnosis may not be necessary if the clinical examination indicates the prognosis is poor with due regard to the welfare and economics of the patient.

Neurological signs are caused by a diverse range of conditions including some metabolic diseases (e.g. hypomagnesaemia), chemical poisons (e.g. lead), plant poisons (e.g. ragwort), bacterial infections (e.g. *Haemophilus somnus*), bacterial exotoxins (e.g. botulism), traumatic lesions (e.g. riding injuries), and genetic disorders (e.g. progressive ataxia of Charolais).

The clinician should not focus wholly upon the nervous system until information has been assessed from the general physical examination, as the involvement of other systems may be overlooked. For example, icterus in association with neurological signs may indicate a primary hepatic condition as the most likely cause.

The *primary aim* of the neurological examination is to identify the presence of clinical signs which are associated with the nervous system. A full neurological examination is recommended. However, many experienced clinicians select signs to be examined to confirm or rule out differential diagnoses generated from initial findings. The progression from clinical signs to differential diagnosis may go through an intermediate step which is the localisation of the lesion within the nervous system. The differential diagnosis may therefore be based either on the constellation of clinical signs that are detected or on the conditions that explain the localised lesion.

Important questions to consider during the clinical examination are the following:

- Is the condition a neuropathological disorder (e.g. spastic paresis), a metabolic disorder (e.g. nervous ketosis), or a musculoskeletal condition (e.g. white muscle disease)?
- Are the signs primarily neurological (e.g. cerebrocortical necrosis) or a consequence of disease in another organ system (e.g. hepatoencephalopathy) or due to extension of disease from another lesion (e.g. spinal abscess, otitis media, sinusitis)?
- Are the signs generalised (e.g. milk fever) or can they be localised to a division of the brain (e.g. cerebellar hypoplasia), a part of the spinal cord (e.g. trauma) or a peripheral nerve (e.g. obturator and sciatic paralysis)?
- Is the condition confined to one animal in a group (e.g. peripheral nerve paralysis) or is it a herd outbreak (e.g. lead poisoning)?

Signalment

Many neurological conditions are specific or more common to certain ages or classes of animal. The signalment alone may enable the initial list of differential diagnoses to be small. Some examples are as follows:

Age – septicaemia with meningitis and encephalitis or cerebellar hypoplasia is more commonly seen in calves, whereas clinical bovine spongiform encephalopathy is confined to cattle over 2 years of age.

Breed – the weaver syndrome is a condition of the Brown Swiss breed and progressive ataxia a condition of the Charolais breed

Sex – nervous ketosis is a condition of high yielding dairy cattle in early lactation, and milk fever is a condition of high yielding dairy cows in the periparturient period.

Class – cerebrocortical necrosis and ruminal acidosis are more common in intensively fed beef cattle.

History

The time of onset, the signs observed and the clinical progression of the condition should be established. Congenital conditions are likely to have been present since birth, whereas traumatic lesions such as traumatic spinal injuries are usually acute in onset with the animal's condition either stabalising or improving. Untreated infectious causes may be acute (e.g. listeriosis) or chronic (e.g. brain abscess) in onset and are usually progressive. A history of the recent introduction of bovine viral diarrhoea (BVD) into the herd may be relevant when presented with a calf with signs of cerebellar hypoplasia. The sequence of events is important to establish; for example, did a recumbent animal show any signs of paresis before going down?

Some important neurological conditions are associated with feeding practices and changes in nutrition. A sudden increase in concentrate feeding may be related to an outbreak of ruminal acidosis or cerebrocortical necrosis. Lack of energy density in the diet of high yielding dairy cows may result in an increase in the incidence of primary ketosis. Incorrect feeding during the dry period in dairy cattle may result in a high incidence of milk fever. Lack of magnesium supplementation may cause hypomagnesaemia which may become apparent following stress. Extreme malnutrition may result in hypovitaminosis A.

Protocols for navel dressing and the possibility of failure of passive transfer of protective antibodies should be checked if there is a high incidence of neonatal calf mortality due to meningitis. Associations with routine procedures may be significant such as tetanus immunisation following castrations or assisted calvings.

The morbidity rate, mortality rate, prevalence and incidence of the problem should be established. These parameters define the extent, severity and dynamics of the problem and assist in compiling differential diagnoses. For example, a dairy herd that has an incorrect mineral content during the dry period may have a serious problem with milk fever in the periparturient cows. The morbidity rate is likely to be high but with a low mortality rate, assuming treatment is given promptly. The prevalence will be low but the annual incidence will be high, even with seasonally calving herds as the disease has a short duration and the cows do not calve concurrently.

Examination of the environment

The environment in which the animals are currently kept and were kept in the recent past should be carefully examined for the presence of toxic material. Examples include rubbish dumps, old flaking paint on disused buildings, degraded engine oil, partially buried batteries, poisonous plants, and access to water supplies contaminated with the blue green algae *Microcystis aeruginosa*. Examination of silage quality may indicate excessive soil contamination with an increased risk of listeriosis.

The examination

Evaluation of the mental status of the animal can be

important in trying to decide if the lesion involves the brain, spinal cord or peripheral nerves.

Animals with lesions of the spinal chord or peripheral nerves usually have a normal mental status and are bright and alert, at least in the early stages of the disease. However, these lesions may be associated with pain, and these animals may be dull and depressed.

Signs of brain involvement include dullness, depression, coma, abnormal behaviour, head pressing, aggression, seizures, circling, blindness, facial asymmetry, nystagmus, strabismus, head tilt, intention tremor and ataxia.

Observations

Ideally, the affected animal(s) should be observed within its (their) group. Abnormalities of social interactions, such as separation or aggression (e.g. BSE), grazing behaviour (e.g. ketosis), posture (e.g. obturator paralysis) and locomotion (e.g. spastic paresis), may be observed. Hyperaesthesia (e.g. hypomagnesaemia), frenzy (e.g. lead poisoning) and compulsive self licking (e.g. nervous ketosis) may be self-evident. Extreme manifestations such as recumbency, dogsitting posture, seizures and opisthotonos will be obvious.

There may be abnormalities of the *head carriage* such as tilt or aversion. A *head tilt* is rotation around the long axis of the midline. This may indicate otitis media, otitis interna or vestibular nuclei damage. The lesion is usually ipsilateral to the lower ear. *Aversion of the head* is a lateral, upward or downward deviation and may be seen with cerebral lesions such as cerebrocortical necrosis. *Head tremor* may be seen (e.g. cerebellar hypoplasia). With cerebellar involvement there is a wide-based stance and ataxia, but without muscle weakness.

Compulsive circling in an unrestricted space may be observed (e.g. listeriosis, space-occupying lesions) and indicates a lesion in the brain stem or cerebellum on the side to which the animal turns, or a cerebral lesion that is usually on the opposite side to the turn.

Visual or auditory deficits may become apparent when the animal is approached, although depression or dullness may also produce a delayed response. A recumbent animal will attempt to rise on approach and further abnormalities such as paresis may be observed.

Forcing the affected animal or group to move at a slow walk will enable the clinician to detect incoordination (e.g. milk fever), ataxia (e.g. hypomagnesaemia), spasticity (e.g. tetanus), or tremors (e.g. hypomagnesaemia, hypokalaemia). *Increasing the pace of movement will reveal any progressive locomotory abnormalities* including hypermetria (e.g. BSE) and knuckling (e.g. traumatic lumbar injuries).

Restraint in a box and the availability of a crush facilitate a more detailed examination.

Examination of the head

Head pressing (e.g. nervous ketosis, listeriosis) and compulsive walking (e.g. lead poisoning, nervous ketosis) may be observed in the confined space of the box. The latter should not be confused with circling.

Facial paralysis (Fig. 14.1)
This is most commonly caused by listeriosis or trauma to the vertical ramus of the mandible. The condition is caused by a lesion in the medulla or damage to

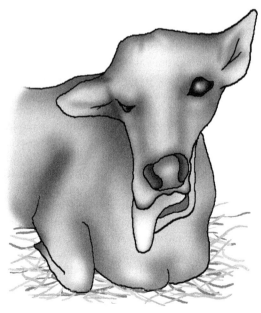

Figure 14.1 Facial nerve and hypoglossal nerve paralysis. Dropped ear, eyelid and jaw, flaccid lip, head aversion and tongue paralysis.

the peripheral facial nerve. It can be detected by observing the symmetry of the head. On the affected side, there is bulging of the cheek due to retention of food, and drooping of the ear and eyelid.

Nystagmus

This is an oscillatory movement of the eyeballs. It consists of a slow movement in one direction with a rapid return to the original position. The direction of the movement relative to the head may be horizontal, vertical or rotatory. Nystagmus occurs with lesions of the pons, midbrain, cerebellum or inner ear.

Strabismus

This is the persistent deviation of the eye within the orbit and may be ventrolateral due to damage to cranial nerve III or dorsolateral due to damage to cranial nerve IV. It is rare but may also occur in some cases of cerebrocortical necrosis. Cranial nerves II, IV and VI are involved either directly or indirectly due to lesions in the cerebellar or vestibular system.

Vestibular eye drop response

In cattle, the eye remains in the original position if the head is tilted upwards, thus giving the impression that the animal appears to look down: this is not abnormal and is known as the vestibular eye drop response.

Animals with loss of vision

These may show over-reaching of the limbs with a goose stepping gait (hypermetria) and are reluctant to move in a strange environment. When forced to do so they bump into the walls, although spatial adaptation occurs quite quickly. An obstacle course can be helpful, although sighted animals may knock objects over when stressed. The fixation, menace response and photomotor reflexes may be helpful in assessing the presence or absence of vision. The pupillary light reflex may help locate the lesion. These reflex tests require restraint. The operator should always be alert in case the patient moves its head unexpectedly. An abnormality in the reflex may be due to a lesion anywhere in the neurological pathways involved.

Fixation reflex (Fig. 14.2)   The head and eyes move towards a moving object such as a falling handkerchief. Repeated attempts are often not diagnostic as cattle fail to respond due to adaptation. (Pathway: retina, optic tract, rostral brain, posterior cerebrum, cranial nerves II, IV, VI and / or cervical nerves.)

Menace response (Fig. 14.3)   Threatening the eye with the hand causes a blink. To ensure it is the moving hand and not the blast of air preceding it, a piece of rigid transparent plastic should be interposed between the hand and the eye before the test. (Pathway: retina, optic tract, anterior brain-stem, posterior cerebrum and cranial nerve VII.)

Palpebral reflex   When the periocular skin is touched the normal animal will close the eyelids. The facial nerve (VII) innervates the muscles which close the eyelids and the trigeminal nerve (V) provides periocular sensation. The absence of this reflex indicates a lesion to one or both of these nerves or their

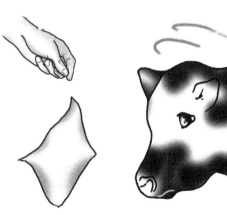

Figure 14.2 Fixation reflex: movement of the head and eyes towards a moving object.

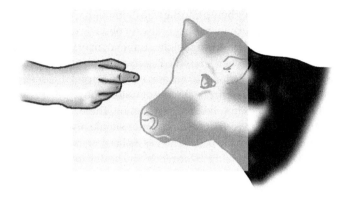

Figure 14.3 Menace response: threatening the eye causes a blink.

nuclei on the affected side. To rule out damage to the trigeminal nerve (V), facial skin sensation can be tested using a pair of haemostats.

Photomotor reflex Closure of the eyelids when a bright light is shone into the eye. (Pathway: retina, optic tract, anterior brain-stem, posterior cerebrum and cranial nerve VII.)

Pupillary light reflex The animal should be placed in a darkened environment for several minutes before performing the test. The direct and indirect responses of both eyes should be tested.

To perform the test a light is shone directly into one of the eyes only. The *direct response* results in constriction of the pupil of the eye which is illuminated. The *indirect or consensual response* results in the constriction of the pupil of the eye which is not illuminated. Animals that are blind due to diffuse damage to the cerebral cortex involving the occipital visual cortex will have normal direct and indirect pupillary light reflexes because the reflex pathways are unaffected. If the animal is blind but has dilated pupils which are non-responsive to light, then the lesion is in the retina, optic tract or brain-stem. Cows with severe milk fever have dilated pupils which are unresponsive to light due to flaccid paralysis of the iris.

Cornea reflex If the cornea is touched, the eyeball is retracted and the nictitating membrane comes across the eye. (Pathway: rostral brain-stem, cranial nerves III and VI.)

Ophthalmoscopy

Ophthalmoscopy of the lens may reveal cataracts in a calf (e.g. BVD). Examination of the retina may reveal thrombosis and haemorrhage of the retinal vessels (e.g. thromboembolic meningoencephalitis). Examination of the optic disc may reveal papilloedema (e.g. vitamin A deficiency, increased intracranial pressure).

Clinical signs associated with cranial nerve lesions

The clinical signs that may be observed with the dysfunction of the cranial nerves are as follows: loss of smell (I, olfactory), loss of vision (II, optic), pupil dilatation and ventrolateral strabismus (III, oculomotor), dorsolateral strabismus (IV, trochlear), loss of facial sensation and motor function of the muscles of mastication (V, trigeminal), medial strabismus and unable to withdraw the eyeball deeper into the orbit (VI, abducens), loss of motor function to the muscles of facial expression (VII, facial), loss of hearing (cochlear) and/or nystagmus and head tilt (vestibular) (VIII, vestibularcochlear), dysphagia (IX, glossopharyngeal; X, vagus; XI, accessory), tongue paresis or tongue atrophy (XII, hypoglossal).

The tongue should be examined to determine its strength and coordination by putting the hand through the diastema and grasping the tongue. Care should be taken to avoid damage to the tongue by the incisor teeth. This is achieved by exteriorising it through the diastema. Cattle have very strong tongue muscles and it should be difficult to maintain the tongue in the examiner's grasp. A limp tongue that remains exteriorised once released is a sign of hypoglossal paralysis or (if more general signs of paresis are present) botulism. Animals that have difficulty swallowing may present with saliva and food material around the muzzle. These animals are prone to aspiration pneumonia and may cough frequently.

Manipulation of the head and opisthotonos

Manipulation of the head in cattle with cerebellar disease may cause opisthotonos which presents with spasm of the neck and limb muscles, causing recumbency with hyperextension of the head and neck and extensor rigidity of the limbs (Fig. 14.4). Opisthotonos is also seen in tetanus, cerebral disease and hypomagnesaemia.

Examination of the neck

The symmetry of the neck and pain on manipulation should be evaluated. The presence of muscle atrophy, peripheral sensation or sweating should be noted.

Clinical signs associated with lesions of the cerebrum

Signs may be caused by diffuse (e.g. cerebrocortical necrosis, hypomagnesaemia, nervous ketosis, lead poisoning), localised (e.g. traumatic injury) or space-occupying lesions (e.g. brain abscess or tumour).

The animal may be dull and depressed. Head pressing and compulsive behaviour such as self licking may occur. There may be blindness with normal

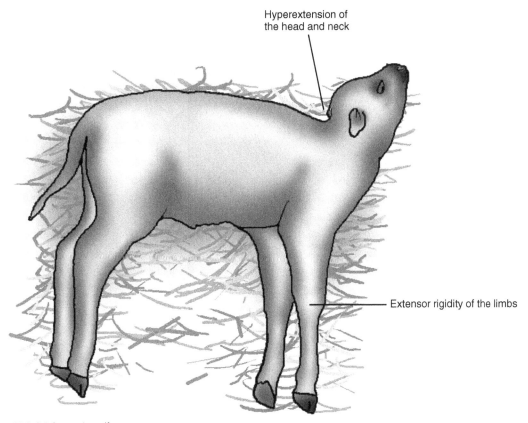

Hyperextension of the head and neck

Extensor rigidity of the limbs

Figure 14.4 Opisthotonos in a calf.

pupillary light reflexes. There may be abnormal vocalisation.

Localised seizures may cause abnormal regional muscular activity and movement, and the animal may remain standing. With generalised seizures the animal is recumbent with exaggerated paddling movements of the limbs or, in more severe cases, thrashing.

The gait is usually normal but movement may be slow and weak. Lesions affecting only one cerebral hemisphere may cause aimless circling or leaning towards the affected side with contralateral proprioceptive deficits.

Clinical signs associated with lesions of the cerebellum

The cerebellum coordinates all skeletal muscle activity. Cerebellar disease is characterised by jerky head movements, head tremor, intention tremor, head bobbing, a wide-based stance and ataxia with a high stepping gait and over-reaching with preserved muscular strength (Fig. 14.5). There may be loss of the menace response and nystagmus is occasionally seen. The head may be elevated. Opisthotonos may occur or be induced by raising the head. The most common cause of cerebellar hypoplasia is calves infected *in utero* with BVD.

Clinical signs associated with lesions of vestibular disease

The most common condition causing vestibular disease (and brain-stem lesions) is listeriosis. Otitis interna and/or otitis media may result in vestibular damage. Manifestations of vestibular disease include ipsilateral head tilt, circling, nystagmus and a staggering gait.

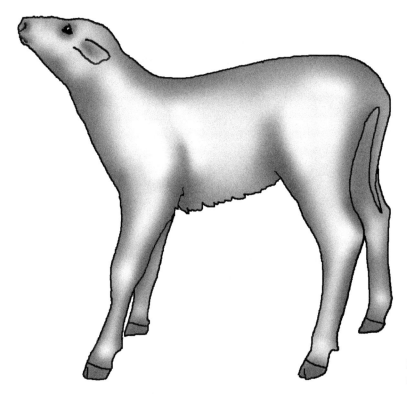

Figure 14.5 Cerebellar disease: wide-based stance and an elevated head position.

Clinical signs associated with upper motor neuron (UMN) lesions and lower motor neuron (LMN) lesions

Loss of upper motor neurons (UMN)

This results in the loss of proprioception (spatial awareness of limb position), weakness or paralysis, increase in extensor tone (hypertonia) causing spasticity, exaggerated or normal reflexes and sometimes abnormal reflexes such as the crossed extensor reflex.

Lower motor neuron (LMN) lesions

These result in loss or reduction of muscle tone and flaccidity, decreased or absent reflexes, weakness and paralysis, with rapid and severe muscle atrophy specific to the skeletal musculature affected.

Localisation of spinal cord lesions

Reflexes, postural reactions and propioception can be easily be assessed in calves, but may be difficult in fractious adult cattle.

Conscious perception of skin sensitivity

This can be tested by applying forceps to the skin and observing a behavioural response that indicates the integrity of the peripheral sensory nerve and spinal cord. A transition from hyperaesthesia to hypoaesthesia or analgesia when moving in a caudal direction indicates of the site of the lesion.

Interpretation of reflex test responses

Normal reflex   This indicates that the spinal cord segment where the LMN is located for that reflex and the peripheral nerve are functional. Reflexes are usually normal if the lesion is caudal to the reflex arc.

Depressed reflex   This indicates the lesion is in the region of the reflex arc.

Hyperactive reflex   This indicates the lesion is cranial to the reflex arc.

It must be remembered that animals with muscle damage, severe systemic conditions or hypocalcaemia may have weak or absent reflexes. Muscle damage may be the result of ischaemic muscle necrosis caused by ischaemia in downer cows or white muscle disease or muscle rupture.

Reflex tests (Fig. 14.6)

Pedal reflex   Applying firm pressure to the interdigital skin fold results in limb withdrawal, usually with a cerebral response. The safety of the operator must be considered when performing this test.

Panniculus reflex   A pinprick over the body results in contraction of the panniculus muscle which is observed as a flinching or twitching of the skin at the test site.

Patellar reflex   With the animal in lateral recumbency and upper hind limb partially flexed, the

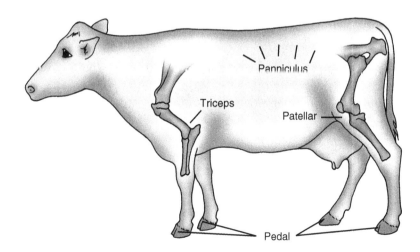

Figure 14.6 Pedal, panniculus, patellar and triceps reflexes.

straight patellar ligament is tapped with a firm object such as a pair of hoof testers or pliers. This causes a rapid extension of the stifle in the normal animal.

Triceps reflex   With the animal in lateral recumbency, the upper forelimb is flexed slightly. The triceps tendon is struck just above the elbow, resulting in contraction of the triceps muscle and extension of the elbow.

Crossed extensor reflex   Flexion of one limb causes extension of the other paired limb. This is normal in the young calf but abnormal in adults, and indicates a UMN defect.

Spinal cord lesion localisation
Lesions C1 to C6   These cause UMN deficits to the fore- and hind limbs.

Lesions between C6 and T2   These affect the LMN to the forelimbs and the UMN to the hind limbs. Affected animals therefore have weakness or paralysis of the forelimbs with poor or absent reflexes and hind-leg weakness (milder than forelimb) with normal or exaggerated reflexes.

Lesions between T3 and L3   Affected animals will have normal forelegs but weakness or paralysis in the hind legs with normal or exaggerated reflexes. These animals may adopt a dog-sitting position, supporting weight on their forelegs (Fig. 14.7).

Lesions L4 to S2   These animals will have LMN deficits to the hind legs only and may adopt a dog-sitting position. In addition, there may be reduced anal tone, bladder paralysis and decreased perineal sensation.

Lesions S1 to S3   These animals will have normal limbs but anal sphincter and bladder paralysis.

Coccygeal nerve damage   This can result from over zealous tail raising or pulling, and may cause loss of tail and anal tone.

Generalised and diffuse disorders

Severely ill and depressed animals are also extremely difficult to evaluate neurologically, as overall reduction in responses may not be due to neurological deficits but to overall weakness.

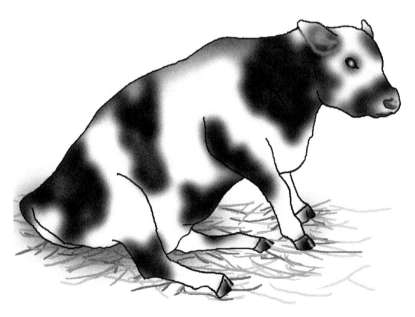

Figure 14.7 Dog-sitting position.

Conditions which produce generalised and sometimes diffuse presentations include hypocalcaemia, botulism, tetanus and hypomagnesaemia.

Hypocalcaemia – reduces neuromuscular transmission and the force of contraction of skeletal, cardiac and smooth muscles. The clinical signs include mydriasis, a dry nose, flaccid paresis, gut stasis, urinary retention and tachycardia.

Botulism – botulinum toxins interfere with the release of acetylcholine at the neuromuscular junction which results in generalised weakness progressing to flaccid paralysis. Clinical signs include ataxia, recumbency, weak tongue retraction and mydriasis.

Tetanus – results in generalised muscular rigidity with exaggerated responses to external stimuli. This is caused by tetanospasmin producing disinhibition.

Hypomagnesaemia – results in uncontrolled muscular contractions of increasing severity due to an increase in nerve transmissions. The signs may include hyperaesthesia, ataxia, recumbency, convulsions, opisthotonos, extensor rigidity, nystagmus and chomping of the jaws.

Examination of gait and posture

Paresis, ataxia (incoordination), hypermetria, hypometria (reduced flexion) and a wide-based stance are evaluated. Differentiation of proprioceptive deficit and motor neuron dysfunction from observations of gait may not be possible. Sensory or propioceptive deficits may include

- stumbling
- circumduction of the outside leg when circled
- scuffing the toe when advancing the leg
- heavy placement of the foot on the ground
- hypermetria.

Observing the standing animal may indicate a wide-based stance or a narrow-based stance. *If the animal is halter trained it should be walked in a straight line, circled and backed up.* Normally on turning the animal crosses the hind legs over neatly and without contact. Stumbling or falling with lack of crossing over of the hind legs on circling is abnormal. Reluctant backing

up with the hind legs being placed too far forward underneath the abdomen are significant findings. The animal should be led over a kerb to test conscious limb placement. Blindfolding or movement up and down a slope may result in ataxia becoming more obvious. The flight of each limb should be carefully assessed for abnormalities (dysmetria).

A calf with unilateral spastic paresis will have hyperextension of the hock within several steps of progression following rising (Fig. 14.8). In severe cases the toe may not touch the ground during forward progression. If there is bilateral involvement, the gait will be stiff with goose-stepping if locomotion is possible.

Evaluation of proprioception

Tests to evaluate proprioceptive deficits to define abnormalities of the upper motor neuron pathways are difficult, if not impossible, to perform on adult cattle. In calves the placement and hopping tests may be helpful.

Placement test
The foot is knuckled over or placed in an abnormally wide or narrow position under the body. The normal animal will either object strongly to the limb positioning or will quickly replace the foot in the normal position. The knuckling test is the best in young calves as they normally have a wide-based stance and may not reposition the limb as expected.

Hopping test
The test is performed by lifting a limb and pushing the animal laterally so that the animal has to hop with the standing leg to support the relocated torso. With proprioceptive deficits the animal fails to hop and may fall if unsupported. In calves this assessment can be achieved by straddling the animal and pivoting so that the animal is moved with one leg raised in an arc towards the supporting contralateral leg. The forelegs and hind legs are evaluated in turn.

Wheelbarrow and hemiwalking tests
Other tests for conscious proprioception are the wheelbarrow test and the hemiwalking test. These can only be performed on young calves. The wheel-

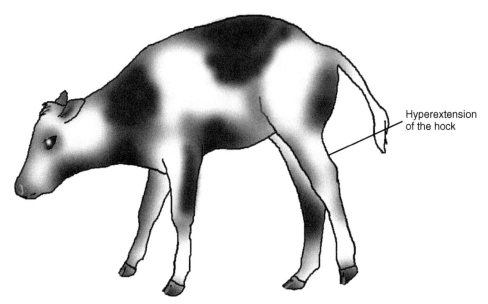

Hyperextension
of the hock

Figure 14.8 Spastic paresis.

barrow test is performed by raising the hind legs or forelegs off the ground and forcing the animal to walk. The hemiwalking test is performed by holding up the thoracic and hindlimb on one side and forcing the animal to move laterally in the opposite direction.

Peripheral nerves

Disorders of peripheral nerves are relatively common in cattle and are usually traumatic in origin or caused by pressure neuropathy to the peripheral nerve. Damage to the spinal roots may also cause localised peripheral nerve paralysis, but this is relatively rare. Signs include weakness or paralysis, poor muscle tone, muscle atrophy in chronic cases, decreased or absent reflexes, and loss of skin sensation.

Forelimb
Suprascapular nerve (spinal nerve roots C6 and C7) Damage may occur when the animal is attempting to pass through a narrow opening or be caused by extreme confinement of the neck. The action of this nerve is to extend the shoulder joint. Paralysis results in abduction on weight bearing during progression, causing the limb to circumduct or swing outwards.

The shoulder joint is dropped at rest and there may be a reluctance to bear weight. There is no area of skin sensitivity supplied by this nerve. In chronic cases atrophy of the infraspinatus and supraspinatus muscles is seen.

Radial nerve (spinal nerve roots C7, C8, T1) (Fig. 14.9) Damage may occur during prolonged lateral recumbency on hard ground or by direct trauma. The radial nerve extends the elbow, carpus and digits. Paralysis results in the inability to extend the elbow carpus and digits. The affected elbow is dropped and the leg is dragged, causing excoriation of the skin of the dorsal aspect of the digits. The radial nerve provides skin sensitivity on the lateral aspect of the elbow to the carpus and the cranial aspect of the carpus and digits.

Median and ulnar nerves (spinal nerve roots C6, C7 and C8; T1 and T2) Damage to these nerves is rare and usually arises due to traumatic damage or overstretching of the brachial plexus in the axilla. These nerves are responsible for flexion of the carpus and digits, and the skin sensitivity of the caudal aspect of the leg. When walking there is a goose-stepping-like action of the affected leg due to the predominance of the extensor action without the counterbalance of the flexors.

Brachial plexus (spinal nerve roots C6 to T2) Damage may occur due to trauma of the axilla by excessive traction on the forelimbs of the calf at parturition, or in adult cattle that have become suspended over a fence or gate with a foreleg(s) caught over the fence and the animal's weight supported by the obstacle in the region of the axilla. Nearly all the innervation of the forelimb passes through the brachial plexus and the outcome depends upon which nerve has been damaged and to what degree.

Hind limb

Femoral nerve (spinal nerve roots L4, L5 and L6) (Fig. 14.10) Femoral nerve paralysis is caused by pressure or overstretching of the nerve, and may be unilateral or bilateral. Overstretching of the nerve may occur when recumbent cows attempt to rise, but more commonly occurs in neonatal calves following a stifle lock or 'hip lock' in anterior presentation. Intervention or abnormal forces during parturition cause hyperextension of the nerve or vasculature, resulting in femoral nerve paralysis. The femoral nerve

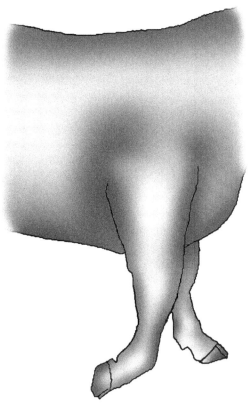

Figure 14.9 Radial nerve paralysis.

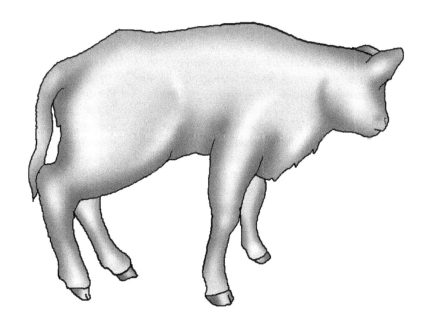

Figure 14.10 Femoral nerve paralysis.

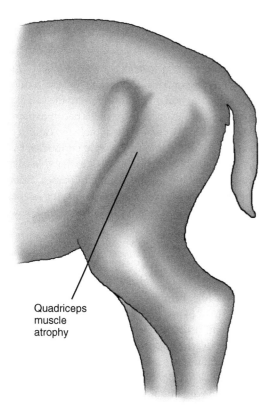

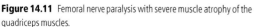

Figure 14.11 Femoral nerve paralysis with severe muscle atrophy of the quadriceps muscles.

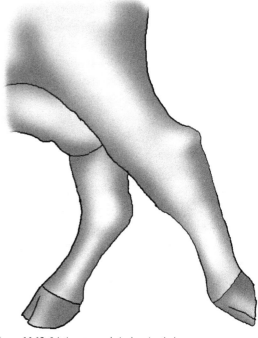

Figure 14.12 Sciatic nerve paralysis: dragging the leg.

extends the stifle and flexes the hip, and provides skin sensitivity to the medial aspect of the stifle and hock. The affected calf may be recumbent or stand with a frog-like posture. Severe neurogenic atrophy of the quadriceps muscle is observed (Fig. 14.11).

Sciatic nerve (spinal nerve roots L6, S1 and S2) (Fig. 14.12)   The sciatic nerve bifurcates to form the peroneal nerve and tibial nerve which are discussed below. The nerve roots of the sciatic nerve can be damaged together with the nerve roots of the obturator nerve by pressure during parturition and may contribute to calving paralysis. Sciatic nerve paralysis is most commonly seen in a young animal following incorrectly placed intramuscular injections into the gluteals or biceps femoris. Complete paralysis is rare. At rest there may be knuckling, and as the animal walks the limb is dragged forward along the

dorsal surface of the fetlock by flexion of the hip only. The position of the hock is dropped with increased flexion when compared with the normal hind limb. The sciatic nerve is responsible for skin sensation with the exception of the medial aspect (saphenous branch of the femoral nerve).

Peroneal nerve (spinal nerve roots L6, S1, S2) (Fig. 14.13)   Peroneal nerve paralysis is commonly observed in cattle that have been recumbent for some time. It is a particular problem in postparturient downer cows. The peroneal nerve in the lower leg is susceptible to pressure neuropathy at a point where the nerve courses over the lateral aspect of the proximal tibia. The peroneal nerve extends the digit and flexes the hock, and is responsible for skin sensitivity over the cranial aspect of the tarsus and metatarsus. The affected standing animal has hyperflexion of the fetlock joint with an inability to extend the phalanxes and overextension of the hock. The foot may be dragged along on its cranial aspect.

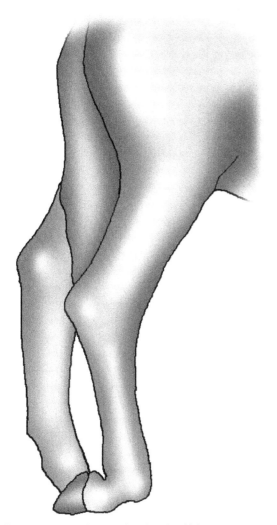

Figure 14.13 Peroneal nerve paralysis: digit is knuckled over onto dorsum; hock is not dropped.

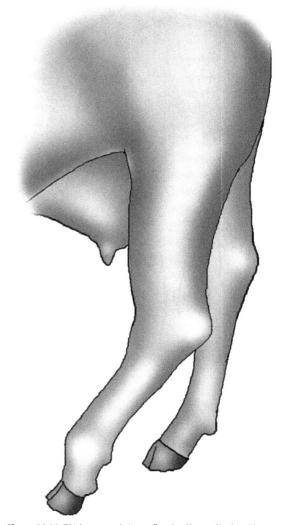

Figure 14.14 Tibial nerve paralysis: overflexed and lowered hock position; the metatarsophalangeal joint is buckled.

Tibial nerve (spinal nerve roots L6, S1 and S2) (Fig. 14.14) Prolonged recumbency or poor injection technique into the caudal muscles of the thigh may cause tibial nerve paralysis. The action of the tibial nerve is to flex the digit and extend the hock, and to maintain skin sensitivity over the caudal aspect of the metatarsus and digits. Affected animals have hyperflexion of the hock and partial forward knuckling of the fetlock joint. The foot is not dragged on the floor and the hooves stay flat on the floor.

Obturator paralysis (spinal nerve roots L5 and L6) (Fig. 14.15) This term is often used synonymously with calving paralysis, but in most cases the L6 root of the sciatic nerve is also affected. During passage of the calf through the pelvic canal, compression neuropathy of the nerve roots L5 and L6 can occur. The action of the obturator nerve is to adduct the hind limb. The sciatic nerve also supplies the abductors, semimembranosus and semitendonosus. The inability to adduct the hind leg(s) predominates in calving

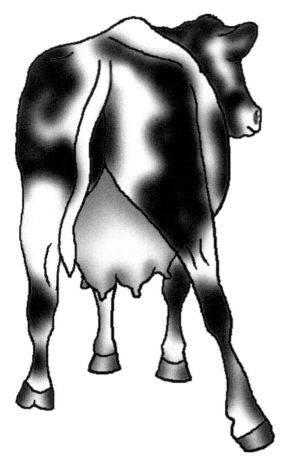

Figure 14.15 Obturator nerve paralysis: abduction of limb.

paralysis. Nerve paralysis is often bilateral, although one side is often more severely affected. The clinical signs depend on the severity of the neuropathy and include hind-leg weakness, ataxia, abduction of the hind leg(s) and recumbency. The obturator nerve has no skin sensitivity associated with it.

The sensory innervation of the skin by the peripheral nerves in the foreleg is shown in Fig. 14.16 and in the hind leg in Fig. 14.17.

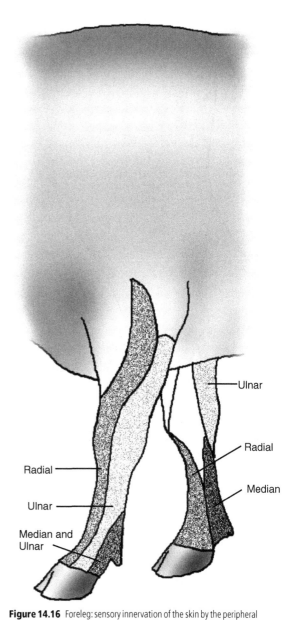

Figure 14.16 Foreleg: sensory innervation of the skin by the peripheral nerves.

Further investigations

Cerebrospinal fluid (CSF) tap

If CNS involvement is suspected, then a CSF sample may assist in reaching a diagnosis. In addition, a post-mortem CSF sample may help to confirm or rule out hypomagnesaemia as a cause of death. Samples can be obtained from either the cisterna magna or the lumbosacral space. The cisterna magna site requires deep sedation with the animal in recumbency, while the lumbosacral site can be sampled in the standing

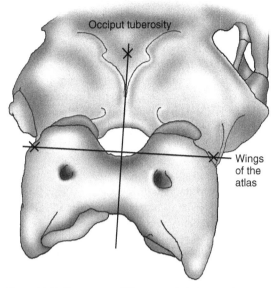

Figure 14.18 Cisterna magna CSF tap: anatomical reference points to locate the puncture site.

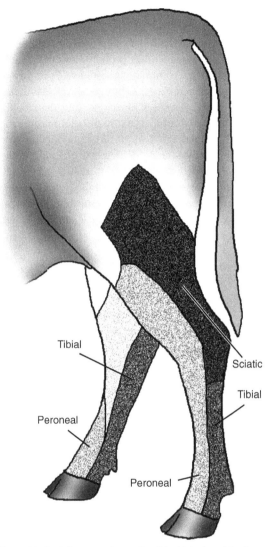

Figure 14.17 Hindleg: sensory innervation of the skin by the peripheral nerves.

animal but requires restraint facilities. Other factors, such as the condition of the patient, should be considered before a site is selected. The site closest to the suspected lesion should be selected as these samples are likely to be the most useful if a lesion is localised. The cisterna magna site can be used to obtain post-mortem samples for magnesium evaluation. CSF samples may indicate spinal trauma, spinal abscessation, meningitis/encephalitis and the presence of bacteria.

Cisterna magna

The animal is deeply sedated and placed in sternal recumbency. The head is flexed until it is perpendicular to the ground to maximise the space between the occiput and the atlas. The site is located in the midline at the level of the widest part of the wings of the atlas which can be palpated (Fig. 14.18). The site is clipped and aseptically prepared. A small amount of local anaesthetic is infiltrated subcutaneously. Sterile gloves should be worn by the operator. A 9 cm 18 BWG (1.20 mm) spinal needle is used in an adult and a 9 cm 20 BWG (0.90 mm) needle in a calf. The needle is angled slightly forwards and advanced through the space between the atlas and the occiput. The distance required to reach the cisterna varies depending on the size of the animal. A full grown animal will the need the full length of the needle, whereas a calf may only require 3 cm. The clinician should feel a pop and a decrease in resistance as the needle goes through into the cisterna. The stylet is then removed to check for the presence of CSF. Time should be allowed for the CSF to flow up the needle. If no CSF appears a sterile syringe should be attached to the spinal needle hub and gentle negative pressure applied. Sometimes entry into the cisterna is not easily perceived. In this case, the needle should be advanced for a short distance with the stylet in place before removing the stylet again to check for CSF. This process is repeated until CSF is obtained. Samples should be taken into EDTA for cytology and into a plain tube for culture. A glass slide smear can be prepared for immediate cytological assessment. If a syringe is used, removal of the CSF should proceed relatively slowly to avoid sudden changes in pressure.

Lumbosacral space

In recumbent animals this procedure can be performed in sternal recumbency, or in small calves in lateral recumbency with the forelegs and hind legs brought together to flex the spine. This maximises the entry into the lumbosacral space. The site is the midline at the level of the depression between the last palpable lumbar dorsal spine (L6) and the first palpable dorsal spine (S2). Another anatomical marker for this site is a transverse line between the each ilium wing (Fig. 14.19). The site is clipped and aseptically prepared. Local anaesthetic is infiltrated subcutaneously at the site. A 9 cm 18 BWG (1.20 mm) spinal needle is used in an adult and a 9 cm 20 BWG (0.90 mm) spinal needle in a calf. The needle is advanced at a right angle to the vertebral column. A 'pop' and loss of resistance is felt on entry into the subarachnoid space. Collection of the CSF is as described for the cisterna magna.

Evaluation of the CSF sample

The gross appearance of the sample can be informative. The formation of a stable foam on shaking the sample indicates a high protein concentration indicative of an inflammatory response. Turbidity indicates an increase in the white cell count. White clots indicate the presence of fibrinogen (purulent meningitis). Xanthochromia (yellow discolouration) indicates haemorrhage 1 to 10 days previously. More detailed analysis may include specific gravity, protein concentration, leukocyte count, differential leukocyte count, leukocyte morphology, presence of erythrocytes, magnesium concentration. Table 14.1 gives CSF values for normal cattle and cattle with bacterial encephalitis.

Post-mortem tissue samples

Post mortem, gross pathology and histopathology are extremely useful in providing definitive diagnoses in neurological cases. Analysis of post-mortem tissue samples may enable the diagnosis of a toxicological condition such as lead poisoning. Post-mortem samples of urine and vitreous humour of the eye are useful in the absence of a CSF sample to check for low magnesium levels. The magnesium content of aqueous humour is less stable than that of vitreous humour. Concentrations below 0.55 mmol/l in vitreous humour within 48 hours of death is a diagnostic marker for hypomagnesaemia.

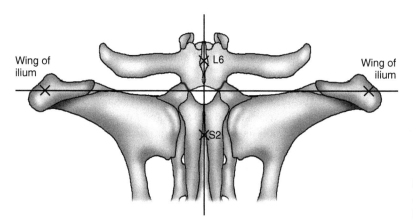

Figure 14.19 Lumbosacral CSF tap: anatomical reference points to locate the puncture site.

Table 14.1 Cerebrospinal fluid values for normal cattle and cattle with bacterial encephalitis

	CSF	
	Normal	Bacterial encephalitis
Specific gravity	1.004–1.008	Increased
Colour	Colourless (non-clotting)	Turbid (yellow/red)
Protein (g/l)	20–40	Increased >200
Albumin (g/l)	10–22	Increased
Globulin (g/l)	2–8	Increased
Leukocyte cell count		
$\times 10^6$/l	0–3	>30
Leukocyte differential	95% lymphocytes	Mainly neutrophils
Magnesium (mmol/l)	0.86	0.86

Blood samples

Blood samples may be analysed to rule in or rule out hypocalcaemia, hypomagnesaemia, hypophosphataemia, hypo- or hyperkalaemia, thiamine (B1) deficiency (erythrocyte transketolase), hypovitaminosis A and ketosis. Haematology can be useful in defining an inflammatory response.

Radiography, electromyography and electroencephalography

In referral centres, radiography, electromyography and electroencephalography have been diagnostically useful.

PHYSICAL SIGNS OF DISEASE ASSOCIATED WITH THE NERVOUS SYSTEM

N.B. Some of these physical signs are also associated with diseases of other body systems and regions.

Demeanour
  Dull
  Depressed

Mental state
  Coma
  Convulsions
  Hyperaesthesia

Generalised states
  Paralysis
    Spastic paresis
    Flaccid paresis
  Opisthotonos
  Tremors
  Convulsions

Behaviour
  Head pressing
  Circling
  Deafness
  Blindness
  Intention tremor
  Aggression
  Vocalisation

Isolation from the rest of the group
Frenzy
Compulsive self licking
Compulsive walking
Dysphagia

Posture
  Recumbency
  Dog-sitting position
  Wide-based stance
  Narrow-based stance

Head and neck
  Facial asymmetry
  Retention of food in buccal cavity
  Eyelid drooping
  Ear drooping
  Head tilt
  Aversion of the head
  Head tremor
  Tongue paralysis
  Intention tremor/head bobbing
  Head elevated and turned skywards
  Dry nose
  Champing of jaws
  Trismus

(*Continued on p. 216*)

PHYSICAL SIGNS OF DISEASE ASSOCIATED WITH THE NERVOUS SYSTEM   *CONTINUED*

Eyes
  Nystagmus
  Strabismus
  Prolapse of the third eyelid
  Fixation reflex absent
  Menace response absent
  Palpebral reflex absent
  Photomotor reflex absent
  Pupillary light reflex absent
  Retina
    Papilloedema
    Haemorrhage
  Lens
    Cataract
  Pupil
    Miosis
    Mydriasis

Gait
  Slow and weak
  Reluctant to move
  Ataxia
  Hypermetria
  Hypometria
  Staggering
  Stumbling
  Knuckling of hind legs

Limbs
  Weakness
  Paralysis
  Muscle
    Atrophy
    Hypertonia (spasticity)
    Hypotonia (flaccidity)

Reflexes
  Exaggerated
  Decreased
  Absent
Loss of proprioception
Loss of sensation

Forelimb
  Swinging outwards (circumduction)
  Reduced weight-bearing
  Dropped shoulder joint
  Dropped elbow
  Leg dragged
  Excoriation of dorsum of digits
  Goose-stepping action

Hind limb
  Straight hocks
  Hyperextension of the hocks
  Frog-like posture
  Knuckling
  Limb is dragged
  Flexion of hock
  Hyperflexion of fetlock joint
  Inability to extend digits
  Hyperflexion of the hock
  Forward knuckling of the fetlock joint
  Abduction
  Weakness

Tail end
  Tail paralysis
  Bladder paralysis
  Loss of peroneal sensation
  Loss of anal reflex
  Pump-handle tail

Part III

Sheep

Clinical Examination of the Sheep

Introduction

The general principles and methods of clinical examination in sheep resemble those of cattle which are fully described in Part II.

- Owner's complaint
- Signalment of the patient
- History of the patient(s)
- History of the farm
- Observation of the environment
- Observation of the animal at a distance
- Detailed observations of the animal
- Examination of the animal
- Further investigations – if cost effective.

Owner's complaint

The accuracy in relation to the real problem may vary greatly with the knowledge and experience of the owner. Most sheep are kept in large groups with knowledgeable owners, but others are kept singly or in small groups as pets. The owner's complaint must as always be taken seriously. However, the *owner's perception* of the loss of a few isolated individuals may be insignificant when compared with a more serious *unrecognised problem* such as endoparasitism or ectoparasitism. In addition, a diagnosis may have already been formed in the shepherd's mind and the observations subconsciously interpreted to fit the diagnosis.

Signalment

Age – some diseases such as watery mouth and lamb dysentery are only seen in young lambs.

Sex – mastitis is seen chiefly in ewes after lambing and after weaning.

Colour – sunburn can be a problem in pale-faced sheep such as the Charollais breed, but is uncommon in dark-faced sheep such as the Suffolk.

Breed – Texels are predisposed to chronic chondritis of the larynx causing partial obstruction of the upper airways.

Genotype – susceptibility to scrapie is related to the genotype.

History of the farm and patient

Local disease information

This may indicate conditions that may be present in the area; an example is louping ill in certain tick areas. *Knowledge of local trace element deficiencies* such as copper or selenium, or excesses such as molybdenum may also be relevant. The *presence of other farm animal species*, the number of sheep on the farm and the groups in which they are kept should be established.

Recent management and husbandry practices

These will occasionally predispose to disease and may include *shearing, tagging, castration, foot trimming* and *dipping*. Post-dipping lameness caused by erysipelas infection may become a problem as a result of the organism gaining access to the joints through superficial injuries sustained during dipping and clipping. If the flock have had their feet trimmed recently, a high incidence of lameness may be observed. Many shepherds are inclined to over-trim their sheep's feet, exposing the sensitive soft tissues. The prevalence of caseous lymphadenitis may increase in an already infected flock following shearing.

Preventative health programmes

It is important to establish what *vaccines*, *fly control products*, *antimicrobials*, *anticoccidials*, *mineral/ vitamin supplements*, *copper injections/boluses* and *anthelmintics* have been administered. The product used, dosages, numbers of treatments, timing of treatments and method of administration should be established. This is particularly important, as some products are obtained from non-veterinary sources. A vaccination programme may have been established to prevent the recurrence of diseases, such as enzootic abortion or enterotoxaemia. It is important to establish whether such a vaccination programme is still operational and whether it is up to date and includes all members of the flock. Many sheep flocks have serious endoparasite problems. A detailed history of anthelmintic administration may indicate inappropriate usage or the possibility of anthelmintic resistance. *Biosecurity protocols* used by the farm should be reviewed in the light of the current problems.

Practice and farm records

Details of current and previous disease problems may be important and relevant to the problem under investigation. Practice records and invoices provide the clinician with an overview of drug usage and historical problems. Clinicians within the veterinary practice may be able to provide an invaluable overview of the farm husbandry methods and problems.

Individual animal identification and detailed record keeping are extremely important, and any such records should be consulted when investigating disease or a suboptimal production problem. *These records may indicate poor lambing percentages, high lamb mortality, poor pregnancy rates, high ewe culling rates, high ewe mortalities, poor growth rates, inappropriate condition scores in relation to the production cycle, a high prevalence of hypocalcaemia, hypomagnesaemia and pregnancy toxaemia.* The animal movement book and the farmer's drug book may provide useful insights into the biosecurity and the range and prevalence of problems on the farm.

Group affected and introductions

It is important to identify the *group of animals affected*. The morbidity and the mortality of the disease should be defined. *Animals recently introduced*, such as those returning from shows and new purchases, may introduce new diseases: foot-rot, caseous lymphadenitis, toxoplasmosis and enzootic abortion are examples.

Diet

Stocking density and pasture management may be relevant to endoparasite control. The ration being fed, access to grazing, how feeding is undertaken, and any sudden change of diet may be significant. The use of conserved forage such as silage or mouldy hay may be associated with an outbreak of listeriosis or ringworm, respectively. Lack of magnesium supplementation to postpartum lactating ewes may increase the risk of hypomagnesaemia. Urolithiasis in male fat lambs can be associated with increased and incorrectly balanced mineral content of the fed concentrate.

Season and weather

The sheep year follows a clearly defined pattern with regard to breeding, pregnancy and lambing. Many diseases are therefore seasonal or cyclical. The class of animal affected, the time of year and the stage of production limit the number of possible conditions. The weather may be a factor in endoparasite numbers and the prevalence of fly-strike. Warm wet wooded pastures are associated with an increased risk of fly-strike. Heavy snows may precipitate pregnancy toxaemia due to reduced energy intake by ewes in the last trimester of pregnancy.

Observation of the environment

An examination of the environment should include where the animals are currently or have recently been kept. This may include pastures, yards or buildings. The supply and quality of food, water and bedding should be ascertained.

Pasture

It is very important to note the quality of pasture and the availability of grass. In dry weather grass growth and quality may be reduced. Sheep eating very close to grass roots may be predisposed to problems such as 'rye grass staggers'.

Supplementary feeding

If supplementary feed is being given during pregnancy it should be ascertained whether there is sufficient trough space for the number of sheep and what quantity of food they are receiving. Pregnancy toxaemia is a very important problem in sheep and is associated with a lack of energy in the diet.

Water quality and quantity

All small ruminants should have access to water, but this may not always be provided for sheep. Water requirement increases dramatically in warm weather and when the intake of dry food is high. The risk of urolithiasis increases with water deprivation.

Foot problems

Foot problems including foot-rot may increase dramatically in damp conditions and through contact of softened feet with stones. Increased rainfall in spring and early autumn increases the risk of a poached and constantly wet environment. In some areas, including East Anglia, sheep are folded onto root crop aftermaths such as sugar beet where these predisposing factors prevail. Housed sheep on wet bedding are also at risk, as are sheep in mountainous areas brought in to more sheltered pasture during the winter and spring with an increased stocking density.

Poisonous plants and endoparasites

Localisation of the affected animal to certain pastures, feeders or water courses may be significant. Fascioliasis may be associated with marshy areas, photosensitisation with the presence of bog asphodel, or blindness with bracken (Fig. 15.1). Lead batteries may have been dumped and buried in a particular field.

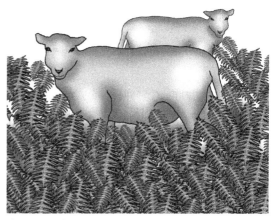

Figure 15.1 Sheep grazing bracken.

Housing

Poor ventilation of housed sheep may predispose them to pneumonia; wet bedding may be associated with a high prevalence of foot-rot.

Other observations

Tags of wool on fence posts and barbed wire suggest a pruritic condition in the flock.

Observation of the affected animals ('over the fence examination')

Sheep are essentially flock animals, finding safety in the presence of numbers of their fellows. If separated they always try to regain contact with their flock, and even if ill they will struggle not to be left behind if the flock is moved on. *Animals that are separate from the rest of the flock should be caught and examined in detail.* Sheep are relatively undemonstrative, and sick animals may show few obvious signs apart from recumbency and isolation.

Feeding behaviour

The grazing or feeding behaviour should be observed. Reluctance to feed may indicate a systemic illness such as pregnancy toxaemia or a localised condition such as a tooth root abscess. Normal faeces in sheep should be pelleted.

Diarrhoea

This is uncommon in healthy adult sheep unless there has been a sudden change onto lush pasture. Diarrhoea will be noted by soiling of the perineal wool, and in summer this may result in concurrent fly-strike. The presence of diarrhoea is normally indicative of an abnormality including parasite infestation, bacterial infection or an unsuitable diet.

Body condition

It is very difficult to assess the condition score of sheep by observation unless recently shorn because of their thick fleeces, and this should be delayed until the clinical examination. However, sheep with extreme emaciation and weakness will be detected (Fig. 15.2);

in young sheep endoparasitism, and in older sheep chronic wasting conditions, may be responsible.

Respiratory signs

Animals with respiratory disease may present with *coughing, exaggerated breathing, nasal discharges* and *exercise intolerance* which may be parasitic (e.g. *Dictyocaulus filaria*), bacterial (e.g. *Pasteurella*) or viral (e.g. visna maedi virus) in origin.

Skin irritation

Signs of skin irritation include localised loss of wool, biting at the fleece or rubbing (Fig. 15.3). Healthy sheep will occasionally rub themselves when close to a convenient object such as a tree. Persistent rubbing indicates pruritus. This may be observed in only one animal in the group e.g. scrapie. Sheep with scrapie may show persistent rubbing and sustain self

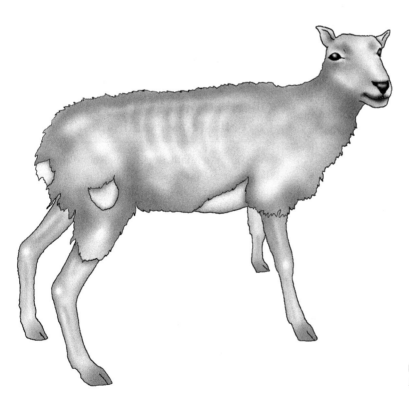

Figure 15.2 Emaciation (resulting from Johne's disease for example).

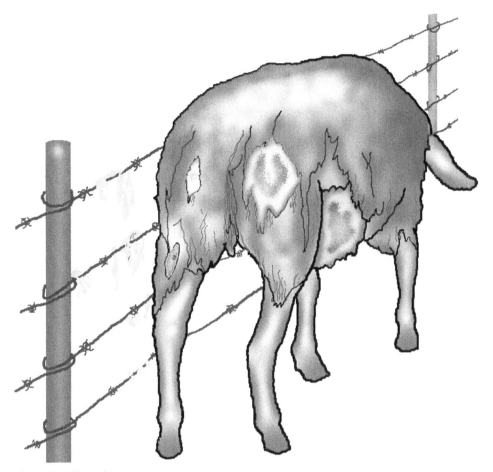

Figure 15.3 Sheep with wool loss and pruritus.

inflicted injury. If a number of animals are affected external parasites should be considered, especially sheep scab caused by *Psoroptes ovis*. Generalised hair loss without pruritus is called wool break or wool drop, and may occur as a result of stress, malnutrition or a febrile disease either in an individual or in a group. In newly shorn sheep, cutaneous swellings associated with superficial lymph nodes and sometimes with green purulent discharges, may indicate caseous lymphadenitis.

Lameness

Any animal with abnormalities of gait or lameness should be examined in detail (Fig. 15.4). These signs are often associated with foot problems such as foot-rot. Foot-and-mouth disease sometimes causes lameness in sheep. In ewes with lambs at foot, apparent lameness may be caused by a painful udder as a result of mastitis. The ewe may not allow the lambs to suckle and enlargement of the udder may be observed. Swelling of the joints is mostly seen in lambs or growing sheep suffering from septic arthritis, and several animals in the flock may be affected.

Nervous signs

Common nervous signs detectable from a distance include circling, head pressing, unilateral facial paralysis, apparent blindness and depression. Animals with listeriosis, gid or pregnancy toxaemia may show some of these signs.

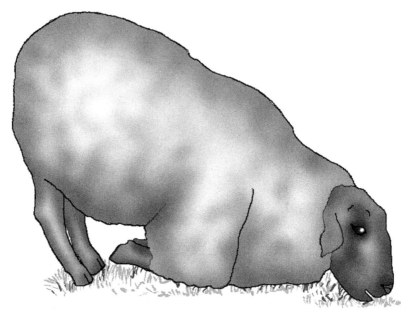

Figure 15.4 Posture of a sheep with foreleg lameness (foot-rot).

Ocular discharges

The presence of several animals with excessive ocular tear staining may suggest an outbreak of infectious keratoconjunctivitis.

Tenesmus

Straining (tenesmus) while attempting to urinate should suggest the possibility of urolithiasis.

Abnormal abdominal contours

Viewing the abdomen from the side and the rear may reveal abnormal abdominal contours. Animals with frothy bloat will have distension of the left dorsal quadrant. In a male animal, a swelling on the ventral abdomen may indicate a ruptured urethra. This is called water belly and is caused by subcutaneus cellulitis and oedema (Fig. 15.5). Rupture of the prepubic tendon results in a dropped ventral abdomen which may reach the floor. A rupture of the suspensory ligament of the mammary gland will present as an asymmetrical dropped udder.

Clinical examination

Separation of animals from the flock for inspection can be facilitated by the careful use of the sheep dog, sheep crook and the strategic placement of mobile hurdles. When dealing with large numbers of animals, particularly those with lambs at foot, great care is required to avoid situations that may lead to crushing and smothering. Adult sheep can die due to compression in a group in a confined space.

The clinical examination should be methodical and comprehensive as in other species. The sheep is restrained by a halter or an assistant holding the animal under the lower jaw and restrained in a corner. *The skin should not be grasped as this is painful for the sheep and causes extensive bruising.* Care must be taken with sheep to ensure the fleece is not damaged, either when catching the animal or if it struggles to escape.

General inspection

Normal sheep should be bright, alert and reactive and resist being caught. Depression characterised by dull-

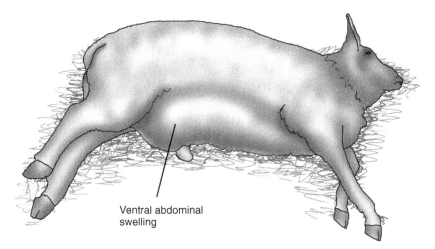

Figure 15.5 Urolithiasis: ruptured urethra (water belly).

ness and indifference to handling may indicate hypocalcaemia, pregnancy toxaemia, endotoxaemia or uraemia. Blindness is seen in cerebrocortico necrosis and bracken poisoning. Persistent skin irritation, even when caught, may indicate myiasis. Extreme excitation may be seen in hypomagnesaemia.

Condition score

This is checked for each animal. Scores are awarded in the range 1 to 5 and there are target figures in sheep for various situations, e.g. a score of 2.5 to 3.0 is considered ideal for pregnancy. Assessment is made by palpating the transverse and spinous processes of the lumbar vertebrae and noting the amount of muscle and fat palpable beside and above the dorsal spinous processes. All parts of the lumbar vertebrae are readily palpable in animals with condition score 1 which have very little muscle (Fig. 15.6). With a score of 5 it is difficult to palpate any lumbar vertebral processes because they are covered in muscle tissue and fat deposits (Fig. 15.7).

Temperature, pulse, respiratory rate, mucous membranes and lymph nodes

Respiratory rate and heart rate

These increase greatly in warm weather, especially in fully fleeced animals. They also increase greatly, as

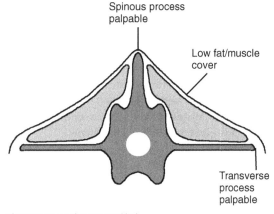

Figure 15.6 Condition score 1 (thin).

does the pulse, when the animal is rounded up and caught. The rate and character of respiration should therefore be assessed at rest before the animal is caught. The normal resting respiratory rate is 20 to 30 breaths/minute. The pulse is taken at the femoral artery or by auscultation of the heart during the examination. The normal resting heart rate is 70 to 90 beats/minute.

Temperature

The normal temperature is 38.5 to 40.0°C.

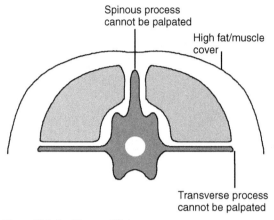

Figure 15.7 Condition score 5 (fat).

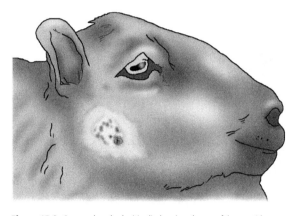

Figure 15.8 Caseous lymphadenitis: discharging abscess of the parotid lymph node.

Mucous membranes

These should be salmon pink in colour and can be conveniently assessed at the ocular, oral (if not pigmented) or the vulval mucosal membranes in females. The mucous membranes may appear pale with anaemia, icteric as a result of intravascular haemolysis or hepatic dysfunction, or hyperaemic and congested with febrile or toxaemic states. Cyanosis is only found with severe conditions of the respiratory and cardiovascular systems.

Capillary refill time

CRT should be less than 2 seconds. It is assessed on a non-pigmented part of the gums and lips or, in the female, on the vulval mucous membranes. Extended CRTs indicate poor peripheral perfusion.

Superficial lymph nodes

These are the submandibular, parotid, retropharyngeal, prescapular, precrural and supramammary glands. They are palpated for enlargement and compared with the opposite member of the pair if palpable. Special attention should be paid to the parotid lymph nodes, the submandibular lymph nodes and the cervical chains in the neck. In recent years these have been found to be an external predilection site for caseous lymphadenitis (Fig. 15.8). Confirmation of infection is by culture of the light green pus found in abscesses associated with infected lymph nodes.

Skin

Skin lesions and/or loss of hair may be the result of mycotic, bacterial and/or viral infections, pruritus caused by ectoparasites, head fly or scrapie infection.

The fleece prevents direct examination of the skin of sheep unless it is first parted by the clinician's fingers. In clipped sheep, visual examination of the skin is straightforward. Visual and manual examination of the entire skin surface is carried out looking for areas of hair follicle non-function, areas of damaged or thickened skin, and for the presence of specific diseases.

Abscess formation – subcutaneously on the poll of rams, often caused by fighting, is not uncommon.

Hair loss over the brisket – may also be seen in rams caused by mounting and serving ewes.

Caseous lymphadenitis – should always be considered when a discharging abscess is found in the proximity of a superficial lymph node and the purulent material is green.

Ectoparasites

In sheep the possible presence of sheep scab and other ectoparasites should always be checked when there is pruritus and/or hair loss (Fig. 15.9). Signs of sheep scab include yellow, crusty, pruritic lesions, especially on the dorsum of the back. Confirmation of the disease is achieved by examining scrapings microscopically for the presence of *Psoroptes ovis*.

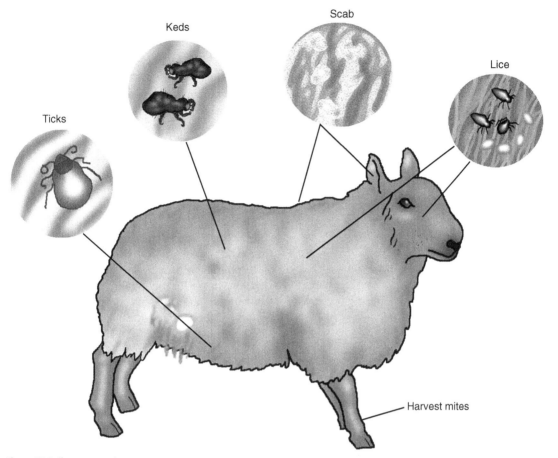

Figure 15.9 Sheep ectoparasites.

Ked and lice infestations are increasing with the reduction in usage of organophosphorous compounds. *Keds* can be easily seen with the naked eye; they are brown in colour. *Louse infestation is increasing in association with injectable ectoparasiticides.* Lice may be observed using a bright light, but patience is usually required. *Lice* and lice eggs attached to the wool can be more easily seen with a magnifying glass. Engorged female ticks are easily seen usually on the ventral part of the body. *Trombicula autumnalis* is found on the distal limbs and may cause intense localised pruritus.

Flies

Blow-fly strike is an ever present hazard during spring and summer unless animals have received recent prophylaxis.

A common site is around the perineum, sometimes in association with diarrhoea (Fig. 15.10). In very early cases small damp areas appear on the coat; the animal appears distressed and is unwilling to move. Areas of reddened skin with visible blow-fly eggs and/or larvae follow. Penetration of the skin and excavation of subcutaneous tissues can occur and signs of generalised shock with skin loss are seen in severe cases. Soiled wool is clipped away with dagging shears to allow better access to the skin.

Headfly may provoke self trauma of the skin of the head, particularly in horned breeds. Hypersensitivity (atopy) to culicoides may present with pruritus and loss of hair around the face and ears with scabby lesions in summer and autumn.

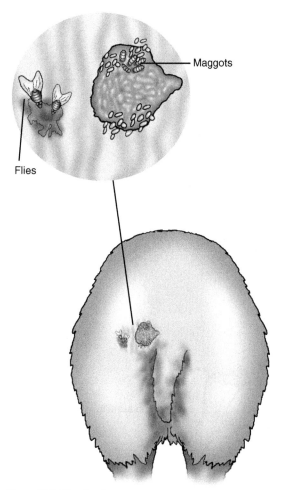

Maggots

Flies

Figure 15.10 Blow-fly strike.

Viral and bacterial infections

Orf causes crusty lesions on the lips (Fig. 15.11). Oral lesions are occasionally seen in lambs. Lesions of orf are also found on the udders and teats of ewes. Affected animals should be handled with care as the disease is an unpleasant zoonotic. Diagnosis is confirmed by identifying parapoxvirus in the vesicular fluid under fresh scabs using electron microscopy.

Matting of the wool may indicate infection by *Dermatophilus* or if stained yellow/green by *Pseudomonas*. *Dermatophilus* infections can also produce red fulminating lesions in the skin of the lower legs, sometimes in association with orf.

Staphylococcal dermatitis and *actinobacillosis* can produce scabby, pustular, necrotic granulomatous lesions at various sites, but particularly on the head.

Staining of the fleece by the sebaceous glands should not be mistaken for abnormality. The eight glands are the infraorbital glands of the head, the interdigital glands of the feet and the inguinal glands of the inguinal folds.

Head

Conformation of the head

This is examined for symmetry. Unilateral facial paralysis will result in flaccid paralysis of the lip, cheek, eyelid, nostril and ear. Accumulations of fluid may occur in the intermandibular space as a result of endoparasites causing hypoproteinaemia. Generalised oedema of the face is seen in photosensitisa-

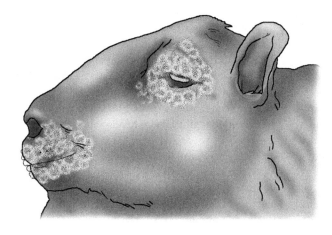

Figure 15.11 Orf: periorbital and mouth lesions.

tion. Thin animals may have an over- or undershot jaw which limits prehension and mastication. Dentigerous cysts and tooth root abscesses can present as bony swellings on the lower jaw. Focal thinning of the skull may indicate the position of a coenurus cerebralis cyst.

Eyes

External examination This may reveal *keratitis* and *epiphora* with *hyperaemia of the conjunctiva*. These signs are features of infectious keratoconjunctivitis (Fig. 15.12) or a foreign body. To facilitate examination of the conjunctival fornices under the eyelids and behind the third eyelid, a few drops of a topical ophthalmic local anaesthetic can be placed in the eye. A pair of fine artery forceps can be used to examine these areas in detail.

Iritis may be seen in sheep due to superficial infection with listeria, usually in association with silage feeding.

Hypopyon is rare and indicates a septicaemia or an infected local traumatic injury.

The *menace response* will be absent in blind animals: checking the pupillary light response may indicate if the blindness is central in origin.

Internal examination Examination of the eye by ophthalmoscope is seldom necessary, although is *useful to confirm bright blindness* caused by chronic bracken poisoning, with narrowed retinal blood vessels and hyper-reflective tapetum lucidum. Papilloedema, a swelling of the optic disc, indicates an increased intracranial pressure. The optic disc in some sheep is often indistinct, even though vision is normal.

Ears

Tears caused by tags becoming caught and being pulled out are common. *Haematomata* of the pinnae are becoming increasingly common in sheep and may be due, in some cases, to parasitic infestation in the ears. In animals with light coloured heads, exposure to sunlight may predispose to proliferative lesions caused by *squamous cell carcinoma* on the pinna and adjacent areas of the head. *Photosensatisation may cause crusting and peeling of the skin of the pinnae.* Abnormal ear carriage, often unilateral, may be seen in some cases of listeriosis, causing *facial paralysis.*

Nares

Nasal discharge may accompany some upper and lower respiratory infections and is occasionally seen in some cases of chronic sinusitis in older ewes. Infestation with *Oestrus ovis* can also cause a nasal discharge, as can turbinate damage or neoplasia. *The*

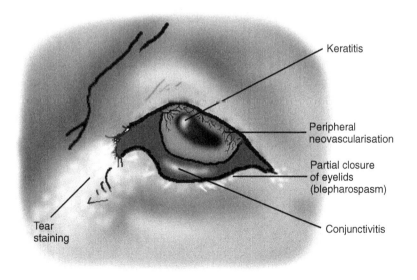

Figure 15.12 Infectious keratoconjunctivitis.

Keratitis

Peripheral neovascularisation

Partial closure of eyelids (blepharospasm)

Conjunctivitis

Tear staining

breath should always be smelled in case there is evidence of ketosis, confirmation of which is by urine or blood analysis.

Mouth

Examination of the mouth is greatly resented by sheep. A sheep gag or a Bayer gag are probably the safest and most useful (Fig. 15.13). If a detailed examination is planned, sedation should be considered.

The *incisor teeth* can be easily examined by pushing the lower lip down with the mouth closed. The broad permanent teeth are easily differentiated from the small deciduous ones. Lambs are born with variable numbers of deciduous teeth erupted. All four pairs of deciduous teeth have usually erupted by 8 months of age. The permanent teeth erupt at 1 year 3 months (central), 1 year 9 months (medial), 2 years 3 months (lateral) and 2 years 9 months (corner). Sheep with loss, breakage or excessive wear of incisors are said to be broken mouthed (Fig. 15.13). It is not uncommon for an animal to have no incisor teeth by the age of 5 years, depending on its diet. The *premolar and molar teeth* can be palpated through the cheek from outside the mouth, allowing gross abnormalities to be detected. They can also be inspected with the aid of a pen torch inside the mouth by holding the mouth open with a gag, helped by sedation or by finger pressure in the diastoma. A long pair of forceps enables them to be palpated for looseness in safety. Sharp points, especially on the first premolar and the last molar, may prevent apposition and cause pain when eating. The caudal part of the mouth *must never* be palpated in the ungagged animal. Molar and premolar teeth may be lost due to periodontal disease, which may result in the cud impacting in the cheek or saliva drooling.

In foot-and-mouth disease, vesicles may be present on the dental pad or tongue, but this is not a con-

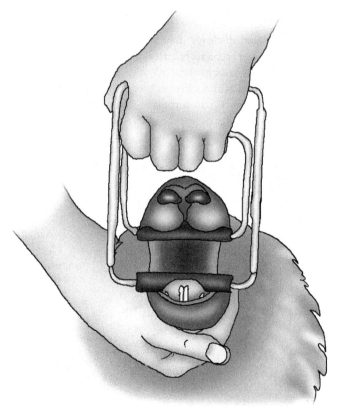

Figure 15.13 Oral examination using a gag in a sheep with some incisor teeth missing (broken mouth).

sistent finding. Focal blanching of the mucous may be the only oral lesion. Oral lesions can occur in orf which may make differentiation difficult. Pustular and/or scabby lesions around the mouth are likely to be present in orf infections. Puffing of the cheeks during respiration usually indicates respiratory distress. This may be caused by upper airway obstruction by, for example, a retropharyngeal lymph-node abscess or severe lower respiratory tract infection.

The *pharynx* and *larynx* may be inspected and the injury visualised using a laryngescope, a gag and an illuminated tubular cattle vaginal speculum or a small-bore PVC pipe and a pen torch. *Traumatic injuries to the pharynx* may be caused by an incorrectly used balling gun. There may be local swelling at the throat caused by cellulitis. Saliva drooling, dysphagia and a necrotic smell may also be present.

Neck

Retropharyngeal lymph-node abscessation
This causes a progressively worsening upper airway obstruction with increased inspiratory noise or stridor. The enlarged abscess can sometimes be felt by external deep palpation, or delineated by ultrasonography or radiography. Endoscopic examination of the pharynx and larynx may reveal the reduced airway and the occluding mass. In most adult sheep the nasal passages, pharynx and larynx can be inspected in the sedated animal using a standard 11 mm fibreoptic endoscope. In smaller animals a paediatric endoscope can be used if available. The instrument is passed carefully along the ventral meatus of the nasal cavity. The trachea, oesophagus and cardia of the rumen can also be inspected.

Laryngeal paralysis and chondritis
Laryngeal paralysis is seen occasionally, especially in rams, and *chronic laryngeal chondritis* in the Texel breed. Affected animals show a fairly sudden onset of stertorous breathing with palpable vibration of the larynx. Loud sounds are audible when the larynx is auscultated, and the volume of sound is greater at this point than in the chest. Endoscopic examination can confirm the diagnosis.

Thrombophlebitis
The jugular vein, which often has a variable position along the jugular furrow, should be examined for signs of *thrombophlebitis* if there is a recent history of intravenous injection.

Foreign body obstruction
Palpation of the oesophagus is performed if foreign body obstruction is suspected in sheep with excessive salivation, free gas bloat, teeth grinding and apparent quidding. An obstruction may be confirmed by attempting to pass a stomach tube down the oesophagus by mouth with a gag in place, or passing a nasogastric tube down the oesophagus via the ventral meatus of a nostril.

Thorax

The respiratory system is examined by auscultation of the lung field which has a similar distribution to that in cattle. Percussion is restricted in unclipped sheep by the presence of fleece. Auscultation is performed by parting the fleece with the fingers and applying the stethoscope to the chest wall. Increased harsh lung sounds are frequently heard in normal sheep immediately after they have been caught. In healthy sheep, further examination after a rest period of 5 minutes usually reveals that the lung sounds have returned to normal. Abnormal lung sounds are as described in Chapter 7. *Chronic respiratory conditions in sheep include maedi, jaagsiekte, lungworms and the visceral form of caseous lymphadenitis. Serology* can be useful to confirm exposure to maedi. The *wheelbarrow test* can be used to support a diagnosis of jaagsiekte. The hind legs of the suspect sheep are lifted from the floor. In sheep with jaagsiekte copious quantities of clear fluid drain from the nares (Fig. 15.14). *Faecal samples* can be used to confirm the presence of lungworm larvae. *Radiology* and *ultrasonography* have proved useful to demonstrate multiple focal abscesses within the lungs in visceral caseous lymphadenitis.

The normal heart sounds can be heard at the 4th or 5th intercostal space behind the foreleg on either side. Cardiac disease is relatively uncommon in sheep, and examination is made by using the same techniques as described for cattle.

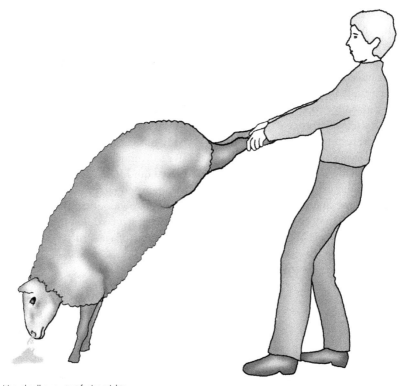

Figure 15.14 A positive wheelbarrow test for jaagsiekte.

The chest can be assessed radiographically. In unclipped sheep the presence of wool reduces the clarity of the resulting radiograph.

Abdomen

Examination is similar to cattle, but on a smaller scale.

Ruminal function is best assessed by auscultation using a stethoscope. The dorsal sac of the rumen is smaller than the ventral sac (the rumen has a 'cottage loaf appearance'). Auscultation directly over the left sublumbar fossa may not always, for this reason, immediately reveal evidence of ruminal movement. Pointing the stethoscope in an anterior direction just under the caudal left ribcage usually permits detection of movement in the dorsal sac. Movements occur at a rate of 1 or 2 per minute. Samples of ruminal fluid are taken and examined in the same way as in cattle. The fullness of the rumen can be ascertained by direct palpation through the left sublumbar fossa.

Bloat is less common in small ruminants than in cattle, and abomasal disorders are rarely diagnosed except in lambs. The rare condition of distension of the abomasum may be palpable on the right in some cases. Ballottement may indicate the presence of large amounts of fluid in the abdomen. A ruptured bladder results in the accumulation of urine in the peritoneum. The caudal abdomen can be readily examined through the flank by ultrasound, allowing assessment of intestinal content and function, the presence of excessive fluid and uterine content. A rectal probe can be used for further examination of the uterus. *Rectal examination* in sheep is limited to digital examination, which enables faecal samples to be obtained. Normal sheep faeces should be pelleted.

Urinary system

To collect a urine sample in the ewe two people are required. One person restrains the sheep in the standing position and temporarily closes off the nostrils. The second operator must be ready at the rear end to collect the urine in a specimen bottle as the sheep squats (Fig. 15.15). If no urine is produced and the sheep is becoming distressed after 30 seconds, the nostrils must be released. Alternatively, the urethra can be catheterised using a dog catheter with the sheep in the standing position. The catheter is gently introduced along the floor of the vagina guided by a gloved finger into the urethra opening, avoiding the more caudal diverticulum. An illuminated canine vaginal speculum or a pen torch can be useful.

In the male, the bladder cannot be catheterised. A urine sample can sometimes be obtained by gentle 'tickling' of the preputial opening with the gloved hand or a piece of straw.

Gross examination of a urine sample may reveal red urine, indicating haematuria or haemoglobinuria; a brown urine indicates a myoglobinuria. If pyelonephritis is present, the sample may contain blood and pus. Analysis using urine 'dipsticks' may indicate a high level of ketones, which may confirm a case of pregnancy toxaemia in the ewe.

If a *ruptured bladder* is suspected, biochemical analysis of the blood may confirm uraemia. Potassium, creatinine and phosphorous may also be useful prognostic indicators. Ultrasonography and abdominocentesis can be diagnostic.

External genitalia in the male

Scrotum

Examination should be performed in the standing position and then in the 'up ended' position. Visual inspection and palpation of the scrotum, including the spermatic cord, may reveal abnormalities of size, texture

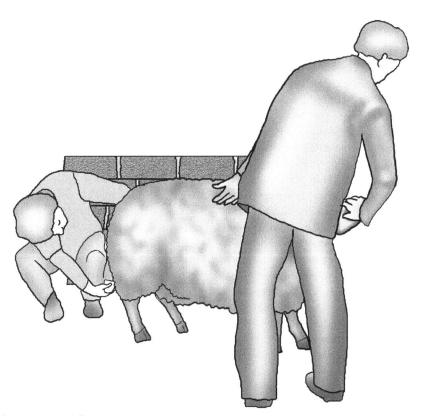

Figure 15.15 Collecting a urine sample from a ewe.

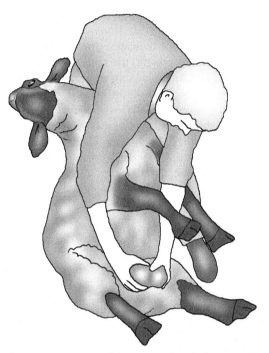

Figure 15.16 Examination of the scrotum in a 'tipped up' ram.

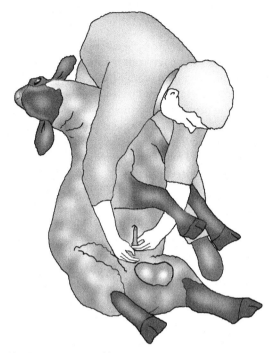

Figure 15.17 Extrusion of the penis in a ram.

and symmetry (Fig. 15.16). Prolapse of intestines through the inguinal ring can occur following open castration.

The contents of the scrotum should be bilaterally symmetrical. The scrotum is palpated to ensure both testes are of equal size and consistency, and are mobile within the scrotum. They should have the consistency of a ripe tomato. The total scrotal circumference in a breeding ram should be approximately 33 cm. Painful, enlarged and hard testicles are found in orchitis. Testicular atrophy may indicate a previous inflammatory episode. Inguinal hernias may be detected by visual inspection and confirmed by palpation or ultrasonography. The epididymes should be attached to the testes and should be soft to the touch. Enlargements or irregularities may indicate an infectious epididymitis. Asymmetry of the spermatic cords with enlargement is found with varicocoeles. If a ram has been vasectomised, scars in the skin of the scrotal neck can usually be found. Further assessment of the testes and epididymes can be carried out by ultrasound scanning.

Penis and prepuce

Examination of the penis and prepuce may form part of a fertility examination, in which case it includes semen collection and evaluation. *To extrude the penis* the ram is placed sitting on his hindquarters with his back supported in as upright a position as possible. The penis is grasped just anterior to the scrotum and is pushed up towards the prepuce to extend the sigmoid flexure. The prepuce is pushed downwards at the same time and the penis is extruded (Fig. 15.17). This is only possible in adult males as the penis is adherent to the prepuce in prepubertal animals. In castrated males extrusion can be difficult, and the penis may have to be grasped using padded forceps. Inflammation and ulceration of the penis (balanoposthitis) is readily identified on extrusion.

In sick male sheep *the patency of the urethral process should always be examined to ensure there are no obstructive uroliths present.* This condition can easily be overlooked because specific signs such as abdominal pain and straining are not always present. The end of the penis is carefully checked to ensure that the urethral process is free, intact and patent. The presence of uroliths within the urethral process is normally quite clearly visible. If a blockage is present further tests, including scanning of the abdomen for a full bladder or excessive fluid in the abdomen and measurement of blood urea and creatinine, are carried out as in the bull. A digital rectal examination may reveal pulsation of the urethra as it runs along the pelvic floor if a blockage is present. If rupture of the bladder is suspected, a sample of peritoneal fluid is taken using a 19 BWG (1.10 mm) needle. Creatinine levels higher than those of the blood indicate the presence of urine within the peritoneal cavity. The preputial opening should be routinely examined for the presence of ulcerative posthitis or pizzle rot. Inflammation associated with this condition may cause occlusion of the preputial opening.

Udder

To examine the udder in detail, the animal should be tipped up into the sitting position to rest on its haunches with its back leaning against the examiner's legs.

Visual inspection of the mammary glands may reveal abnormalities of the suspensory apparatus, abnormal swellings and discolouration of the skin. *Palpation* of the udder will identify oedema, inflammation, fibrosis, scarring or abscessation.

Mastitis in sheep is relatively common and may be localised to the mammary gland or result in endotoxaemia. Udder pain and swelling may initially cause a stiff gait or lameness. The affected udder is initially warm and painful to the touch. Pyrexia is usually present. Milk may be discoloured (including blood-stained) and clotted. In cases of acute severe mastitis, part of the udder may become cold, necrotic or gangrenous. In affected animals the disease can be life-threatening, and animals with areas of ventral subcutaneous oedema just anterior to the udder have a particularly poor prognosis (Fig. 15.18). Systemic signs of endotoxaemia may be present. Gangrene may involve the teat on the affected side, and extensive sloughing may occur. In more chronic cases the affected mammary gland may be non-functional and feel small, hard and fibrosed on palpation.

Small, painful crusty lesions are found on the

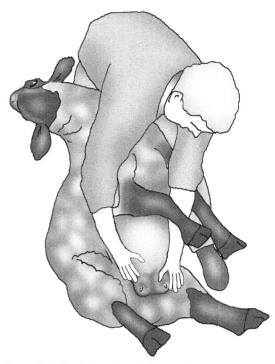

Figure 15.18 Examination of the udder in a ewe with severe acute mastitis.

udder and teats of animals suffering from orf. The infection readily spreads to the mouths of lambs.

Vulva

Visual inspection of the vulva during pregnancy may reveal a *vaginal eversion* or *prolapse, sometimes with a concurrent rectal prolapse caused by straining* (Fig. 15.19). The vulva may be swollen with erosions in ulcerative vulvitis. Orf lesions can also be seen on the vulva. *Uterine prolapse* may occur following parturition, with the uterus hanging down the perineum through the vulval lips. *Prolapse of the intestines* through a ruptured dorsal vaginal wall postpartum is observed on occasion soon after or during parturition. *Vaginal discharges* are observed postpartum. Purulent discharges postpartum indicate an endometritis. Offensive bloody discharges accompanied by endotoxaemia are seen in acute severe metritis. *Normal lochia* following an uncomplicated birth is reddish brown and odourless, and may

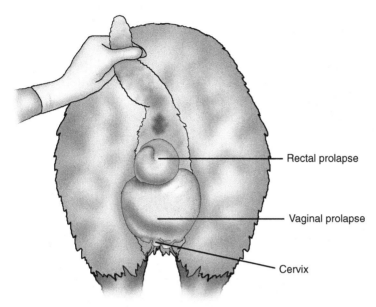

— Rectal prolapse

— Vaginal prolapse

— Cervix

Figure 15.19 Vaginal and rectal prolapse in a ewe.

be discharged for a period of 1 to 3 weeks. The caudal vagina can be inspected by parting the vulval lips. Visualisation may be assisted by the use of a pen torch and a small speculum. Small necrotic plaques are sometimes seen following assisted lambings.

Limbs and feet

Locomotor problems are common in sheep. Lameness and abnormalities of gait may result from infectious and non-infectious conditions affecting the nervous and musculoskeletal systems.

Identification of the affected limb(s) may be facilitated by observing the weight bearing while standing and at the walk. Gross swellings should be noted. Once the affected limb is identified it should be carefully examined and compared, if necessary, with the opposite leg. Severe lameness of a single limb which is unable to bear weight is found with bone fractures. Gentle manipulation may reveal abnormal movement, pain and crepitus. Stethoscope auscultation can assist in revealing this.

Detailed examination is facilitated by 'up ending' the sheep. The foot is washed and closely inspected. The horn of the hoof and wall, the interdigital space and the coronet should be visually inspected, palpated and manipulated to identify abnormalities. Hoof testers can be used to help identify the seat of pain.

Conditions of the foot causing lameness are common in sheep (Figs 15.20 and 15.21). Overgrown horn should be removed and the remaining horn carefully examined for erosion and penetration by underrunning infection which occurs in foot-rot. The quality of the horn should be noted. The white line should be inspected for integrity and signs of impaction and penetration. All infected or compromised horn is carefully pared away and further inspection is made to ensure the third phalanx (P3) is not exposed.

The *interdigital area* is inspected from above and below for signs of interdigital growths, integrity of the skin and inflammation. Skin necrosis and an offensive odour are additional consistent signs of foot-rot. Earth packed in this space and stones lodged between the digits can cause lameness which is relieved by their removal. Soft tissue swelling with or without purulent discharge may indicate an abscess. Swellings and eruptions at the coronary band or the heel may be traced to ascending infections from the white line. Blisters may be found at the junction of the horn and skin around the coronary band, and at the bulbs of the heel in foot-and-mouth disease. If these vesicles have burst, a ragged-edged erosion is

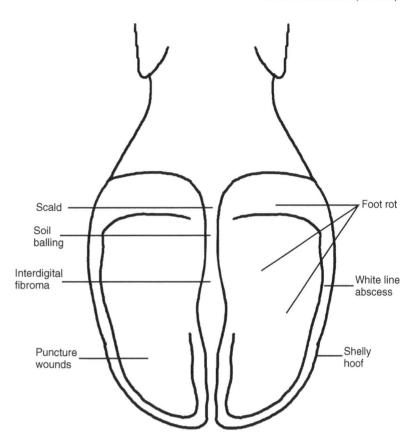

Figure 15.20 Locations of some important causes of lameness in sheep.

left. Gross swelling of a digit in association with acute pain on manipulation may indicate a septic arthritis of the proximal or distal interphalangeal joints; radiography is useful in locating the site and providing further diagnostic detail.

The *limb above the foot* is carefully checked. Joints with septic arthritis have distended capsules, are hot and painful, and have reduced movement. The movement of each joint is checked to ensure that the range of movements is comparable to the normal side. The condition can be confirmed by the analysis of joint fluid obtained by arthrocentesis. Erysipelas infection can occur in lambs and adult sheep, and causes some joint swelling and thickening of the epiphyses of affected limbs. There may also be some joint effusion, but this is often less than in cases of septic arthritis caused by *Streptococcus dysgalactiae*. Crepitus may be felt in chronic cases of arthritis. Checks are made on muscles for evidence of atrophy or abnormal swellings and pain. Muscle and tendon

ruptures may be identified. If white muscle disease is suspected, a blood sample can be checked for creatinine phosphokinase, and a urine sample for myoglobinuria. Radiography and ultrasound can also be helpful in some cases.

Nervous system

Sheep are susceptible to a variety of neurological disorders of differing aetiolgies. In many of these conditions treatment of the individual is of limited value, but a rapid and accurate diagnosis is essential to implement appropriate flock treatment control and prevention. This section provides a brief summary of the examination of the nervous system. A more detailed description for cattle is given in Chapter 14.

Neurological conditions

Many common neurological conditions are age related.

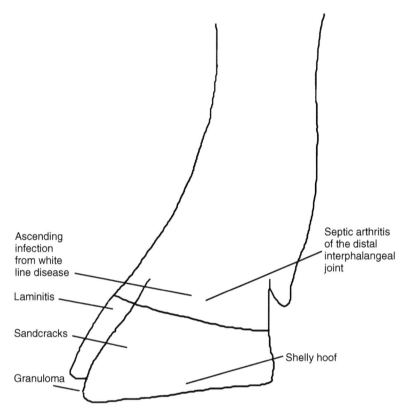

Ascending infection from white line disease

Laminitis

Sandcracks

Granuloma

Septic arthritis of the distal interphalangeal joint

Shelly hoof

Figure 15.21 Locations of some lesions associated with lameness in sheep.

Birth to 7 days of age – border disease (tremors), congenital swayback (ataxia), daft lamb disease (star gazing), bacterial meningitis (depression) and tetanus (spastic paresis).

Seven days to 3 months of age – brain and spinal abscesses (paresis), delayed swayback (ataxia), listeriosis (circling, facial nerve paralysis, head aversion), louping ill (abnormality of gait) and, less commonly, focal symmetrical encephalomalacia (dullness) may be seen in animals.

Three months to 2 years of age – conditions include coenuriasis (circling, head tilt), polioencephalomalacia (recumbency, star gazing, nystagmus) and hepatic encephalopathy (hyperaesthesia, fitting).

Adult sheep – conditions include cervical subluxation (paresis), listeriosis, brain abscesses and scrapie (ataxia, pruritus, loss of weight). *Metabolic conditions in adult ewes* include pregnancy toxaemia (dullness, recumbency, head pressing), hypocalcaemia (weakness, recumbency, flaccid paralysis), hypomagnesaemia (hyperaesthesia, staggers) and kangeroo gait (ataxia).

Examination
Observations may include:

Behaviour – wandering, apprehension, circling, head pressing and fits

Mental state – dullness and depression, hyperexcitability

Head position – aversion, tilted, high or low head carriage

Head coordination – intention tremors.

Movement of the flock will *reveal*

- recumbency
- intention tremors
- loss of balance
- incoordination
- ataxia.

Abnormalities of head carriage in sheep can provide important diagnostic information.

Exaggerated attentiveness may be caused by hyperaethesia or defective vision.

Head tilt, which is a rotation about the long axis, may indicate inner- or middle-ear infection or a lesion in the upper medulla ipsilateral to the lower ear.

Lateral deviation of the head may indicate unilateral blindness.

Vertical aversions with the head displaced vertically up or down is seen in conditions causing a raised intracranial pressure, meningitis and cortical lesions of the cerebral or cerebellar lesions.

Head tremors usually indicate a cerebellum or diencephalon lesion.

Head pressing may be observed.

Compulsive circling movements may indicate a brainstem or cerebellar lesion on the side to which the animal turns or a cerebral lesion which is usually on the contralateral side (Fig. 15.22).

Physical examination of the *conformation of the head* may indicate asymmetry. Facial paralysis may cause unilateral bulging of the cheeks by retention of the cud, lingual paralysis, drooping of the ear and/or eyelid. *Nystagmus* is an oscillatory movement of the eyeballs and is associated with lesions in the vestibular apparatus or cerebellum. An *obstacle course* can be used to confirm bilateral or unilateral blindness. The *pupils* should be checked for symmetry. A pen torch can be used to check the pupillary and consensual light response. The menace and palpebral response should be present in the healthy animal. Loss of prehension and saliva drooling may indicate flaccid paralysis.

The animal's *muscle tone* should be tested for spasticity (tetanus) or flaccidity (botulism and hypocalcaemia).

Spinal lesions may result in tetraparesis (cervical vertebrae subluxation in fighting rams) or paraparesis (spinal abscessation in lambs normally at C7/T1) (Fig. 15.23). Localisation and characterisation of the lesion can be achieved by testing proprioception, skin sensation, the panniculus response, deep pain, pedal reflexes, triceps reflex, the patellar reflex, tail tone, the anal reflex, and observing bladder control. Hemiwalking and wheelbarrow tests are less easy to interpret due to submission. The wheelbarrow test is performed by raising the hind legs or forelegs off the ground and forcing the animal to walk. The hemiwalking test is performed by holding up the thoracic and hind limb on one side and forcing the animal to

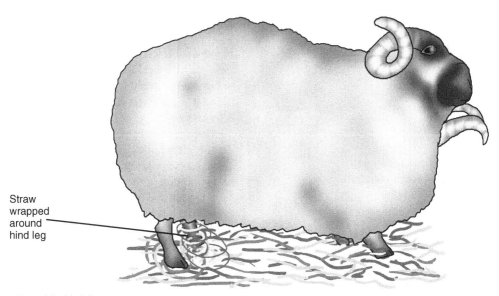

Straw
wrapped
around
hind leg

Figure 15.22 Head tilt with circling.

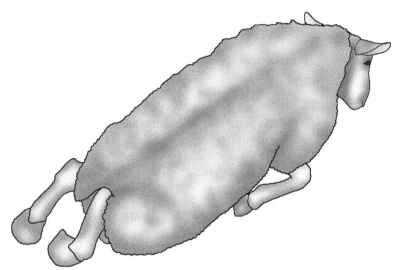

Figure 15.23 Spinal abscess causing paraplegia.

move laterally in the opposite direction. Previously undetected weakness or proprioceptive deficits may become apparent. A wide-based stance indicates proprioceptive abnormality and/or a cerebellar lesion.

The *Taenia multiceps (Coenurus cerebralis) cyst* is usually found in the right or left cerebrum or the cerebellum. The following signs may be present with a cerebellar lesion:

- head tremor
- head tilt
- dysmetria
- wide-based stance
- bilateral blindness
- nystagmus.

The following signs may be present with a cerebral lesion:

- head aversion
- wide circling (lesion ipsilateral)
- tight circles (lesion contralateral)
- depression or excitability
- unilateral blindness (lesion contralateral).

In scrapie and *Psoroptes ovis* infection, rubbing of the back, particularly near the base of the tail, results in the nibbling reflex. If rubbing is continued, some animals may collapse into a trance-like stupor with mild epileptiform fits before recovering.

Further examinations

When economics permit, the use of additional procedures may be justified, such as *abdomincentesis, cerebrospinal fluid tap, tracheal wash, radiology* and *blood, faecal and urine analysis.* Many of the further investigations outlined for cattle are equally applicable to sheep and the relevant chapters should be consulted for detailed descriptions of methodology.

Blood sample collection

Blood is collected from the jugular vein. In sheep the vein may be tortuous, having a constant position only at the angle of the jaw. In clipped and unclipped sheep it is readily raised by a ligature placed carefully around the base of the neck. The position of the vein is confirmed by palpation. Many sheep farmers do not like wool clipped off their sheep if they are show specimens, and the ligature method allows ready location of the jugular vein without clipping by palpation and parting the fleece. Routine haematology and biochemistry are carried out on samples taken in EDTA and heparin, respectively.

Post-mortem examination

Where a number of animals are affected a post-mortem examination may provide useful additional information and samples for analysis. Post-mortem examination may be needed to provide a definitive diagnosis by gross pathology (e.g. pneumonia) or histopathology (e.g. scrapie).

Cerebrospinal fluid samples

These can be obtained from the cisterna magna through the atlanto-occipital space under deep sedation, or from the lumbosacral space. To obtain a CSF sample from the lumbosacral space the sheep is usually placed in lateral recumbency and the spine flexed by holding the four legs together to maximise the lumbrosacral space. The sample can be grossly inspected for signs of inflammation and/or sent for cytological analysis and culture.

Biochemistry

Biochemical analysis of CSF fluid can be used to rule in or rule out *hypomagnesaemia*. Serum, urine and aqueous humour from the anterior chamber can also be used for this purpose. Rotheras tablets or urine dipstick patches can be used to detect ketones in urine, milk or saliva samples, and confirm a diagnosis of ketosis: urine samples are the most sensitive. Blood samples can be used to confirm a diagnosis of hypocalcaemia by measuring the calcium levels and cerebrocorticonecrosis can be confirmed by measuring the erythrocyte transketolase activity.

CLINICIAN'S CHECKLIST – EXAMINATION OF SHEEP

Observations		Jaw	(overshot, undershot)
Behaviour	(abnormal, excitable, depressed, pruritic, separated from flock)	Teeth	(age, losses, broken, condition)
		Eyes	(keratitis, conjunctivitis, foreign body, blindness)
Fleece	(loss, peeling off, perineal faecal staining)		
		Chest auscultation	
Respiration	(dypnoeic, tachypnoeic, hypernoeic, cough, nasal discharge, poor exercise tolerance)	Heart	(rate, rhythm, murmur)
		Lungs	(respiratory rate and depth, abnormal sounds)
		Abdomen	(size, shape, rumen rate, abnormalities on auscultation, palpation and ballottement)
Head carriage	(aversion, tilted, lateral deviation, high)		
Feeding	(inappetent)	Limbs and joints	(pain, swelling, crepitus, angular deformity, abnormally warm, muscle wastage, wounds)
Mobility	(lame, circling, ataxia, recumbent)		
Physical examination			
Ease of catching	(normal resistance, little resistance, abnormally easy)	Vulva/vagina	(discharge, prolapse)
		Perineum	(faecal staining, faecal quality)
Condition score	(1(thin) to 5(fat))	Nervous system	
Temperature	(normal, high, low)	**With animal tipped up**	
Mucous membranes	(colour: pale, icteric, cyanotic, injected)	Male external genitalia	(scrotum, testes, prepuce, penis, vermiform appendage, patency of urethra)
Superficial lymph nodes	(enlarged, abscessation)	Udder	(swelling, fibrosed, lesions, patency, milk quality, teat abnormalities)
Fleece and skin	(wool loss, ectoparasites, myiasis, pruritic, skin lesions)		
Head		Feet	(overgrown, under-running, smell, pain, interdigital growths)
Head	(conformation and position)		
Ears	(discharge, swellings)		

Examination of lambs

History

Farm records should be consulted. The weight of the lambs born, the lambing percentage, the percentage born alive/born dead, the percentage alive at the end of lambing and the percentage sold may identify a problem when compared with national averages for the production system under investigation. *Geographical location* may indicate deficiencies to consider, such as hypothyroidism in Derbyshire. *Previous problems* on the farm may be related to the present problem. Conditions such as swayback caused by copper deficiency, entropion or coccidiosis may be recurrent problems. The *current vaccination programmes*, including diseases causing abortion, clostridial diseases and orf, should be considered. *Prophylactic treatments*, such as antibiotic treatments for watery mouth and the use of anticoccidials, may be relevant to the current problem. *Lack of protocols* for navel dressing may be related to an increase in the incidence of neonatal joint ill.

The clinical signs observed, the group affected, and the morbidity and mortality rates of the current problem should be noted together with possible risk factors. The lamb may have been weak since birth, and there may be a failure of passive transfer of immunity due to lack of colostrum intake. Protracted or assisted births can be associated with hypoxia and metabolic acidosis. Meningeal haemorrhages and fractured limbs can result from excessive traction being applied during manipulation. Poor management, housing and the lack of experience of employees at lambing time may contribute towards a high prevalence of hypoglycaemia and hypothermia. Ewes with a poor condition score may also have reduced quantities of milk and colostrum. Poor ewe nutrition, particularly in the second half of pregnancy, results in reduced quantities of colostrum. Inappetence may be present in a variety of painful conditions.

Signalment

Some conditions affecting lambs are *age related*. The onset of hypothermia and/or hypoglycaemia usually occurs during the first 24 hours of life. This may be due to exposure and/or starvation. Watery mouth usually occurs from 5 to 36 hours after birth, and lamb dysentery is usually seen in lambs aged 36 hours and above. Cryptosporidiosis, rotavirus infection and salmonellosis may be seen between 48 hours and 7 days of age. Coccidiosis is most commonly seen in lambs 4 to 6 weeks old. Endoparasitism may be present in 6 to 8 week old lambs at grass.

Some conditions are *breed related*. Daft lamb disease is associated with specific breeds, in particular Border Leicester and Scottish half-bred sheep. The condition known as redfoot is only seen in the Scottish Blackface breed and crosses.

Observations

Useful information can be derived from observations of the affected lamb(s).

Behaviour, demeanour, appearance, response, posture and gait can be assessed. Star gazing with the head held in dorsiflexion may indicate congenital cerebellar atrophy of daft lamb disease. A lamb which has an empty looking abdomen and is tucked up may be starving. A lamb with a bloated swollen abdomen may have watery mouth or abomasal bloat. Abomasal bloat may be observed in lambs reared on *ad libitum* milk units. A depressed neonatal lamb which is weak and unable to stand may be hypothermic and/or hypoglycaemic. Reluctance to walk or a stiff gait may indicate joint ill. A severely lame lamb with a dangling leg may have a bone fracture.

Many clinical signs can be observed from a distance. Coughing in intensive finishing systems may indicate a mycoplasmal pneumonia. Obstructive urolithiasis in fat lambs being intensively reared may present with abdominal straining if the bladder is still intact, or dullness if the bladder has ruptured causing uraemia. The affected animals will be depressed and anorexic, and may have diarrhoea. Uraemia is also a feature of nephrosis in lambs aged 2 to 16 weeks.

Neuromuscular signs are easily recognised. Tremors may be observed in Border disease. Sudden death, trembling, blindness and fitting in growing lambs are signs seen in cerebrocortical necrosis. Growing lambs affected by louping ill may show a wide range of neurological signs including an abnormal bounding gait. Several lambs with hind-leg ataxia that are unable to keep up with their ewes when gently driven, may have swayback caused by copper deficiency in the ewe; however, if only one individual is affected a spinal abscess should be considered. Sudden collapse, stiff hind legs, weakness or breathing difficulties in lambs may be caused by white muscle disease, and an elevated serum creatinine phophokinase in addition to vitamin E and selenium levels may confirm the diagnosis. Stiffness and an unwillingness to move with muscle tremors may be seen in tetanus which is usually associated with a recent wound. This may progress to generalised tetanic spasms with hyperaesthesia.

Physical examination

Lambs can be lifted onto a table or held under the arm by an assistant for examination.

Temperature, heart rate, respiration and mucous membranes

Temperature   *Hypothermia* is a common condition that can be fatal without treatment (Fig. 15.24). The normal temperature in a lamb is 39 to 40°C. Severely hypothermic lambs can have temperatures below 32°C. Lambs with temperatures below 37°C require intensive treatment. Subnormal temperatures may also be found in watery mouth and other conditions causing severe debilitation. The use of incubators and intraperitoneal glucose injections can be life-saving, but poorly supervised use of incubators can result in hyperthermia with fatal consequences. *Pyrexia* is associated with an inflammatory response.

Heart rate and respiration   The heart rate of a normal lamb is 80 to 100 beats per minute and the respiratory rate 36 to 48 breaths per minute. Both may be

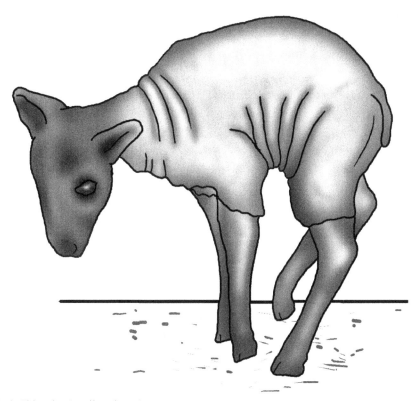

Figure 15.24 A lamb with hypothermia and hypoglycaemia.

elevated with an endotoxaemia and decreased in hypothermic or moribund animals.

Mucous membranes   The mucous membranes of the *eye* and *buccal cavity* should be checked. Pale membranes may indicate anaemia or shock. Jaundice may be present in young lambs given cow colostrum or in older lambs with copper poisoning.

Septicaemia   This may be caused by a variety of bacterial organisms, and affected lambs are dull, weak, unable to stand, pyrexic and anorexic, sometimes with nervous signs.

Skin

Hairy coats may be present in lambs affected with Border disease. *A steely appearance and loss of normal wool crimp* can occur with copper deficiency. *Dehydration* causes a reduction in the skin elasticity which can be most usefully assessed using the skin over the eyebrows and/or ventral abdomen. The skin is raised by pinching the skin between the thumb and the finger. In dehydration the skin remains elevated for more than 5 seconds. The eyes may also be sunken and the lamb weak and depressed.

Head

Palpation of the skull may reveal crepitus associated with a fracture.

Eyes   The eyes should be examined. In septicaemic animals *hypopyon* may be present, with the anterior chamber containing inflammatory material. *Entropion* or inturning of the eyelids is a common condition which may be unilateral or bilateral; *keratitis, corneal ulceration* and *tear staining* may be present as a consequence (Fig. 15.25). *Rupture of the cornea* sometimes occurs. In the absence of entropion the conjunctival recesses beneath both eyelids and the third eye lids should be examined for a *foreign body* such as a grass seed. The application of a topical local anaesthetic and a pair of fine artery forceps facilitate this procedure. *Infectious keratoconjunctivitis* should be considered if no physical cause of conjuctivitis, keratitis and epiphora are found and several animals are affected. *A clear bilateral watery ocular discharge* is seen in cobalt deficiency, in addition to poor growth and anaemia.

Examination of the mouth   A finger should be placed inside the mouth. A strong suck reflex should be elicited. Absence or a weak response is abnormal. *Excessive saliva* around the mouth may indicate the presence of watery mouth (Fig. 15.26). *Pustular or scabby lesions around the mouth* in several lambs with reluctance to suckle may suggest orf infection. Protective gloves are advisable to guard against this painful zoonosis. The mandibles are examined for *over-* or *undershot apposition*. The mouth is opened

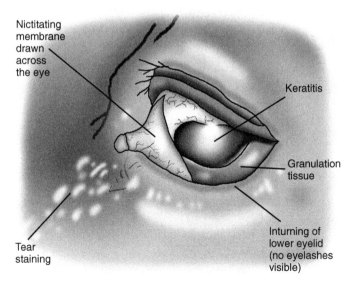

Nictitating membrane drawn across the eye

Keratitis

Granulation tissue

Tear staining

Inturning of lower eyelid (no eyelashes visible)

Figure 15.25 Entropion of the lower eyelid.

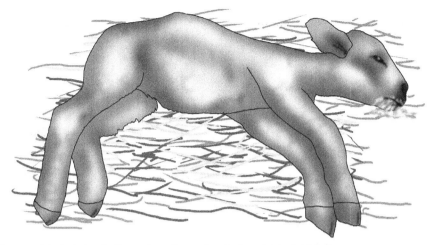

Figure 15.26 Watery mouth in a lamb: the animal is recumbent with excessive salivation and abdominal distention.

and examined using a pen torch. The hard palate is checked for the presence of a *cleft palate. Holly leaves* are occasionally found lodged in the pharynx and cause choking; however, these animals are usually found dead.

Chest

Fractured ribs may be a cause of abnormal breathing rhythm due to pain; palpation and radiography (if justifiable) can be used to confirm the diagnosis.

Auscultation of the heart should be performed; the *presence of a murmur* may indicate a congenital heart defect such as a ventricular septal defect or a vegetative endocarditis from another septic focus such as joint ill. The lamb may have poor exercise tolerance with tachypnoea and tachycardia. A linear ultrasound probe may identify valvular vegetations.

Abdomen

The abdomen should be palpated and auscultated with a stethoscope. An enlarged abdomen in a lamb 7 days old and above which is otherwise alert may indicate *atresia ani*. In a sick lamb with *abdominal distension, auscultation with palpation or ballottement may indicate fluid and gas in a static abomasum*. This is likely to be *rattle belly* or *watery mouth* caused by *Escherichia coli endotoxaemia. Abdominal pain* is recognised by extreme tensing of the abdomen and groaning on palpation. Abdominal pain is present in other

conditions such as lamb dysentery and coccidiosis. *In male lambs with obstructive urolithiasis, a urine-filled distended bladder may be palpated or visualised with ultrasonography.*

The *umbilicus should be carefully palpated and visually inspected.* Infection may be present with a distended, hot and painful navel. The infection may extend internally, affecting the congenital umbilical structures and liver. This septic focus may also give rise to bacteraemia and/or septicaemia causing joint ill, meningitis and internal organ abscessation. Umbilical hernias may be visually identified, and palpation will reveal whether the contents are reducible or not. On some occasions there is an intestinal prolapse through the umbilical region which will be obvious.

Limbs

The feet, joints and bones of all four legs should be systematically examined by manipulation and palpation. Previous observations may indicate upon which leg to focus or which joint should be more carefully examined.

Feet The condition and integrity of the horn of the hooves should be checked and any swellings investigated. Complete detachment of the horn from the sensitive laminae is seen in the condition 'redfoot'. Interdigital abscesses are relatively common in lambs and affected animals present with severe

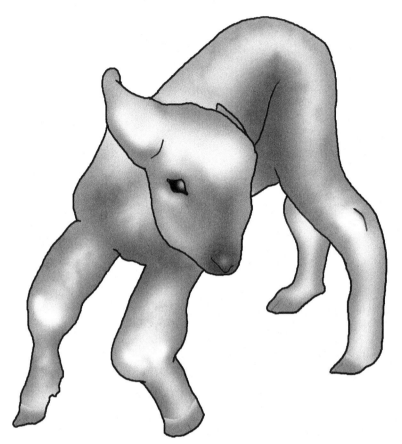

Figure 15.27 Joint ill in a lamb: the animal has enlargement of the carpal and hock joints.

lameness with a hot and swollen claw. Manual pressure may cause an abscess to exude purulent material which will confirm the diagnosis.

Legs The examination then proceeds up the leg. Each bone should be palpated, and if a fracture suspected the site should be gently manipulated to check for crepitus. Applying a stethoscope to the area on manipulation may increase the chances of auscultating crepitus. Radiology, if economically justified, will confirm the diagnosis and detail the type of fracture. Extreme protein deficiency and a dietary imbalance of phosphorous and calcium may result in osteodystrophy, causing deformities such as an inward or an outward bowing of the forelimbs.

Joint ill This is a relatively common condition in lambs and previous observations may increase the suspicion of this condition. The animal may also be depressed and febrile. The *fetlocks, carpi, hocks and stifles may be hot and painful, with joint capsule distension causing fluctuating swellings* (Fig. 15.27). Confirmation may be achieved by arthrocentesis. The skin over the enlarged joint capsule is aseptically prepared and a sample of joint fluid obtained using a sterile needle and syringe. The gross appearance of the sample may confirm a diagnosis of suppurative arthritis; if not, cytology may be helpful. Bacteriological culture of the sample may characterise the aetiological agent. *Streptococcus dysgalactiae, Escherichia coli, Erysipelothrix rhusiopathiae* and, in tick areas, *Staphylococcus aureus*, are common causes. A *vegetative endocarditis may also be present*. Hind-leg paralysis may result from spinal trauma or a spinal abscess.

Anal area

The presence of a patent anus is confirmed when the temperature is taken.

The position of the constricting ring to remove the distal section of the tail can be checked to ensure sufficient length of tail is retained in female lambs intended for breeding. The tail remnant should cover the vulva.

The presence and type of faeces should be assessed. There may be staining of the perineum by diarrhoea, and scouring may be observed during defaecation following or during placement of the thermometer in the rectum. *The association between diarrhoea, endoparasitism and fly-strike should be considered with lambs at grass, and the skin around the tail examined for the presence of maggots.* With lamb dysentery the lamb is severely ill and the faeces are bloody. *In older lambs with watery dysenteric faeces, coccidiosis should be considered. The possibility of a ruptured bladder and/or nephrosis should be considered when presented with a depressed (male) lamb with diarrhoea.* Check that the rubber ring has not been incorrectly placed around the neck of the scrotum ensnaring part of the urethra.

Further investigations

A *post-mortem examination* may be justified where there is a high morbidity. Gross pathology may indicate the cause such as in obstructive urolithiasis or pulpy kidney. Alternatively, samples may be tested to confirm or rule out a tentative diagnosis such as nephrosis or copper poisoning.

Blood samples can be used for a variety of purposes. The ewe can be tested for copper status which may help confirm an outbreak of swayback. Blood testing the lambs may confirm cobalt deficiency or a low vitamin E and/or selenium status. In young lambs in which sampling may be required for estimation of blood glucose, the jugular vein is readily raised under the short fleece by digital pressure.

Electron microscopy can be used to confirm a diagnosis of orf.

Faecal samples from a representative group of animals can be screened for rotavirus, *Escherichia coli*, *Clostridium perfringens* Type B, endoparasites and coccidiosis.

Ultrasonography is extremely useful for visualisation of internal structures.

Part IV

Pigs

Clinical Examination of the Pig

Introduction

As in other species, diagnosis of disease in pigs is based on an assessment of the following:

- owner's complaint
- history of the farm and the patient
- signalment of the patient
- detailed observation of the patient, the other pigs in the group and their environment
- comprehensive clinical examination.

A provisional diagnosis is made. Further clinical tests, clinical pathology and possibly a post-mortem examination may be employed to confirm or refute the provisional diagnosis. Because many pig diseases are infectious and pigs are often kept intensively in large groups, the health of other pigs in the group must be considered. The importance of a comprehensive clinical examination and an accurate diagnosis in these circumstances cannot be over-emphasised. It enables a targeted programme of treatment and preventative medicine to be mounted.

Special features of clinical examination of the pig

The natural tendency of the pig to try to escape from any restraint or confinement limits the way in which it can be restrained, handled and examined. Its tendency to squeal when restrained makes some aspects of the examination such as auscultation of the chest difficult, but seldom impossible. Sows with litters and breeding boars are potentially aggressive and dangerous. Their pens should not be entered in the absence of a stockperson.

Attempting to examine one or two sick pigs in a group of twenty others can be difficult. Individual pigs can be taken out of the pen briefly for examina-tion, but they must be reintroduced carefully as the returning pigs may be set upon, attacked or even killed by their pen-mates. The difficulties of examining pigs can be largely overcome by using a quiet and gentle approach. Patience, quietness and a knowledge of pig behaviour are very important. In general, the greater the restraint of the pig the less effective the clinical examination. For some procedures such as blood sampling and X-ray examination, restraint and possibly sedation are essential. In every case the clinical examination should be as thorough and detailed as possible.

Preservation of high health status when visiting a pig farm

Visits to elite 'disease-free' pig farms cannot be made unless the veterinarian has been in 'quarantine' for at least 3 days before the visit. The veterinarian must always strictly observe the farm's hygiene regulations and make every effort to avoid bringing disease onto the farm. Similar careful precautions should be taken on leaving the farm. The term 'disease-free' should always be clarified. On some farms it does not include freedom from enzootic pneumonia.

Farm records

Computerised records of all aspects of the herd's performance and profitability are an important management tool on many pig farms. Examination of the records is an important part of a routine visit. Records available may also contain *details of the carcase quality* and the *food conversion rate* of recent batches of finished pigs. Poor results may require further investigation. In the breeding herd, details of *reproductive parameters*, for example the farrowing index (mean number of pigs per sow per year) and litter size, will be available for comparison with target figures.

Owner's complaint

Disease problems in pigs often have a sudden and spectacular onset. It is not uncommon to be called to a farm on which a number of pigs in a group have been found dead, others are showing varying degrees of illness and other batches in nearby accommodation are possibly also at risk. The owner is very concerned about losses – of pigs and money – and is anticipating an immediate diagnosis, effective treatment and a programme of preventative medicine. The clinician should ensure that all necessary equipment is taken to deal with the problem.

History

Past history

The past history of the unit may be known to the clinician. The practice may have investigated and treated a number of previous problems. The breed and type of pigs kept will be known as will the type of unit, for example weaner production or bacon pig production. The size of the farm and the approximate numbers of boars, sows, gilts, finishers and other pigs will also be known. The quality of management of the farm will also be known – accommodation, general cleanliness, animal welfare, feeding regime, stockmanship. Other information will include the vaccination policy of the herd and, especially in outdoor units, the worming policy. Ectoparasite control may also be practised. Details of this, including the drugs used and the frequency and success of usage will be known. Reports from previous farm visits may be available.

Knowledge of a unit's history should never be allowed to outweigh the importance of current observation and clinical examination.

If the long-term history is not known, much information can be quickly obtained by observation and questioning the owner or stockperson.

Short-term history

The short-term history of the pigs – especially those that are ill – is also important. The following points are noted:

(1) Are the affected pigs home-bred or were they purchased?
(2) If purchased, how long have they been on the farm?
(3) Where did they come from? Is anything known about the disease status of the farm of origin? Purchased breeding stock are often hybrids of known health status, but disease breakdowns can occur.
(4) Did the pigs (if purchased) appear normal on arrival?
(5) Has there been a recent change in diet? A mild transitory enteritis is seen in many herds when new grain is introduced into the diet after harvest.
(6) Are all the pigs eating? Loss of appetite is often an early sign of illness. This is easily identified if set feeding times are used, and is less easily detected in *ad libitum* systems.
(7) Has this group of pigs had any previous problems?
(8) Have the pigs been treated before by the practice or by the farmer?
(9) What treatment was given and with what response?
(10) What is their vaccination status and is it up to date?
(11) How long have the pigs been ill?
(12) Have any pigs died and when did the deaths occur?
(13) Are the carcases of any recent deaths available for post-mortem examination?
(14) How many pigs are affected?
(15) What signs of abnormality have been seen?
(16) Does the farmer or stockperson have any idea what the problem may be? This can be helpful, should always be noted, but may be misleading.
(17) Have there been any known problems with the power or water supplies?

Signalment

The breed, age and sex of the pig or pigs to be examined will enable particular problems to be checked. For example, common causes of enteritis in piglets include *Escherichia coli* and *rotavirus* organisms which rarely cause disease in adults. Diseases such as mastitis are confined to the sow.

The pigs' environment

The general appearance of the farm may be an indication of the standard of management and cleanliness in the pig unit. A clean accessible foot-dip free from manure and other dirt is a good sign. The housing of the pigs should be assessed in a methodical manner.

(1) *Ventilation* – an immediate assessment can be made by a personal appraisal of the atmosphere. Does the air feel comfortable to breathe? Is it full of dust, causing people entering to cough or experience breathing difficulties? If the atmosphere is unsuitable for people it is also unsuitable for pigs. An intense smell of ammonia indicates damp conditions including inadequate bedding, poor drainage and ventilation. Are air outlets and inlets adequate? Draught may indicate excessive air movement. Are any fans working and clean? Kennel-like shelters for pigs installed within the pen may compromise ventilation.

(2) *Stocking density* – is this satisfactory? Overcrowding compromises welfare and predisposes to disease.

(3) *Ambient temperature* – a comfortable temperature for adult pigs is 19°C; it should be higher for piglets.

(4) *Light* – there should be sufficient light for the stockperson to be able to see and inspect all the pigs at any time.

(5) *Bedding* – is this clean and plentiful?

(6) *Cleanliness of the pigs* – pigs are naturally very clean animals, and dirtiness of housed pigs can be indicative of poor bedding management or overcrowding.

(7) *Dunging area* – faeces are normally passed in one corner of the pen where they can be assessed. Loose faeces may be passed anywhere in the pen if the pigs have diarrhoea. Blood in the faeces may be seen in conditions such as swine dysentery. Slatted floors may allow loose faeces to pass unnoticed from view.

(8) *Abnormal discharges* – such as *blood* and *pus* should not be present in healthy pigs. Blood may indicate haemorrhage through injury or internal blood loss such as may occur in gastric ulceration, dysentery or porcine intestinal adenomatosis (PIA). Fresh blood may indicate injury caused by tail- or ear-biting or through damage sustained by contact with sharp objects. Blood may also be seen in cases of pyelonephritis. *Vomitus* – vomiting may occur in cases of overeating. It may also be seen in cases of gastritis caused by *Hyostrongylus rubidus* and in cases of severe illness, for example peracute and acute erysipelas. In piglets it is seen in 'vomiting and wasting' disease.

(9) *Flooring* – bedding is considered important for pigs' comfort but may not be used in some farrowing pens and in slatted floor units. Floors should be checked for sharp corners and other hazards which can cause foot or pressure point injuries, especially if such injuries are detected during either observation or clinical examination of the pigs. In creep areas, poor quality mesh flooring can cause minor foot or limb injuries which predispose to entry of organisms causing septic arthritis (joint ill).

(10) *Water availability* – where is the source of water? Is the number of drinkers up to the standard required by current welfare codes?

(11) *Feeding facilities* – those found will depend on whether twice daily wet feeding or *ad libitum* dry feeding is used. Pigs on a twice daily feeding regime should empty their trough within 10 minutes of being fed. If any food has been left in the trough, is it in good condition? If *ad libitum* dry feeding is used, are the food quality and availability satisfactory? If an automatic feeding system is used, is there any evidence that it is not working properly? Is there sufficient trough

space for the number of pigs in each pen? Is an analysis of the food available?

(12) *Fitments* – are these in good condition? Are there any sharp projections on feeders which might cause injury to the pigs?

(13) *Outdoor environments* – are increasingly used for breeding stock. Does the environment appear satisfactory? Are the water supply, fencing, wallows and shade for hot weather satisfactory? Is the field free from old bricks and other debris which might predispose to foot or other orthopaedic injuries? Is there any evidence of vermin? Shiny areas on posts might suggest pruritus caused by mange infestation.

(14) *State of repair of premises and equipment.*

Observation of the pigs

Initial observation of the undisturbed pigs

At this stage, the clinician is looking for any obvious signs of abnormal behaviour and general signs of ill health which may later require further detailed investigation. Individual pigs may be clearly unwell (Fig. 16.1.)

The house, pen or field should be entered as quietly as possible to avoid disturbing the pigs. Ideally, they should first be observed without their being aware of the presence of the observer. The clinician should look carefully to see if any departure from the normal is evident.

Pigs naturally spend much of their time sleeping, and it is not unusual, especially in younger animals, to find a group lying comfortably huddled together. Usually one member of the group is keeping an eye open. Huddling may also be a sign that pigs are cold. If sleeping pigs are suddenly alerted, healthy animals often make a short sharp barking noise which sounds as if they are clearing their throats. They also often make this same noise if new straw has been added to the pen and they are galloping around in an excited fashion. When new bedding is added the pigs will spend time rooting around in the straw eating some of it. Recently weaned and mixed groups of pigs will spend much time fighting or sham fighting until their hierarchy is established. Signs of tail biting (Fig. 16.2) and other vices may be seen.

The whole group should be observed to see if there are any pigs who are behaving unlike the rest of the group. Any pigs that are not with the main group and are standing or lying away from them may be unwell. *Inspection of all the pigs on the farm* is also an essential part of the routine visit and one for which the veterinary surgeon is particularly well qualified. The clinician must *look in every corner of each pen* to ensure no ill pigs are there. Any sick pigs should receive a full clinical examination.

Response of the pigs to people
Pigs are often initially startled by the arrival of the

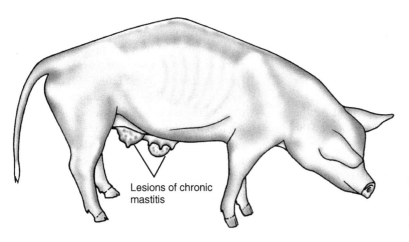

Lesions of chronic mastitis

Figure 16.1 Thin sow syndrome: the animal is in very poor condition showing ribs and backbone; she also has two lesions of chronic mastitis.

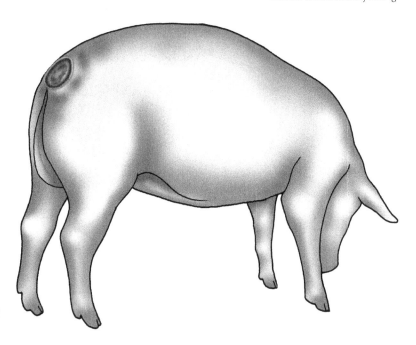

Figure 16.2 Tail bitten pig: the tail has been completely eaten away with additional perineal damage. Haematogenous spread of infection may lead to spinal damage.

clinician or any unusual activity in their environment. They quickly come to investigate and may attempt to nibble the clinician's clothing and equipment. Some pigs in the group will be bolder than others and make the first approach. Individual pigs will enjoy being rubbed or tickled while others remain wary of human presence. Instruments, cases and other equipment should never be placed on the floor as they may be rapidly damaged by the pigs. Excessive interest in boots may be seen in pigs suffering from *iron deficiency anaemia*. Affected piglets often have very pale skins and search vigorously for sources of iron including fragments of soil. *Very sick pigs* in a group may completely ignore human presence. Such pigs may also be bullied or attacked by other members of the group.

Specific signs of disease noted at this stage may include poor bodily condition, respiratory abnormalities including coughing, sneezing or laboured breathing, neurological signs, lameness, diarrhoea, pruritus and abnormal body shape.

Condition score

Group members should be approximately the same size, weight and show similar bodily condition. Any pigs who are smaller than the rest may always have been runts, but others may have lost condition through illness. Small ill-thriven pigs may have longer body hair than those in better condition. In extremely thin pigs the backbone and ribs may be clearly visible (Fig. 16.3).

Observation of the sow and piglets in the farrowing house

The sow and her litter should be considered as one unit, since illness in the sow may affect the piglets and *vice versa*. The clinician should be aware of normal porcine behaviour and interaction in the farrowing house so that abnormalities can be recognised and investigated. When not being fed by the sow, the piglets will mostly lie and sleep in the creep area under their lamp. If hungry, the piglets will stay close to the sow making a high pitched rather disgruntled sound. They may nuzzle the sow with their snouts, trying to encourage her to lie on her side and feed them. If unsuccessful they may attempt to root the floor and to drink any spilled water from the sow's trough or, if desperate, her urine. When not feeding her piglets, the sow usually lies in sternal or less commonly in lateral recumbency. If her udder is uncomfortable, e.g. with mastitis–metritis–agalactia (MMA) syndrome, mastitis, or if the unclipped

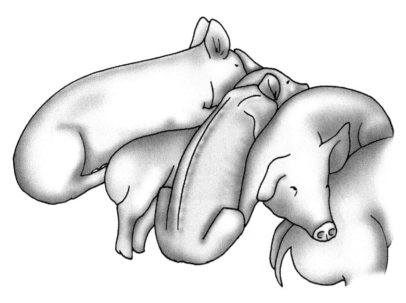

Figure 16.3 Group of young pigs showing one pig (third from left) in much poorer condition that its fellow pigs.

piglets' teeth are causing her pain, the sow may remain in sternal recumbency, refusing to lie on her side. If all is well the sow will call her pigs to feed at intervals of 1 to 2 hours throughout the day. The call to feed is an intermittent medium-pitched sound.

Observation of piglets' appearance and movement

The piglets should be watched as they come out to feed: are any left behind in the creep area? Occasionally, an individual will be so deeply asleep that the sow's call is not heard. Mostly failure to come out to suckle indicates that the piglet is either unable to walk, e.g. with severe joint infection, or is too weak to respond to the sow's call through disease or malnutrition. The piglets should be observed to see if any are scouring. Affected animals often look empty and have yellow or green faecal material running down their perineal area. Coughing or snuffling may be heard as the piglets start to move, and may indicate the presence of a dusty environment or of respiratory disease.

Observation of piglet feeding

The piglets normally respond to the sow's call and approach the udder and start to nuzzle the sow's udder and teats with their noses, making a squeaking noise. Each piglet then seeks its own teat; there may be some fighting and quarrelling amongst them until each is settled on its own teat. The bigger, stronger piglets are usually found on the anterior pectoral teats, with the smaller piglets placed more caudally. Piglets usually remain on the same teat throughout their suckling period. If the litter size is small and also after part-weaning, individual piglets may adopt and feed from two or even more teats.

Once milk let-down begins the sow makes another sound – intermittent grunts short in duration and slightly lower pitched than her call to feed sound. This 'milk let-down' sound is sometimes referred to as the sow 'talking to her pigs'. If milk let-down is successful, the piglets stop nuzzling and hang back on their teats with their ears held against their shoulders (Fig. 16.4). Their throat movements indicate they are swallowing milk. If a piglet is briefly detached at this point from its teat and the teat is milked, milk will squirt out under pressure as it does at farrowing time under the influence of oxytocin but not at other times. In a multiple sow farrowing house, the sound of one sow calling and then feeding her pigs will often cause the other sows to follow suit. Milk let-down seldom exceeds periods of 60 to 90 seconds. After feeding, the piglets usually root at the sow's udder in the hope of stimulating further milk

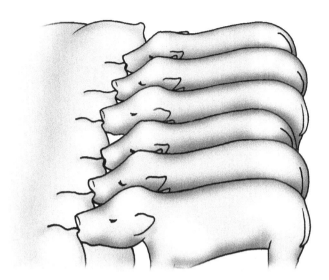

Figure 16.4 Group of piglets drinking from the sow at the time of milk let-down. See text for details.

let-down. They then settle down to sleep near the sow or return to their creep area. They should have a full, contented appearance. The appearance of a sick sow and her litter is very different (Fig. 16.5).

Assessment of the sow in the farrowing house

If approached quietly in the farrowing house, the sow in recumbency will normally remain lying down. Gently massaging her udder will encourage her not to rise. If disturbed or if food is offered she will normally roll into sternal recumbency and get to her feet, her front end rising first. The sow may be aggressive towards strangers and make an angry short 'barking' noise when approached; she will occasionally snap at people within range. If sick, the sow will often be disinterested in food and may exhibit difficulty in getting up, especially when attempting to raise her rear end. Rising may be especially difficult if the sow is confined in a farrowing crate. If stimulated to rise, the sick sow may utter a thin, weak, reedy squeal of protest. This is usually a bad sign, indicating severe illness requiring urgent assessment and treatment.

Clinical observation

Because of the normal temperament of the pig, it is important to complete as much of the clinical exami-

nation as possible by careful and methodical observation before proceeding to a physical examination. Initial observation has included both the overall appearance of the group and of individual pigs, especially those that appear unwell. Having observed the pigs without disturbing them they should now be subjected to closer scrutiny to enable them to be properly and methodically inspected. Abnormalities observed at this stage can be followed up in greater detail when the pig is physically examined. Further observation is made when the pigs get to their feet. The points to note, which should include assessment of behaviour and environment mentioned above, are as follows.

Breathing

Are any pigs showing rapid or exaggerated breathing movements? If so, and especially if coughing or sneezing is heard, respiratory disease may be present. Open mouth breathing is an ominous sign of severe respiratory disease. The respiratory rate of individual pigs can be measured at this stage.

Neurological signs

Individual pigs showing incoordination, ataxia, tremor, head tilt or fitting may be spotted at this stage. Sleeping pigs may occasionally show muscle tremors, but these disappear when the pig wakes.

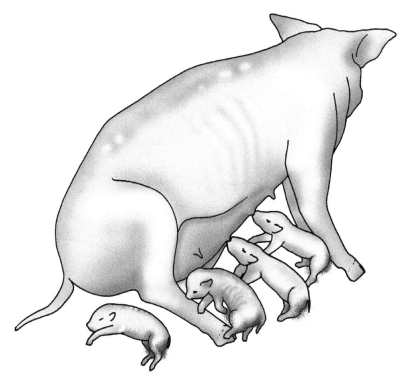

Figure 16.5 Sow who is unwell failing to feed her piglets. Note her reluctance to lie in sternal recumbency. One piglet is dead, another thin and malnourished, and several show signs of enteritis. Compare with Fig. 16.4.

Fitting   Together with other signs such as nystagmus and opisthotonos, fitting is seen in cases of *meningitis* caused by *Streptococcus* and *Haemophilus* species (Fig. 16.6). Intermittent fitting may be seen in cases of *water deprivation*. Fitting is also seen in cases of *classical swine fever* together with other signs involving many body systems.

Incoordination   This may be seen in *bowel oedema* where the pig may lose the ability to use its forelimbs (Fig. 16.7). In this condition the pig also shows signs of general depression (Fig. 16.7). If disturbed it may utter a bubbly squeal: this is caused by laryngeal oedema.

Ataxia   This may occur with spinal injury or abscessation.

Tremor   Various forms of *congenital tremor* are seen in piglets.

Head tilt   This is often seen in cases of *middle ear* or *vestibular disease* (Fig. 16.8). If such cases deteriorate the pig may become unable to balance and will repeatedly roll onto the same side.

Lameness

- Are any pigs obviously lame?
- Which limb is affected and how severe is the lameness?
- How many pigs are affected?
- Can the animal take any weight on the affected limb?

Total inability to bear weight may indicate a *fracture*. Mild lameness may disappear if the pig is frightened but reappear later when the animal is not stressed.

- Can any *joint swelling* be seen?
- Does *joint movement* seem restricted?

Such changes may be present in acute or chronic arthritis.

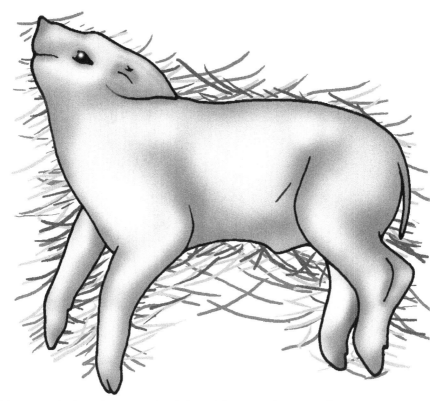

Figure 16.6 Piglet meningitis showing opisthotonos. Note the piglet's extended head and neck and extended forelegs.

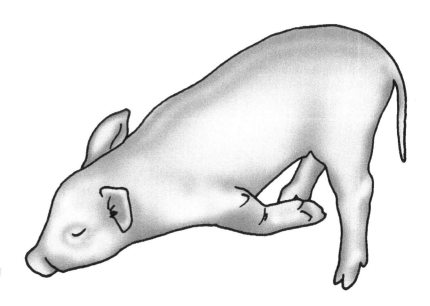

Figure 16.7 Young pig with bowel oedema. Note the closed upper eyelid and the pig's inability to extend its forelegs.

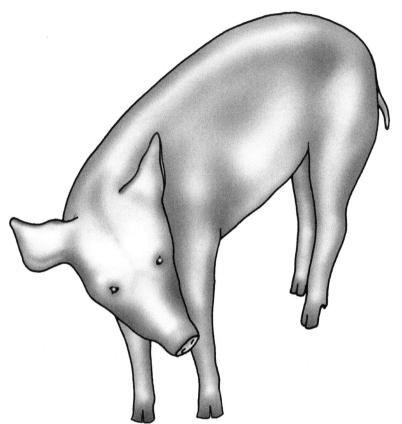

Figure 16.8 Pig with middle ear disease. Note the animal's head tilt to the right as a result of vestibular damage.

- Is there any obvious swelling of the feet?

Painful swelling of one digit may be seen if the foot or toe is infected, e.g. in 'bumble-foot'. In *foot lameness* the pig may frequently attempt to place the affected foot on the ground, but repeatedly snatch it away when it experiences pain.

Diarrhoea

- Are any pigs showing signs of diarrhoea?

In severe enteritis, faecal staining around and below the anus may be seen. Chronic diarrhoea may be associated with weight loss.

- What colour are the faeces and do they contain blood?

Dark faeces staining the perineum are seen in *swine dysentery* (Fig. 16.9).

Pruritus

Pigs normally rub themselves at intervals, but pruritus with frequent rubbing may be caused by ectoparasites, especially in mange or louse infestation.

- Are any skin lesions present?
- Is the skin discoloured or damaged?
- How extensive are the lesions?

Abnormal body shape

Bodily disproportion   Some hereditary conditions such as the *humpy-backed pig syndrome* are associated with gross bodily disproportion.

Abdominal distension   This is an ominous sign, especially when seen in anorexic pigs. The most common cause is *rectal stricture* which can easily be overlooked. This is discussed below under 'Ab-

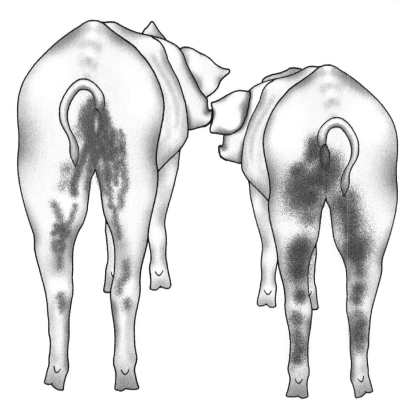

Figure 16.9 Pigs with swine dysentery. Note their poor bodily condition and the characteristic dark faecal staining on the perineum and hind legs.

domen'. Other causes of abdominal distension include ascites (rare in pigs and mostly associated with hepatic cirrhosis), peritonitis and obstruction of the small bowel by ascarid worms.

Twisting and deviation of the nose   This may occur in chronic cases of *atrophic rhinitis*.

Lateral deviation of the spine and swelling of the longissimus dorsi muscles (mostly unilateral)   This may be seen in cases of acute myopathy associated with vitamin E and/or selenium deficiency.

Muscle swelling   This may be seen in some forms of the *porcine stress syndrome* where muscle degeneration or necrosis has occurred.

Abnormal swellings on the body surface
Abnormal swellings on the body surface are common in pigs. Causes include hernias.

Scrotal and umbilical hernias (Fig. 16.10)   These are common in pigs, but provided they are reducible they are often left untreated. Where castration is practised constant vigilance for scrotal hernias is essential. Failure to detect it can have a fatal consequence if the bowel escapes through the opened hernia.

Subcutaneous abscesses   These are very common in pigs and are usually associated with bite wounds or other injury, with *Arcanobacterium pyogenes* being the common bacterial cause.

Haematomata   These are also usually associated with injury and may later become infected.

Aural haematomata   These affect the pinna of the ear (usually unilaterally) and may become so heavy that they cause a degree of head tilting. A common cause of aural haematomata is frequent head shaking which, in turn, may indicate mange infestation in and on the ears by *Sarcoptes scabiei*. Chronically

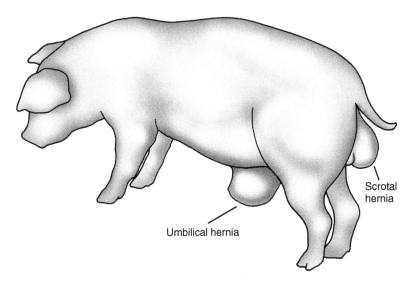

Umbilical hernia

Scrotal hernia

Figure 16.10 Pig with umbilical and scrotal hernias. It is unusual to see the two conditions in the same animal.

affected or untreated aural haematomata become crumpled and deformed – a *'cauliflower ear'*.

Swelling in the prepuce   Male pigs normally have a degree of swelling in the prepuce associated with the large *preputial diverticulum* in this species. This is discussed below under 'External genitalia in the boar'.

Callus formation   Especially over the pressure points of the elbow and hock, callus formation may be associated with inadequate bedding and poor hygiene. Secondary infection may be a complication of such lesions.

Clinical examination

Restraint for examination

To be effective and stress-free, the clinical examination must be carried out with minimum restraint of the patient. Some degree of confinement and prevention of escape will be necessary in many cases. A board can be used for this purpose (Fig. 16.11). Small piglets can be picked up by a hind leg and held for examination. If firm restraint is required, e.g. for blood sampling, restrain with a snare or a line around the upper jaw (Fig. 16.12). Large groups of pigs can be moved to smaller areas for detailed clinical examina-

tion. If the pigs are not anorexic their attention may be distracted by offering a little food whilst the clinical examination is performed. Individual pigs from weaners to adults can be restrained for taking temperature, looking at feet, and brief auscultation of the chest, by holding them by their tails (Fig. 16.13). This is not possible in docked animals. Feeding stalls or weighing crates can be useful to restrain single or groups of pigs.

Sedation of the pig

This may be necessary in some circumstances. *Azaperone* (Stresnil – Janssen Animal Health) is the only sedative licensed for use in pigs. The dose is 0.5 to 2.0 ml per 20 kg bodyweight; see datasheets for details. Given by intramuscular (i.m.) injection, the animal must be left undisturbed until the drug takes effect. Response to treatment is variable.

A more reliable and longer lasting (but unlicensed and expensive) combination of sedative drugs is as follows:

- detomidine 50 to 100 µg/kg by i.m. injection given in the same syringe as
- butorphanol 0.2 mg/kg by i.m. injection
- ketamine 3 to 5 mg/kg by i.m. injection given 5 to 10 minutes later.

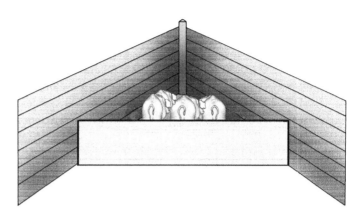

Figure 16.11 Board used to restrain a group of young pigs in a corner for examination and treatment.

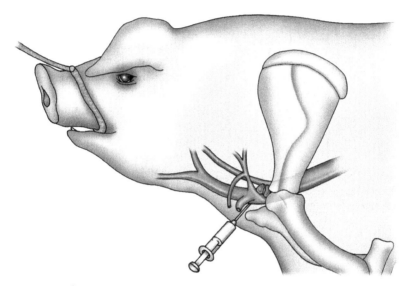

Figure 16.12 Pig restrained by a snare for blood sampling from the anterior vena cava. The snare is placed around the upper jaw as far back as possible and is tied to a fixed object such as a post. The needle is inserted at a point halfway between the shoulder joint and the manubrium of the sternum.

Emergency reversal of this combination is by i.m. injection of atipamazole 50 mg/kg.

Azaperone at a dose of 2 mg/kg may be substituted for detomidine in the above combination. Ketamine may be included in the same syringe as butorphanol and detomidine or azaperone.

Adult pigs

Temperature, pulse and respiration

Respiration Unless the pig is lying quietly or is ex-
tremely dyspnoeic, counting the respiratory rate can be difficult. In the less severely ill pig the respiratory rate changes frequently whenever the pig is disturbed or finds something interesting to smell or investigate. The *character* of porcine respiration is more important than the rate. The character and frequency of coughing and sneezing should also be noted.

Slow breathing with an intense inspiratory and expiratory effort may be seen in cases of rhinitis in which the pig – which is reluctant to breath through

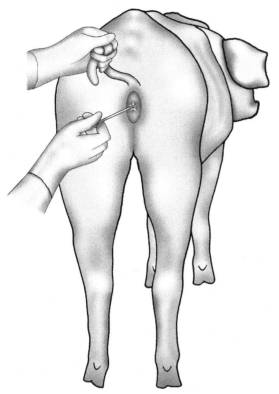

Figure 16.13 Tail hold for restraining a pig. The tail is looped round the first finger. Growing and adult pigs can be restrained for short periods using this technique. Here the pig is being held whilst its temperature is taken.

its mouth – experiences difficulty in forcing air through the congested and obstructed nasal passages. Rapid breathing with increased expiratory effort is seen in cases of enzootic pneumonia, for example, affected animals sometimes being termed 'panters'. Rapid breathing with cyanosis of the skin (white pigs) or mucous membranes (all pigs) indicates either severe cardiac disease, e.g. endocarditis, mulberry heart disease, or extremely poor lung function, e.g. as seen in advanced pneumonia and pleurisy. Open-mouthed breathing indicates severe respiratory distress (Fig. 16.14).

Temperature This is an extremely important parameter in pigs. The pig's normal temperature is 39°C (102.5°F) and any departure from this figure either up or down can be significant. The pig's temperature can rise rapidly in the presence of infection, and temperatures of 41°C may be seen with conditions such as subacute erysipelas, and 42°C with meningitis. *Heat stroke* is not uncommon, and body temperature can rise to 43°C (110°F). A temperature below 39°C is not a good sign, suggesting that the pig is unwell either through advanced disease, toxaemia or a metabolic disorder. Hypothermia can also occur in very sick pigs exposed to cold conditions. Further examination and tests may be necessary to elucidate

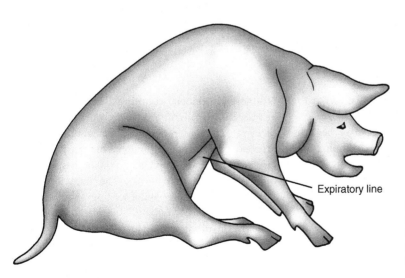

Expiratory line

Figure 16.14 Pig with severe respiratory distress. Note open mouth breathing, dog-sitting position and the expiratory line caused by intense muscular contraction as the pig tries to force air out of its lungs.

the cause of the problem. It is important to check that the thermometer is in contact with the rectal wall if a low temperature is recorded. Sudden movements of the pig backwards or sideways and other members of the group pushing between the clinician and the patient, can result in damage to the thermometer.

Pulse Occasionally in a quiet, thin pig it is possible to palpate the femoral artery pulse, but in most cases reliance is placed upon measuring the heart rate by auscultating the heart. The tendency of the pig to move when the stethoscope is placed on the chest means that in many cases the pulse can only be counted for brief periods of 10 seconds or so, and the pulse rate per minute is calculated from this brief observation. The normal pulse rate for adult pigs is approximately 100 beats/minute.

Mucous membranes

These can be inspected in a quiet pig by examining the ocular conjunctivae. Tickling the pig behind the eye with the finger and very quietly advancing the finger to depress the lower eyelid will allow brief but effective inspection and evaluation of the mucosa. In sows and gilts the vulval lining provides an alternative and easier access to the mucous membranes. Capillary refill time (normally 2 to 4 seconds) can be taken here. Pallor of the mucosae is seen in anaemia, yellow colouration in jaundice, and petechial haemorrhages in some cases of septicaemia.

Carcase lymph nodes

These cannot normally be palpated in pigs unless they are grossly enlarged, because they are both deeply buried and surrounded by fat. In some cases of *anthrax* one submandibular lymph node may be enlarged: see below under 'Neck'. Occasionally, in all ages of pig from 1 week to several years, *multicentric lymphosarcoma* is seen, with some or all of the lymph nodes being grossly enlarged, readily visible and palpable.

Skin

An overall assessment of the skin is made visually and then manually noting the following:

Skin colour This is important in white pigs. The skin may be red, inflamed and tender to the touch if *sunburned. Dark purple blotches* may be seen in cases of severe *toxaemia* and *septicaemia* resulting from toxic mastitis, for example. This is an ominous sign of life-threatening illness. Such areas are mostly seen on the lower surface of the neck, behind the elbows, on the caudal surface of the thighs and on the perineum (Fig. 16.15). *Skin pallor* is seen in cases of anaemia in a litter in which the iron injection has been missed. *Jaundice* is relatively uncommon in pigs, but can

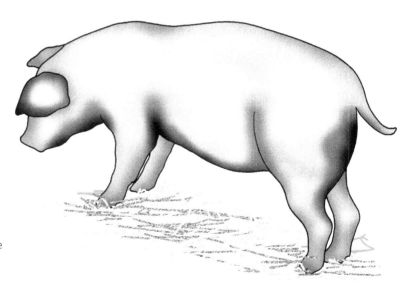

Figure 16.15 Skin discolouration in a pig with septicaemia. Dark purple blotches may be seen on the ear-tips, jowl, belly, behind the forelegs and on the caudal aspects of the thighs.

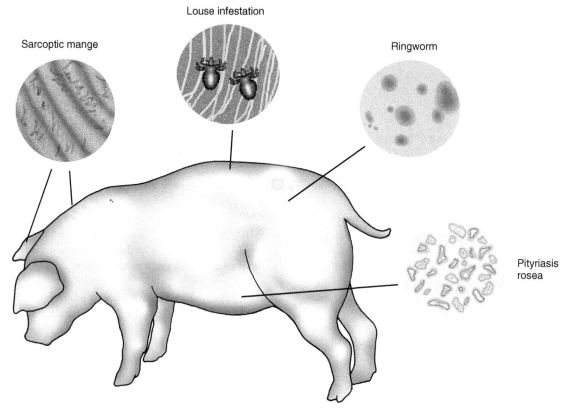

Figure 16.16 Skin diseases in pigs. Sow showing gross lesions and common sites of sarcoptic mange, louse infestation, ringworm and pityriasis.

occur in *Leptospira interrogans* (*Leptospira icterohaemorrhagica*) infection and in some cases of hepatic cirrhosis. It also occurs in some cases of postweaning multisystemic wasting syndrome (PMWS).

Ectoparasites The large dorsoventrally flattened *pig louse, Haematopinus suis*, is occasionally seen and may cause pruritus (Fig. 16.16). A more common condition is *sarcoptic mange*. Pruritic pink lesions are seen in early cases; thickened pruritic lesions on the head, back, flanks and hindquarters are seen later (Fig. 16.16). Mites are difficult to find in chronic cases where allergy-related skin changes are the dominant feature. *Sarcoptes scabiei* mites can occasionally be seen by eye in the dark wax of an infested ear, or identified microscopically: see below under 'Ears'.

Skin texture The skin of the dorsal part of the body is normally thick and immobile. On the ventral surface, the skin is normally quite thin and mobile. Generalised thickening of the skin may be seen in the rare conditions of zinc deficiency (*parakeratosis*) and vitamin B deficiency.

Skin turgor This can only be effectively assessed on the eyelids or on the ventral surface of the body. Turgor is increased in dehydrated animals, for example.

Skin lesions The *raised, diamond-shaped lesions* of acute and subacute *swine erysipelas* may be visible and palpable, especially on the dorsal surface of the neck and over the thoracic walls (Fig. 16.17). Initially the lesions are pink, but they become red and then black as the lesions age. Occasionally in neglected cases much of the thick skin of the dorsal surface of the body sloughs off leaving exposed subcutaneous tissues. In black pigs the lesions are palpable but

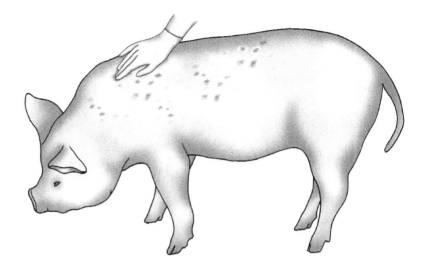

Figure 16.17 Sow with subacute swine erysipelas showing the characteristic diamond-shaped lesions on her skin: the lesions may be palpable before they are visible.

difficult to see. In other pigs they are palpable for some hours before they are visible. In adult animals the clinician's hand should always be run over the skin of the dorsal surface of the body, specifically feeling for erysipelas lesions, especially in febrile animals (Fig. 16.17).

Skin injuries such as *bite wounds* are very common and if caused by a boar's tusks may be both deep and extensive (Fig. 16.18). *Subcutaneous abscesses* are also common, being seen as raised, warm, fluctuant lesions of varying size: to confirm diagnosis a needle is inserted, releasing pus. *Pressure sores* may be seen over the elbows and just below the hocks. *Haematomata* are also commonly seen, and puncture by needle releases serum.

Variable hair growth is seen on the dorsal parts of the skin. Increased hair growth may be seen in ill-thriven animals.

Ringworm is common, especially in some outdoor herds; most cases are caused by *Trichophyton mentagrophytes* and large light brown irregular lesions are seen (Fig. 16.16). Much more common than true ringworm is the condition of unknown aetiology, *pityriasis rosea*, seen in individual growing pigs. Slightly elevated and irregular lesions are seen, especially on the ventral surface of the body (Fig. 16.16). The condition disappears as quickly as it appears.

Head
This is examined methodically noting the following:

Shape of the head In ill-thriven pigs, the nose may be very long and the head looks larger than the body. Also see below under 'Nose'.

Ears These should be checked for *bite wounds*, *haematomata* and *damage* sustained through loss of ear tags. The outside of the pinna should be examined for signs of *sarcoptic mange* such as crusty pruritic lesions, which are often also on the poll; the proximal ear canal should be examined for evidence of the dark wax also present with this infestation. In very good light it may be possible to see pin-head-sized mites moving in this wax. The pig's hearing should be checked by the animal's response to clapping hands. Foreign bodies in the ears and eyes of pigs are very uncommon.

Eyes The pig's eyes are seldom involved in disease. Vision should be checked. It may be compromised in some oriental breeds by skin folds over the eyelids. Signs of *nystagmus* may be seen in cases of meningitis. The eyes may quickly sustain *corneal damage* if the pig has struggled in lateral recumbency for some time. The eyes may be sunken in dehydrated ani-

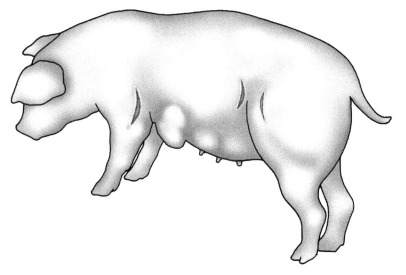

Figure 16.18 Sow showing bite wounds on her foreleg and flank. The swelling behind her left foreleg may be a haematoma or an abscess.

mals. Protrusion of the eyes giving an *exophthalmic appearance* is seen in the uncommon condition of *mediastinal lymphosarcoma*.

The *eyelids* may be swollen and oedematous in cases of *bowel oedema* (Fig. 16.7).

Ocular discharge may be seen in some respiratory infections with tear staining on the cheeks of affected animals.

Mouth   The mouth is difficult to examine in an unsedated subject, but is rarely involved in abnormalities. Excessive growth of the tusks may be seen in boars. In the unsedated animal the mouth can be examined by restraining the pig on a snare and prizing the mouth open with a smooth piece of wood.

Nose and nostrils   Asymmetry or deviation of the nose may be seen in cases of *atrophic rhinitis*. Nasal discharge, often mucopurulent, may be seen in cases of *rhinitis*. Snuffling breathing sounds may be heard from one or both nostrils in such cases.

Neck

This is short and fat, and it is impossible to see or raise the jugular vein. Swellings and oedema around the submandibular lymph nodes and larynx are seen in some cases of *anthrax*. *Nodular swellings* may be seen on the neck immediately behind ears caused by reaction to previous subcutaneous injection.

Heart

Auscultation of the heart can be difficult other than in quiet or very ill animals. The stethoscope is placed behind the shoulder joint at the level of the 5th rib. When possible, both sides of the chest should be auscultated. Gross cardiac abnormalities may be audible, e.g. a *murmur* over the tricuspid or mitral valve in some cases of *endocarditis*. When these animals are exercised a marked increase in heart rate is noted and the heart rate is slow to return to normal. A cardiac *apex beat* may be palpable in young, thin animals or anaemic animals where cardiac enlargement has occurred. Percussion of the porcine chest is usually unrewarding. *Fluid sounds* are occasionally heard in cases of *pericarditis* and *mulberry heart disease*.

Lungs

Auscultation of the lungs is unrewarding in many cases due to movement of the pig, noise from the patient, its fellows and the environment. In many cases, brief contact with the stethoscope on the chest wall is all that is possible. The lung field extends from the shoulder back to the 13th rib dorsally and ventrally back to the 7th rib. In advanced cases of *enzootic pneumonia* increased lung sounds, squeaks and bubbling sounds may be heard in the dependent portions of the lung lobes. In cases of *pleuropneumonia* abnormal sounds may also be present in the dorsal areas of the lung. *Pleuritic rubs* can be heard in some cases. Very little movement of the chest wall is seen during normal respiration. In cases of dyspnoea, there is increased movement in the abdominal muscles at inspiration and especially expiration.

Abdomen

A pig that is eating well should have a full appearance. Detailed palpation of the abdomen is resented and usually not tolerated by most pigs. In recumbent sows in late pregnancy, fetal presence and fetal movement may be detected. Gross abdominal distension may be caused by a *rectal stricture* in adult pigs. Suspicion of the presence of this lesion must be checked by digital rectal examination with a gloved, lubricated finger (Fig. 16.19) to see if a stricture is present about 2 cm anterior to the anus. An early indication of this condition is the difficulty experienced when inserting the thermometer. Affected pigs may be tympanitic and have some perineal faecal stain-

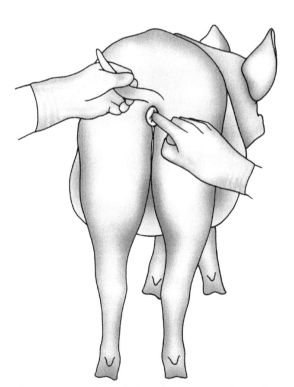

Figure 16.19 Pig with a rectal stricture. The pig is in poor condition and has a grossly distended abdomen. A digital rectal examination is essential to confirm the diagnosis.

ing, and also show intermittent flatus. Borborygmi are audible via the stethoscope in quiet animals, and suggest normal bowel movement. Percussion of the abdomen may reveal evidence of *ascites* in animals with pear-shaped enlarged abdomens and tympany in cases of rectal stricture or peritonitis. Ascites in pigs is usually associated with hepatic disease, especially cirrhosis.

Perineum

This is an important area. In scouring animals *faecal staining* around the anus and down the perineum may be seen. *Rectal and vaginal prolapses* are quite common, especially as farrowing approaches. Great care must be taken by inspection and palpation to determine which structure is (or whether both are) prolapsed.

External genitalia in the sow

The *vulva* should be inspected. The vulva is red and slightly oedematous during *oestrus*, at which time the sow will stand still when pressure is placed on her back. At other times such pressure would normally cause her to run away. *Vulval tears* are commonly seen and are mostly associated with bite wounds. *Vulval haematomata*, usually involving one lip of the vulva, are seen in postparturient sows. A white or yellow *vaginal discharge* may be seen in cases of MMA and also (without necessarily being abnormal) during pregnancy. *Metritis* may be part of the MMA syndrome, but can occur without signs of mammary abnormality. A *severe toxic metritis* with an associated unpleasant odour may follow retention of dead piglets at farrowing or following abortion. The discharge may contain fetal and placental remnants. A vaginal examination should be performed to confirm a suspicion of piglet retention. *Uterine prolapse* is often associated with fatal haemorrhage or severe shock. One or both horns may be completely or partially prolapsed.

Rectal examination in the sow

This can be carried out with a well-lubricated gloved hand. The dry faeces of the sow and her narrow pelvis make the procedure less informative than in the larger farm species. The caudal genital tract, the bladder, the blood vessels within the pelvis and sometimes the ovaries can be palpated. It may be possible to palpate the caudal pole of a grossly enlarged left kidney.

External genitalia in the boar

The *testes* are situated just below the anus. They should be of equal size and on palpation have the consistency of a ripe tomato. Softening and reduction in size may be seen in cases of testicular degeneration. The skin covering the scrotum is often damaged by fighting injuries. Vasectomy wounds, if present, will be found in the inguinal region. The *penis* can be palpated within the prepuce and the spiral anterior pole is found 10 cm from the anterior end of the prepuce. The *sigmoid flexure* of the penis in boars is anterior to the scrotum and in thin boars is palpable subcutaneously between the hind legs. The presence of the large fluctuant *preputial diverticulum* (Fig. 16.20) in boars has been mentioned above. Squeezing this swelling will usually cause foul smelling fluid to exude from the prepuce. The diverticulum can easily be mistaken for an abscess or hernia, with dangerous consequences. The clinician is advised to wear gloves when handling this area.

Bleeding from the prepuce may occur at or after service, and the erect penis should be examined at mating for evidence of wounds or other damage. Cases of *suspected infertility* are investigated as in the bull (see Chapter 11).

Udder

This must be examined in adult females or in gilts coming up to service: 14 teats should be present. In gilts some *teats may be inverted*. Some of these will evert with pregnancy and the onset of lactation. Each mammary gland should be examined. Each teat has two small orifices, and it is normal only to be able to squeeze out a bead of milk from each unless the sow is farrowing or feeding her piglets.

In *acute mastitis* one or more – but seldom all – of the glands are affected. They are hot, reddened and sometimes extremely hard and slightly oedematous (Fig. 16.21). In such cases life-threatening toxaemia may ensue. The temperature is initially elevated but may fall as the sow's condition worsens.

Chronic mastitis is seen mostly in dry sows with one or more mammary glands being replaced by chronic fibrous tissue, sometimes with purulent tracts (Fig. 16.1).

Bite wounds from other sows, the boar or her piglets may also be present. In *mastitis–metritis–agalactia* (MMA) syndrome. In this condition the whole udder is mildly indurated and a firm ridge is palpable on the lateral surfaces of the udder where it merges with the body wall (Fig. 16.22). In most MMA cases there is a white mucopurulent vaginal discharge and the body temperature is either normal or subnormal. In any case of agalactia the piglets rapidly show signs of hunger

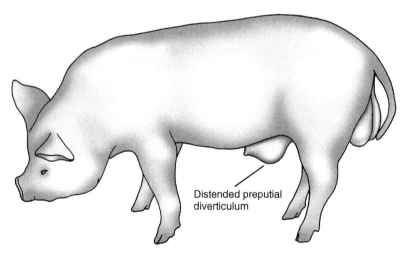

Distended preputial diverticulum

Figure 16.20 Young boar with a distended preputial diverticulum. See text for details.

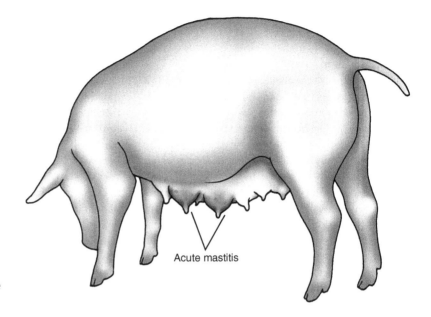

Figure 16.21 Sow with acute mastitis involving two mammary glands. The affected glands are inflamed, swollen, extremely hard, and may be painful to the touch.

Acute mastitis

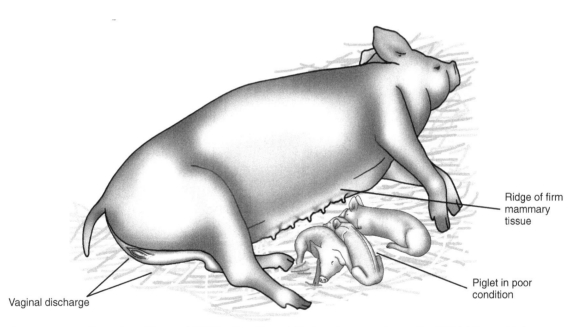

Ridge of firm mammary tissue

Piglet in poor condition

Vaginal discharge

Figure 16.22 Sow with mastitis–metritis–agalactia (MMA) syndrome. The sow is lying in semisternal recumbency, a ridge of slightly indurated udder is palpable, and the sow has a slight vaginal discharge. The few piglets present are depressed and one is in poor condition.

and decline – observation of this may indicate disease in the mother.

Urinary system

Pyelonephritis is sometimes seen in sows and gilts a few days after service. Boars are less commonly affected. The condition should always be considered and a urine sample from dull animals, examined, especially from those in the post-service period. The animal is initially mildly febrile, but in untreated cases the temperature soon falls and the animal becomes toxaemic and uraemic. Examination of a urine sample will confirm the condition by the presence of pus, blood and cellular debris. The sow can be encouraged to pass a urine sample by stimulating the vulval skin in the standing patient. If this is not successful a catheter can be digitally inserted into the external urethral orifice, which is palpable on the pelvic floor, and passed forwards into the bladder.

Limbs and feet

Lameness and reluctance to get up and to move often indicate problems with the limbs. Visual inspection will allow the clinician to compare an abnormal limb with the opposite side. Gross lesions such as *broken claws* or *swollen joints* may be hidden by bedding or mud. Each limb is examined methodically starting with the foot. *Overgrown hooves* which become cracked may be painful and cause lameness. Unsedated pigs usually resent attempts to pick up their feet: hence, it is best to examine them when the pig is recumbent. Massage of a quiet sow's udder may encourage her to remain in lateral recumbency while her feet are examined (Fig. 16.23). In cases of lameness in adult pigs, it is advisable to examine the foot in detail before attempts are made to persuade the patient to stand. The solar surface of the digits is examined for evidence of injury, erosion or infection (Fig. 16.24). Defects in the hoof can be caused by injury or biotin deficiency. *Infection in the white line* is sometimes seen (Fig. 16.25) and may extend to the coronary band. Infection just above the coronary band with severe swelling in the fetlock area has been termed *bumble-foot* and is so painful that although the pig is able to put its foot down it is very reluctant to do so. Skin lesions of vesicle formation and subsequent ulceration are seen in cases of *foot-and-mouth disease*, *swine vesicular disease* and also through contact with

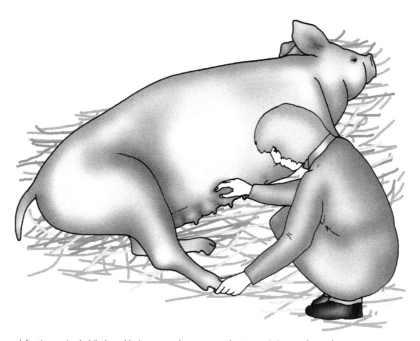

Figure 16.23 The sow's foot is examined whilst her udder is massaged to encourage her to remain in sternal recumbency.

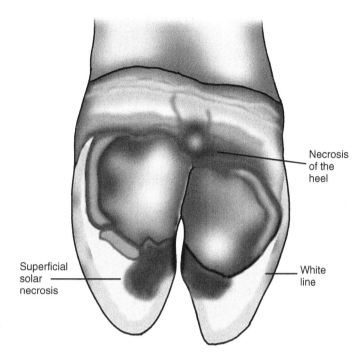

Figure 16.24 Pig's foot showing areas of necrosis in the sole and heel.

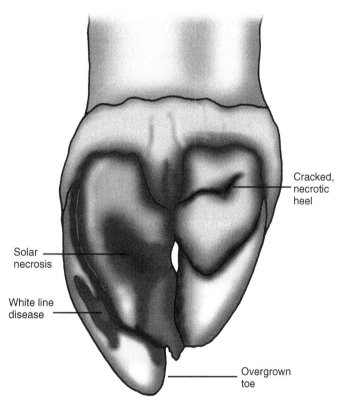

Figure 16.25 Pig's foot showing overgrowth of the lateral toe, white line disease and some necrosis of the sole and heel.

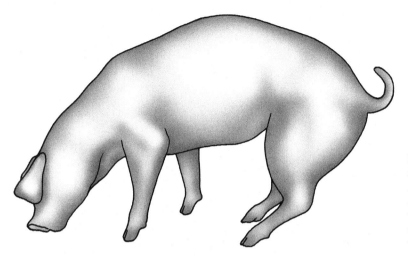

Figure 16.26 Growing pig showing signs of polyarthritis caused by *Mycoplasma hyosynoviae*. Note the distended hock joint and the hind feet placed abnormally far forward. The animal is trying to take weight on its nose in an attempt to reduce the weight on its painful forelegs.

corrosive chemicals, which may include concentrated disinfectant.

Joints The joints should be examined: heat, swelling and distension of the joint capsules may be seen in cases of *septic* or *mycoplasma arthritis* in which one or more joints may be affected (Fig. 16.26). In chronic cases, severe swelling of the joints may be seen, with involvement of the surrounding tissues including the bones. The exact pathology may only be determined by X-ray examination. In some cases there is little bony involvement, but in others severe destructive *osteomyelitis* is present. Affected joints can become completely or partially ankylosed with severe reduction in movement. Streptococcal, *Arcanobacterium pyogenes*, mycoplasma or *Haemophilus* infections may be involved. *Chronic arthritis* associated with erysipelas is often associated with exostosis formation in the distal radius and tibia, and proximal metacarpus and metatarsus, with little increase in joint fluid. Collecting samples of joint fluid for cytology requires sedation of the patient. Tendon damage is relatively uncommon in pigs.

Fractures These often occur as the result of injury and may involve the long bones, especially the femur and humerus of fast growing pigs. Affected limbs are non-weight bearing, but palpation of the fracture can be difficult as a result of the thick surrounding musculature. Crepitus may be palpable or can be heard

through the stethoscope. *Slippage of the epiphyseal head of the femur* is seen in young boars and gilts. It results in severe lameness in which the animal is able but reluctant to bear weight. Muscle wasting around the affected area rapidly develops. Confirmation of this diagnosis requires radiography of the anaesthetised animal. This lesion is part of the *osteochondrosis leg weakness syndrome*. In other cases of the syndrome, cartilage abnormalities may lead to *degenerative joint disease* and bowing deformity of long bones. An X-ray and sometimes a post-mortem examination may be used diagnostically.

Muscle rupture This is sometimes caused by the animal slipping. Damage to the adductors of the hind limbs occurs when both hind limbs slip laterally on a slippery surface. Affected animals are unable to get to their feet without help, but complete resolution may occur with time.

Piglets

Piglets can easily be picked up for close examination. Lifting them quietly by a hind leg will often enable them to be picked up and examined in silence. Holding them around their thorax will mostly cause squealing, and if one piglet in the litter objects noisily the others will usually do the same when picked up. Squealing by piglets can provoke aggression in the sow, and if treatment of the piglets is proposed it is

The piglets are examined visually all over, checking the entire body for signs of abnormality. As they are picked up *febrile piglets* may feel very warm to the touch and in joint ill cases the joints, especially the hocks, may also feel very warm. Temperature and pulse may be higher than in older pigs. Neonatal piglets are susceptible to *hypothermia*. *Pericarditis* is a complication of some neglected cases of *iron deficiency anaemia*, and auscultation of the chest in such cases may reveal muffling of heart sounds and other cardiac pathology. Sudden death can occur when such patients are handled.

General examination of piglets is as for adult pigs with the following additional features:

Skin

This is delicate and easily damaged in piglets. Large subcutaneous *haematomata* can also arise from crushing injuries caused by the sow in which subcutaneous haemorrhage occurs. Superficial bite injuries on the snout arise as a result of fighting with other piglets for teats. Skin infections such as *greasy pig disease* (exudative epidermitis) caused by *Staphylococcus hyicus* may be seen on the face and body (Fig. 16.27). *Skin abrasions* may be seen, especially over the carpus and lower forelimb, if the floor surface is not smooth. Abscesses may also be seen.

Head

Inclusion body rhinitis may cause snuffling in very young piglets. The canine teeth of piglets are very sharp and are usually clipped at birth. If this has been badly done, foul smelling infected lesions may be found at the base of these teeth and involving the gums. *Necrotic stomatitis* lesions, which are diphtheritic and foul smelling, may be seen on the tongue or cheeks. A number of *congenital abnormalities* may involve the head, including macroglossus and microphthalmia. *Conjunctivitis* is seen in a number of conditions including classical swine fever.

Abdomen

Abdominal distension in piglets is often caused by an *imperforate anus*, and the anus should be carefully checked for patency in such cases. *Scrotal* and *umbilical hernias* may be visible in early life (Fig. 16.10).

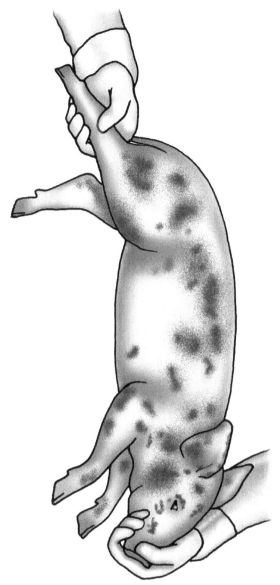

Figure 16.27 Piglet held by the hind leg with the mouth closed. Dark, crusty lesions of greasy pig disease are seen on many parts of the skin.

best to remove them from the sow into a box or the creep area for safety. Squealing is high pitched and intense, but the volume can be effectively reduced by holding a noisy piglet's mouth closed during the examination (Fig. 16.27). This should not be done if there is evidence of respiratory distress.

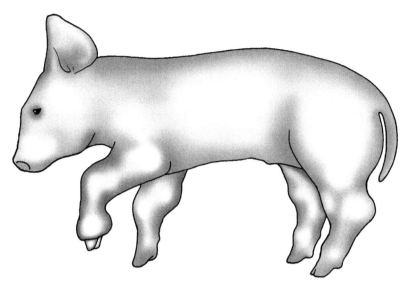

Figure 16.28 Piglet with polyarthritis (joint ill). Note distension of the carpal, hock, elbow and fetlock joints. The gross distension of the lower left forelimb may be caused by arthritis or local abscess formation.

Joints

Joint swelling and heat is seen in cases of *septic arthritis*, which is a common cause of lameness in piglets (Fig. 16.28). Chronic changes including joint ankylosis may develop in untreated animals (Fig. 16.29).

Crushing injuries inflicted by the sow involving the limbs can cause severe lameness in piglets.

Feet

Bruising of the feet and *sole erosions* are quite common in baby piglets and may be caused by unsuitable flooring.

Diarrhoea

This is a very common sign in piglets and is often associated with severe depression and dehydration. *Escherichia coli enteritis* often causes a yellow scour and may be accompanied by *rotavirus* infection. Many of the viral infections such as *transmissible gastroenteritis* (TGE) produce a green scour. In both these conditions the piglets are thin and empty looking.

In *Clostridium perfringens* infection, diarrhoea is heavily contaminated with blood. Affected animals often look plump and well-fed, but death can occur very rapidly. Laboratory assistance is required to determine the cause of enteritis.

Other diagnostic aids

Careful and patient observation and examination of the porcine patient will normally result in a provisional diagnosis of the disease. Other aids such as radiography and ultrasonography are also helpful. When ultrasonography is used, great care must be taken to prevent the patient or its fellows from damaging the expensive and delicate instrument. The cost of such procedures should be carefully considered and discussed with the farmer. Sacrifice of a severely affected animal for post-mortem examination may be useful as a diagnostic aid. A complete post-mortem examination may be carried out on the farm. Samples are taken for serology, haematology, microbiology, virus isolation or histopathology as required. Examples include faecal samples for culture and skin scrapings. Diagnostic samples may be collected after slaughter at the abattoir. These include lungs and snouts to determine the extent of diseases such as enzootic pneumonia and atrophic rhinitis.

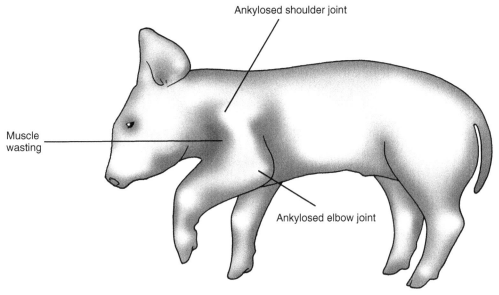

Muscle
wasting

Ankylosed shoulder joint

Ankylosed elbow joint

Figure 16.29 Piglet with chronic arthritis of the left shoulder and elbow joints. The joints are ankylosed and there is severe muscle wasting on the upper limb.

CLINICIAN'S CHECKLIST – CLINICAL EXAMINATION OF PIGS

Careful observation should precede clinical examination
Observe and preserve health status of the farm
Owner's complaint
History – long term and short term
Signalment – breed, age and sex of the pig or pigs
Pigs' environment – observation and inspection
Observation of the pig or group of pigs
   Behaviour
   Clinical observation
Clinical examination
   Temperature, pulse and respiration
   Inspection of mucous membranes
   Palpation of carcase lymph nodes – often not palpable
   Skin

Head and neck
Heart and lungs
Abdomen, including digital rectal examination if abdomen
   distended
Udder
Perineum
External genitalia of the sow
External genitalia of the boar
Urinary system
Limbs and feet
Special features of clinical examination of piglets
Clinical pathology (if required)
Post-mortem examination (if required)

Part V

Goats

Clinical Examination of the Goat

Introduction

Goats are kept individually or in small groups as pets. Small and large herds of goats are kept for milk, fibre or meat production. Goats are often classified with sheep as small ruminants, but although there are some similarities between the species there are also important differences.

Many owners are very experienced and knowledgeable, but others may have little knowledge of caprine husbandry and disease. Illness may not be recognised until the disease has reached an advanced stage.

Although happy to graze, goats are by choice browsing animals and require secure fencing. Goatlings are able to jump over fences exceeding their own height. Goats can reach high branches, including those of toxic plants. Many goats can tolerate regular exposure to small quantities of toxic plants. They are adversely affected by larger amounts of such plants or by sudden exposure to them.

Production records

These may be available in milk producing herds. Many commercial doe goats are only bred once in two years.

Owner's complaint

This can be helpful in focusing the clinician to a particular disease syndrome.

History

The long-term and short-term history of the herd and patient should be considered. The background health status of the herd can provide useful information, as can details of parasite control and disease prophylaxis. Parasite levels in pet goats living alone can be very high. Vaccination against the clostridial diseases, including booster vaccination, is not always practised. Some herds are vaccinated against *Chlamydia* and *Toxoplasma* abortion. Imported goats may bring in exotic diseases. Recent attendance at shows allows contact between different groups of animals and the possible transmission of diseases such as mange and ringworm.

Signalment

The breed, age and sex of the patient can provide important information. Some conditions are confined to a single breed. The sticky kid syndrome is seen only in male kids of the Golden Guernsey breed. British Saanen goats are heavy milkers and with British Toggenburgs may be particularly prone to production diseases such as ketosis and hypocalcaemia. Maiden milking (milking without a prior pregnancy) and *gynaecomastia* (milk production by the male) are particularly common in British Saanen goats.

Environment

This should be carefully checked for factors that might predispose to disease. Goats do not tolerate cold or wet conditions caused by inadequate shelter, especially in winter. Kids are especially vulnerable to cold. Sunburn may occur on the faces of white goats, and primary or secondary photosensitisation can also produce skin lesions. Although quite fastidious feeders, goats may be tempted to eat poisonous plants. If consumption of such plants is suspected, the pasture and surrounding hedgerows should be checked for their presence. The availability of good food and water should be assessed in every environment. Goats may refuse to eat low quality concentrates or roughage. Zinc and other trace element deficiencies have been seen in some herds. The composition of any concentrate diet, vitamin or mineral supplement should be checked.

Observation of the patient

The goat should be observed as unobtrusively as possible. Healthy goats are usually quite active. They are alert to noise and the activity of other animals. They are inquisitive and usually approach people in a friendly manner. Bleating is heard quite frequently. Some goats are in the habit of 'star gazing'. They look upwards and then rotate their heads through an angle of at least 180 degrees. This movement is repeated quite often and is considered normal. Heart failure in goats is uncommon, but if present and the patient's coat is short, jugular distension can be readily seen and brisket oedema may also be present.

The patient's bodily condition score is best determined when the goat is physically examined. Weight loss may be caused by malnutrition, a high parasite burden and chronic conditions such as Johne's disease. The patient's breathing and any evidence of coughing or diarrhoea may be observed at this stage.

The overall shape of the body should be observed. Distension of the left upper quadrant of the abdomen is seen in cases of bloat. Right-sided distension in the ventral quadrant may occur in cases of vagal malfunction in which abomasal emptying is delayed. Abdominal enlargement occurs in pregnancy and also in pseudopregnancy from which it should always be differentiated (see below). Some elderly but healthy doe goats develop a pear-shaped and rather pendulous abdomen as they lose muscle tone.

Skin diseases in goats are quite common. Some conditions such as sarcoptic mange are associated with intense pruritus. Affected animals may rub or nibble at themselves frequently, and areas of alopecia and excoriation are seen.

Signs of lameness are normally readily detected and enable the clinician to see which leg(s) are involved. Joint swelling is seen in a number of conditions including caprine arthritis encephalitis virus (CAEV) syndrome. Foot lameness is common, and a detailed examination of the feet at a later stage is required.

Disparity between the two sides of the udder may be seen in cases of chronic mastitis. Unilateral orchitis can be suspected if an obvious disparity in size between the testes is observed. Intersex in goats is associated with the polled (hornless) state. In some affected animals gross abnormality of the external genitalia may be seen, but requires a detailed gynaecological examination for confirmation. Vaginal discharge may indicate the presence of a uterine infection or the presence of a genital tumour.

Neurological diseases affecting behaviour, gait and balance include scrapie, listeriosis and gid.

Close observation of the goat

This can be carried out before or after the animal is restrained. When approached, recumbent healthy goats normally rise. If they are very friendly and relaxed or too ill to stand they may not get up. The animal is inspected methodically, commencing at the head or any other convenient point. The coat should be sleek and slightly shiny. Any areas of hair loss, excessive grooming or visibly inflamed skin should be noted for further examination. Obvious swellings or discharges anywhere on the body should also be noted. The eyes should be bright and free from ocular discharge. With the exception of the Anglo-Nubian, the ears are carried in an erect position. Drooping of one or both ears and other signs of ear discomfort may be seen in cases of psoroptic mange (see below). The head and neck are very mobile, and the goat will follow the clinician in an interested manner with its head, sometimes sniffing or making contact with its lips.

The animal should be breathing normally and with minimal effort. The abdomen should look full, but not be abnormally distended. The goat should be weight bearing on its four legs. Faeces are dry and pelleted and are passed with little effort at frequent intervals. In both sexes urination often occurs without effort as the animal is restrained.

Abnormalities of gait and posture may be detected at this stage. Behavioural abnormalities can be associated with specific diseases such as scrapie and the metabolic diseases including hypocalcaemia, hypomagnesaemia and ketosis. A wide range of neurological signs has been seen in cases of scrapie in goats. Cardiac insufficiency and terminal illness may be accompanied by abnormal behaviour.

Clinical examination

The goat should be restrained for clinical examination. If used to a halter or head collar, the patient can be secured by this. If unused to head restraint the animal may fight against it and become distressed. In such cases the goat can be readily restrained by an assistant with one arm in front of the base of the neck and the other around the hindquarters. Horned animals must be held with care to avoid damage being done to the horns or a butting injury being sustained by the clinician.

Temperature, pulse and respiration

Respiratory rate and character should be assessed before restraint, temperature and pulse (from the femoral artery) being taken immediately after the animal is restrained. The normal values are given in Table 17.1.

The *mucous membrane colour* can be assessed in the conjunctival or vulval mucosa; it should be salmon pink. Pallor may indicate *anaemia* which is investigated as in cattle. Causes of caprine anaemia include copper deficiency and a high nematode burden. The membranes may be *yellow* in jaundiced animals and congested in the presence of infectious diseases in which pyrexia is present. In terminal toxaemia the membranes may become pale and pinkish-grey in colour. The *capillary refill time* is taken either at the

Table 17.1 Normal temperature, pulse and respiration rates in goats

Temperature	39–40°C
Pulse rate	70–90 beats/min
Respiratory rate	
Adult	15–30 breaths/min
Kid	20–40 breaths/min

vulval mucosa or in a non-pigmented part of the gum or dental pad. It should be less than 2 seconds and not more than 3 seconds. The *state of hydration* should be checked by raising a fold of skin on the neck or chest wall. In a well hydrated animal the skin should immediately fall back into place.

Carcase lymph nodes

These have approximately the same distribution as in cattle. Lymph node enlargement is normally readily palpated. The parotid and submandibular lymph nodes are frequently the site of infection with *caseous lymphadenitis*. Fluctuant swellings may be present. If these rupture spontaneously or are opened, thick green pus is seen. Abscesses caused by the organism may be located, but are initially symptomless elsewhere in the body including the chest and pituitary gland. Enlargement of other lymph nodes may indicate active or recent local infection.

Skin

This should receive a comprehensive visual and manual inspection over as much of the body as possible. Skin disease is common in goats, and differential diagnosis may require laboratory testing. Skin thickness and mobility are checked and any variation in temperature noted for evidence of local inflammation. The flexor surfaces of normal joints often feel warm to the touch if the goat has recently been recumbent. These areas can also be infested with sarcoptic mange and are one site of seborrhoeic dermatitis in pygmy goats.

Skin health is often a reflection of the general health of the patient. *Chronically ill goats*, including those carrying large intestinal worm burdens, may have dry scaly skin with reduced elasticity and hair growth. Some skin diseases such as orf and ringworm are zoonotic.

The *distribution of skin lesions* is also important. Ringworm lesions, for example, are mostly found on the head.

Self inflicted injuries
These are seen with pruritic skin diseases. Goats with chorioptic mange may nibble at the lesions seen on

the caudal aspect of the lower limb. Perineal lesions are easily accessible to the goat, and any irritation in this area may be the subject of biting and severe secondary damage. During the breeding season male goats frequently urinate on the caudal aspects of their forelegs. This can produce raw inflamed areas which the animal may nibble and rub. Self inflicted skin injuries are also occasionally seen in cases of scrapie. Affected animals may bite at their legs with a manic intensity, producing quite deep wounds.

Common skin diseases

Some of the more common skin diseases of goats are described in summary form below. A number of diseases cause dry crusty lesions with a varying degree of pruritus. In many cases, skin scrapings, bacterial culture and biopsy may be required to arrive at a definitive diagnosis. Wherever possible and subject to economic considerations, samples should be taken early on in the course of the disease and from the youngest lesions present.

Louse infestation   This is a common problem. Both chewing and sucking lice may be seen. They often cause intense pruritus and are usually clearly visible as a result of hair loss in affected areas. The species of louse involved can be identified by microscopic examination of individual lice or those found in skin scrapings. Egg cases are often found adherent to hairs.

Mange mite infestation   All four species of mange mites can cause skin disease in goats (Fig. 17.1).

Sarcoptic mange – dry crusty intensely pruritic lesions are found on the head (especially on the outer surface of the pinnae, around the eyes and the lips and chin). They are also found on the legs, perineum and tail.

Chorioptic mange – is found chiefly on the caudal surface of the lower parts of the legs. Crusty superficial pruritic lesions are seen, and the surface-living mite is normally readily identified in skin scrapings.

Psoroptic mange – is found on the inner surface of the pinnae of infested goats. Some irritation is seen and the affected ear may appear to be uncomfortable. The lesions, which extend into the external auditory canal, are dry, crusty and layered.

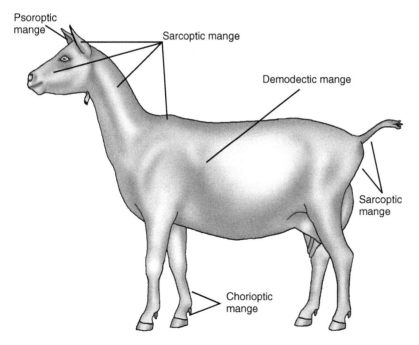

Figure 17.1 Common sites of mange infestation in goats.

Demodectic mange – is found in a pustular form often in the skin covering the patient's ribs. Compression of the slightly pruritic pustules releases small quantities of purulent material in which large numbers of mites can be found.

Fly worry   This may produce raised oedematous urticarial lesions at the site of individual fly bites. *Blow-fly strike* is less common in goats than in sheep. Open wounds and faecal soiling in moribund goats may predispose to infestation. Recumbent goats must be carefully examined all over to ensure blow-fly strike is not present.

Bacterial skin disease   This is seen chiefly in debilitated animals. *Staphylococcus aureus* can produce a pustular dermatitis. Areas of thickened, slightly pruritic crusty skin may be seen in areas, including the chest wall and udder, from which the causal organism can be cultured. *Arcanobacterium pyogenes* is an opportunist pathogen causing subcutaneous abscesses in various parts of the body. It gains access through wounds sustained accidentally. Hard granulomatous lesions up to 4 cm in diameter may develop subcutaneously in goats following clostridial vaccination.

Viral skin diseases   *Contagious pustular dermatitis (orf)* is seen in goats, although less commonly than in sheep. Dry proliferative crusty lesions are seen on their lips and may also be present on the udder, feet and tail. Removal of the crusts reveals painful, inflamed, exudative tissue underneath. The causal parapoxvirus can be identified using electron microscopy.

Foot-and-mouth disease – the virus causes vesicles and then ulcerated areas on the lips, gums, teats, coronary band and the interdigital region of the feet. Affected animals may also be lethargic, pyrexic and anorexic.

Papillomatosis – viral warts can be found on the skin in various parts of the body including the udder and teats.

Ringworm   This is a relatively uncommon problem in goats. Affected animals have a number of dry slightly raised white or grey lesions, very similar to those seen in cattle.

Psoriasiform dermatitis in pygmy goats   This condition of unknown aetiology is seen in certain families of pygmy goat. Affected animals have crusty lesions in the same areas as may be infested with sarcoptic mange. The lesions are less pruritic than those of sarcoptic mange. Histology shows cellular changes similar to those of human psoriasis.

Less common skin diseases   These include the following:

Sticky kid disease – seen only in male kids of the Golden Guernsey breed. Affected kids are normal apart from the skin which fails to dry out after birth. Sebum secretion appears excessive, although its composition is normal. Affected kids may be susceptible to other disease conditions.
Pemphigus foleaceous – this autoimmune disease produces crusty lesions at the mucocutaneous junction of areas including the mouth, eyes and perineum.
Infestation with ticks, keds, harvest mites and Cheyletiella – may produce skin lesions confirmed by isolation of the causal agent. All are capable of producing local irritation which is sometimes worsened by self inflicted damage.

Photosensitisation following consumption of plants such as St John's wort and exposure of non-pigmented areas of skin to the sun can lead to skin lesions. Affected skin has deep fissures, leakage of serum in the early stages and extensive superficial scabs.

Head and neck

The two sides of the head should be compared to see if there is any disparity between them. *Listeriosis* can cause local paralysis of the facial muscles, including those controlling ear movements. In some cases nystagmus is also seen. The *goat's breath* should be smelled – ketone bodies, levels of which are high in cases of *ketosis*, may be detected in this way. They can be more reliably recognised by analysis of milk or serum. *Foul smelling breath* may indicate oral (including dental) or respiratory disease; further examination should confirm whether either is present. The patient's ability to see and hear should be checked.

Excessive salivation is uncommon. It may be associated with oral disease or oesophageal obstruction (choke) and other causes of dysphagia including enlargement of the retropharyngeal lymph nodes. *Salivary cysts* occur chiefly in Anglo-Nubian goats and some are congenital: the cysts are fluid filled, painless swellings seen either in the submandibular area or on the side of the face. Salivary duct damage may lead to oral *mucocoele* formation. *Facial abscesses* may follow injury or tooth root infection. Ultrasonography, radiography and needle aspiration are useful aids to diagnosis. Goats suffering from *tetanus* may show signs of bloat, trismus, hyperaesthesia and uncontrolled tetany of the muscles. *Nasal discharge* is uncommon, but may be seen in cases of sinusitis and upper respiratory infection. The patient's palpebral, menace, corneal and light response reflexes should be tested. Tongue control, swallowing, etc., should also be observed to ensure there are no other *cranial nerve deficits*.

Eyes

The eyes should be examined for any signs of disease. The iris is usually quite pale and surrounds the horizontally oblong pupil. *Infectious keratoconjunctivitis* is seen occasionally and may spread to other animals within a group. The conjunctiva is inflamed and there may be an ocular discharge. The cornea often becomes opaque and vision may be impaired. *Squamous cell carcinomata* occasionally involve the eyelids.

Foreign bodies in the eye are seen, especially when young goats are feeding from an elevated hay rack. Initial unilateral epiphora and blepharospasm may be followed by further inflammation and corneal damage. A foreign body can slip under the third eyelid. The conjunctivae should be thoroughly searched after the administration of a topical anaesthetic. Playful or aggressive butting may lead to *corneal damage*. Deeper lacerations in or around the eye can occur as a result of horning injuries. The exact details of any injury must be determined by a careful and methodical examination under sedation and topical anaesthesia.

Entropion is rare in kids. One or both lower eyelids may be involved. Initially epiphora is seen but in untreated cases severe corneal ulceration may follow.

Mouth

This should be carefully examined. Goats do not like having their mouths opened and it may be necessary to use a gag. The mouth, including the tongue and teeth, should be carefully examined to ensure that no visible abnormalities are present. Deciduous and permanent dental details are summarised below.

Caprine dentition

The arrangement of teeth in goats is given in Table 17.2. The permanent incisors erupt sequentially as follows:

1st (central) incisor	15 months
2nd pair of incisors	21 months
3rd pair of incisors	27 months
4th pair of incisors	33 months

Care must be taken to identify and distinguish deciduous and permanent teeth. After 15 months when the incisor teeth are changing a clear distinction between the two tooth types is readily seen. At first glance there is some similarity between the full mouth of a 12 month old goatling and that of a 3-year-old doe.

Tooth wear is dependent on age and diet. Signs of wear, possible tooth loss and some loosening of teeth are often seen in animals over 5 years of age. The cheek teeth should always be examined, especially if the incisors are showing signs of wear. Gross abnormalities such as missing or overgrown teeth may be palpable through the cheeks. In the relatively un-

Table 17.2 Caprine dentition

	Incisors	Premolars	Molars	Total teeth
Deciduous teeth				20
Upper jaw	0	3	0	
Lower jaw	4	3	0	
Permanent teeth				32
Upper jaw	0	3	3	
Lower jaw	4	3	3	

common condition of *mandibular lymphosarcoma* the incisor teeth may become very loose as mandibular bone is replaced by tumour tissue. The animal may be unable to prehend food, although the teeth themselves may appear normal. X-ray examination of the mandible reveals the extent of bony damage. Spread to other organs may occur. *Giant cell tumours* may also have a predilection site in the mandible.

Cardiovascular system

Heart disease is relatively uncommon. Kids are occasionally born with *cardiac anomalies* which may be incompatible with life or with normal growth and development. In most cases they can be located by auscultation and ultrasonography. Severe vitamin E and/or selenium deficiency may cause *cardiomyopathy* in kids: sudden death or signs of heart failure may be seen. The deficiency is further discussed under the locomotor system. *Congestive heart failure* is occasionally seen in older animals or those with cardiac anomalies. Clinical signs include distension of the jugular veins and brisket oedema. The cause of heart failure can be investigated in detail as in cattle (Chapter 6).

Respiratory system

The animal will usually be examined as a result of difficulty of breathing, coughing and other signs of respiratory distress. Rapid breathing alone is not necessarily a sign of respiratory disease since it may be seen in cases of hypocalcaemia, heart disease, bloat and also terminal diseases of various aetiologies. If other animals are showing similar clinical signs they may all be suffering from the same infection or have been exposed to the same adverse environment, including very hot weather. *Hyperthermia* can cause rapid breathing in affected animals.

Coughing in animals either at or recently brought in from pasture can be caused by infestation by *lungworms*, including *Dictyocaulus filaria* and *Muellerius capillaris*.

Dusty, poorly ventilated buildings can both predispose to respiratory disease and exacerbate the signs of an existing problem. *Vaccination history* is also important: *Mannheimia haemolytica* (*Pasteurella*

haemolytica) is an important respiratory pathogen in goats, and vaccination against the organism is used in some herds. In outbreaks of respiratory disease due to *M. haemolytica* and other bacterial infections, affected animals are often pyrexic and anorexic. Viruses are not currently thought to play a major role in caprine respiratory disease. Pneumonia may, however, be a feature of CAEV infection. Inhalation pneumonia may occur in animals that have been drenched carelessly.

The animal should be watched to see the pattern of respiratory movements and whether inspiration appears more difficult than expiration. *Tracheal collapse* may cause inspiratory dyspnoea, whilst *emphysema* may cause difficulties on expiration.

The chest is examined by auscultation and percussion. Radiography and ultrasonography may also be used. The harsh breathing seen in sheep shortly after restraint is not seen in goats. The upper and lower parts of the respiratory tract are auscultated to determine whether any pathological findings are general or localised. In cases of pneumonia, lung sounds over the whole lung field are increased and abnormal sounds (squeaks, bubbling sounds) are audible in the dependent parts of the lung. Rubbing sounds associated with pleurisy and crackling sounds associated with emphysema may also be heard. Percussion may provide evidence of ventral consolidation of diseased lungs.

Further diagnostic tests may include attempts to isolate causal organisms from nasopharyngeal swabs or by tracheal lavage in the sedated animal. Diagnosis of lungworm infestation may involve larval counts in faeces.

Gastrointestinal system

This is quite frequently involved in caprine disease and is approached as in other ruminants. The history of the patient is of great importance. Changes in diet can cause diarrhoea and colic, as can possible exposure to toxic materials. Details of herd internal parasite control are also important. *Anthelmintic resistance* has been seen in goats. A *history of recent worming* does not mean that helminths can be ruled out from the diagnosis. Patient *signalment* is also important. Alterations in the milk supply to kids is an important cause of diarrhoea. *Coccidiosis* is a major cause of diarrhoea in kids over 4 weeks of age, but may also affect older animals. *Carbohydrate engorgement* can affect goats of any age fed on concentrates.

Changes in appetite

These may be a sign of disease, including those involving the gastrointestinal system. *Idiopathic anorexia* is occasionally seen in goats, possibly following a change of ownership and home. No specific signs of disease is shown and all blood and biochemical parameters may be normal.

Abnormalities in abdominal shape

In *ruminal bloat* the left and subsequently the right side of the abdomen may be distended and the tympanitic rumen is detected by percussion. Ruminal gas can be released by nasogastric tube. Rumen fluid samples for evaluation of pH and normal protozoa can be taken by this route or by paracentesis. Ruminal movements can be monitored by auscultation. The dorsal sac of the rumen is smaller than the ventral sac in goats, and movements may not be heard unless the stethoscope is directed anteriorly just under the last rib on the left side. Normal ruminal contents have a dough-like consistency, but in cases of *ruminal impaction* may be hard and non-compressible.

Vagal dysfunction

In goats this may reduce or increase ruminal movements and interfere with abomasal emptying. Small intestinal activity can be monitored by auscultation in the lower right flank where borborygmi are normally clearly audible.

Transabdominal ultrasonography at this point provides considerable additional information about the content and function of the abdomen. Intestinal movement can be observed, and an increased echodensity and reduced bowel movement are seen in peritonitis. The scan may also reveal increased amounts of fluid in the peritoneal cavity, bladder or uterus. The *liver* is clearly seen underneath the upper last three ribs on the right side and if enlarged it can be palpated behind the last rib. *Hydatid cysts* may be seen in the liver and elsewhere in the abdomen. They are often asymptomatic but occasionally interfere with liver function.

Abdominal discomfort (colic)

This may be indicated by a number of clinical signs. The animal may be dull, bleat anxiously and change position frequently. It may kick at the abdomen, or look at its flanks frequently. Pulse and respiratory rates are increased. Ruminal and intestinal movements may be reduced. Paracentesis should normally produce scant, yellow, non-cellular peritoneal fluid. Increased amounts of fluid with increased cellular content and red colouration may indicate an abdominal catastrophe such as intestinal torsion or intussusception. Further diagnosis may involve laparotomy.

Diarrhoea

This is quite frequently seen in kids, especially following a sudden change in milk quantity or concentration. In older goats it may also follow sudden dietary change. In all age groups diarrhoea can indicate infection or parasite infestation. Details of management and especially feeding must be obtained. Vaccination status is also important: up-to-date vaccination against *Clostridium perfringens* may lessen the likelihood of diseases caused by the various strains of this organism.

Details of accommodation should be reviewed. Kids kept in damp yards with their mothers are more susceptible to coccidiosis than those kept outside. Helminth infestation is very important in animals at grass. Kids over 4 weeks of age are highly susceptible to coccidiosis. Gastrointestinal helminth parasites are especially important in animals in the 4 to 12 week age group but must also be considered in older animals.

Affected animals must receive a full clinical examination to assess their general health and hydration status. Animals suffering from *Salmonella typhimurium* infection may be pyrexic and pass blood in yellow coloured faeces. Cases of mild *carbohydrate engorgement* may show few symptoms, but in more serious cases there may be ruminal stasis, diarrhoea and dehydration.

In all cases of diarrhoea the faeces must be carefully examined. Faeces containing partially digested food are seen in cases of carbohydrate engorgement. Blood and mucus are seen in salmonellosis. Dark changed blood is seen in coccidiosis and cryptosporidium infection. Kids may die of acute coccidiosis before developing signs of diarrhoea. Laboratory investigation is mandatory. Coccidial oocyst counts of over 10 million per gram of faeces may be seen, but may be much lower in very ill kids. Isolation of any cryptosporidial oocysts is thought to be significant. Worm egg counts of more than 2000 eggs per gram of faeces are significant in kids. In older animals quantitative egg counts are of less significance.

Faecal culture is more rewarding than the culture of swabs, and in younger kids examination for *rotavirus* should be performed. The sacrifice of a moribund animal for further investigation should also be considered.

Urinary system

Abnormal function of this system may be detected by abnormalities in urination and the appearance of the urine. General signs of ill health followed by severe depression may be seen in cases of renal failure, the extent of which can be determined by monitoring plasma levels of urea and creatinine. Effective functioning of the renal system is also dependent on adequate fluid intake and good blood circulation. A history of reduced urination, pain at urination, frequent attempts at urination, difficulty in urination or urine abnormalities may alert the clinician to possible problems in this body system.

External signs of urinary problems include the presence of uroliths on the preputial hairs and a bloodstained or purulent discharge at the end of urination. Very occasionally, a grossly enlarged left kidney may be palpable through the right flank. In thin animals a transabdominal ultrasonographic scan of the kidneys may confirm the presence of problems such as hydronephrosis or pyelonephritis. Contrast radiographic studies of the urinary system can also be used in goats.

For further details of the clinical examination of the urinary system, the reader is referred to the section on renal diseases and urinary abnormalities in cattle (Chapter 9). Clinical signs of two specific urinary diseases in goats are summarised below.

Cystitis and pyelonephritis
Ascending infection involving the bladder, the kidney(s), or both, is occasionally seen in doe goats, sometimes associated with recent parturition. In cases of cystitis the goat may urinate frequently, passing small amounts of urine which may be bloodstained or contain pus. Goats suffering from pyelonephritis may also pass abnormal urine, but are often initially pyrexic and anorexic. A urine sample can be taken by catheter from the doe, but not from the buck. Urinalysis may confirm the diagnosis.

Urolithiasis
This is seen mostly in castrated male animals. Diets high in phosphorus or magnesium and low in calcium, a recent urinary infection, or restricted water supply, may predispose to urolithiasis. Common sites for uroliths include the urethral process and the sigmoid flexure of the penis. The patient may make frequent unsuccessful attempts to pass urine and may exhibit bruxism and abdominal pain. Calculi may be seen on the dry preputial hairs and urethral contractions may be felt on digital rectal examination. Further evaluation of the problem should be undertaken to determine whether the bladder or urethra has ruptured. The urethral process is examined for signs of obstruction by sedating the goat and gently pushing the penis out of the prepuce. This is only possible in postpubertal goats. Radiographs of the urethra and bladder can be used to detect the presence and location of radio-opaque uroliths. Ultrasonography can be used to detect the size and intactness of the bladder when this is not possible by palpation. Subcutaneous urine around the prepuce can also be detected. Abdominocentesis can be used to demonstrate the very high levels of urea and creatinine seen in the peritoneal fluid when rupture of the bladder has occurred.

Female genital system

Fertility control schemes are used in larger herds, and the clinician may be asked to examine an individual herd member or a pet doe in which reproductive failure has occurred. The history of such animals is very important as it may direct the clinician to seek specific abnormalities that could be responsible for her problem. For example the young polled doe who has failed to show oestrus might be an intersex. The older doe with a chronic vaginal discharge who has failed to conceive might have a problem with chronic endometritis. Details of the feeding and management of breeding goats are also important.

In every case a full clinical examination must be made with a comprehensive evaluation of the reproductive system. The *possibility of pregnancy* must always be born in mind, especially in animals thought to be suffering from anoestrus.

Clinical examination of the female genital system

This should start with an assessment of the animal's general health. A doe in very poor condition may be in anoestrus as a result of her condition rather than specific reproductive abnormalities. The animal's vulva and perineum should be inspected, and signs of a poor vulval seal or an abnormal discharge noted.

Intersexes

These are quite common in goats. Most affected animals are male pseudohermaphrodites. They are genetically female with an XX karyotype but have a variety of phenotypic appearances. Two main phenotypes are seen:

(1) *Normal vulva and external genitalia* – affected animals have no cervix and a very short vagina. The anogenital space may be over 3 cm and slightly longer than normal. The abnormally short vagina can be demonstrated endoscopically or more simply by inserting a sterile, lubricated rod and comparing the depth of insertion with that possible in a normal doe (Figs 17.2, 17.3).

(2) *A penis-like structure and gonads in a perineal position* – affected animals may have difficulty in passing urine, and in some cases hypospadia is seen (Fig. 17.4).

Freemartinism occurs in goats, but is much less common than other intersex conditions. Affected animals

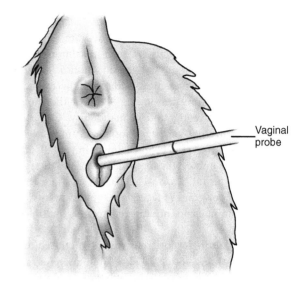

Figure 17.2 Goat intersex: the external genitalia are normal but the vagina is shortened. See also Fig. 17.3.

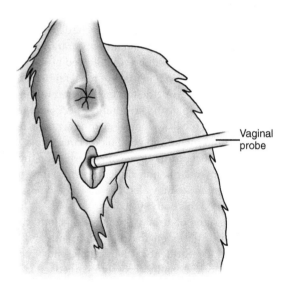

Figure 17.3 External genitalia of normal doe, with probe showing normal vaginal length. See also Fig. 17.2.

may show slight clitoral enlargement and usually have no cervix. Diagnosis requires genetic evaluation when a karyotype reveals that the animal is an XX and XY chimera.

Pregnancy and pseudopregnancy

Pseudopregnancy (also known as pseudocyesis, false pregnancy and hydrometra) This is quite common in goats and must always be considered in animals presented for pregnancy diagnosis or for investigation of abdominal enlargement. Up to 30% of does may be affected during their lives, and the incidence increases with age. It may follow service by a buck or may occur spontaneously after oestrus. Specific signs include progressive abdominal enlargement. The animal appears to be pregnant and mammary development and lactation occur towards the end of pseudopregnancy. A sudden loss of uterine fluid ('cloudburst') occurs approximately 145 days after oestrus or service. This fluid loss may not be witnessed. A sudden reduction in abdominal size and dampness of the vulva, perineum and the patient's bedding may be suggestive of recent pseudopregnancy. Less commonly the fluid is released more slowly in the form of an intermittent vaginal discharge.

Specific tests are required to differentiate pregnancy from pseudopregnancy:

(1) *Transabdominal ultrasonographic scan* – 40 to 70 days post oestrus. In pseudopregnancy the fluid filled uterus is clearly demonstrable. No fetus or fetal membranes are present (as they are in pregnancy), but light marks may be visible caused by overlying of the distended horns (Figs 17.5, 17.6).

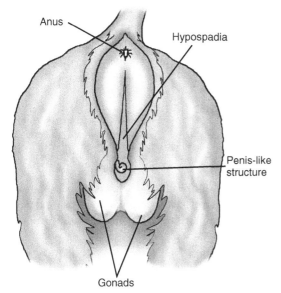

Figure 17.4 Goat intersex showing abnormal external genitalia.

Anus

Hypospadia

Penis-like structure

Gonads

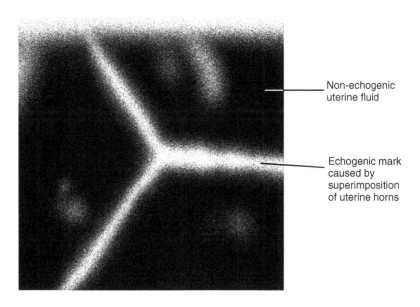

Non-echogenic uterine fluid

Echogenic mark caused by superimposition of uterine horns

Figure 17.5 Ultrasonographic scan of a doe goat with pseudopregnancy. Compare with Fig. 17.6.

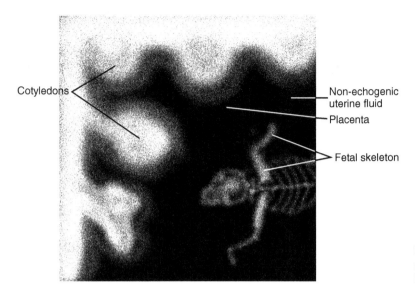

Cotyledons

Non-echogenic
uterine fluid

Placenta

Fetal skeleton

Figure 17.6 Ultrasonographic scan of doe goat at 70 days of pregnancy. Compare with Fig. 17.5.

(2) *Radiographic examination* – no fetal skeletons are visible at 70 to 90 days post oestrus or service as they are in pregnant animals.

(3) *Detection of oestrone sulphate in milk or blood at more than 45 days* – the hormone is present in pregnancy but absent in pseudopregnancy.

(4) *Abdominal palpation* – no fetus is palpable in late gestation in pseudopregnant animals.

Progesterone levels in blood and milk are elevated in both pregnancy and pseudopregnancy.

Investigation of vaginal discharge This should be undertaken, preferably with information concerning the previous breeding records of the affected doe. In the *immediate postpartum period* a vaginal discharge may be associated with retained fetal membranes, a retained fetus, necrotic vaginitis, an acute septic metritis or a low grade endometritis. A manual vaginal examination can be performed in the immediate postpartum period. It must be carried out with great care and may cause discomfort to the doe.

Retained fetal membranes These may be seen hanging from the vulva or palpated within the vagina or uterus.

Retained fetus Multiple birth is common in goats and it is not uncommon for a fetus to be retained after

kidding. A foul vaginal discharge may be seen and the presence of a fetus detected by vaginal examination, abdominal ultrasonography or radiography.

Necrotic vaginitis This may be a sequel to dystocia. A scant vaginal discharge may be seen and the doe is normally quite bright and alert. Plaques of necrotic vaginitis (initially dark red in colour but later green) are visible on the walls of the vagina when the vulval lips are parted.

Acute septic metritis The doe is normally depressed, pyrexic and anorexic. A foul vaginal discharge may be visible at the vulva. The condition is usually seen several days after kidding and a manual vaginal examination may not be possible or desirable. If required, a vaginal examination can most safely be performed using a speculum or by endoscopy.

Endometritis This condition may be seen usually 2 weeks or more after kidding. Affected does are bright and alert, and the only abnormality on clinical examination is a whitish-yellow vulval discharge. A vaginal examination using a speculum or endoscope normally reveals a partially closed cervix with small amounts of purulent material coming through it. The material may be seen pooling on the floor of the anterior vagina. Gross enlargement of the uterus may be confirmed by an abdominal ultrasonographic scan. If the uterus is still intra-abdominal it can be detected and its contents evaluated by scanning.

Chronic vaginal discharge This may be seen in older does, often with a history of infertility. A full clinical and gynaecological examination of such animals may reveal the presence of quantities of purulent material (*pyometra*) in the uterus. The possibility of the presence of *vaginal*, *cervical* or *uterine tumours* must be borne in mind in animals suffering from a chronic vaginal discharge. Such tumours may be visible as firm and irregular structures within the genital tract when the doe is examined with a vaginal speculum. Further evaluation can be made by radiography including intrauterine contrast studies or ultrasonography. A biopsy may be taken via an endoscope for histology. *Vaginal sponges* left *in situ* may provoke a chronic vaginitis and vaginal discharge.

Ovarian dysfunction This occurs in does but is not as well understood or researched as it is in cattle. *Follicular ovarian cysts* may cause short oestrous cycles, and chronically affected animals may show 'nymphomaniac' behaviour. *Luteal ovarian cysts* may cause signs of anoestrus. Hormone profiles, including a milk or blood progesterone assay, may provide useful information. Rectal examination is not possible in does.

Male genital system

The approach to examination of the buck is basically similar to that in the bull. There are important differences between the species and these are summarised below. Entire male goats have an active scent gland just caudal to each horn base which emits a characteristic odour. This may seem initially quite sweet and pleasant, but later may become abhorrent.

Problems involving the genital system are relatively uncommon in bucks. However, bucks are often found to be in poor condition. Loss of condition may be caused by poor feeding or heavy burdens of internal and external parasites. Poor fertility may be a reflection of poor husbandry or the result of an abnormality confined to the genital system.

Examination of the male genital system

This can be divided into the following parts:

(1) clinical examination of the buck and a detailed examination of the genital system
(2) assessment of libido
(3) observation and assessment of service behaviour
(4) semen collection and evaluation
(5) further diagnostic tests if required.

(1) Clinical examination of the buck

A full clinical examination should be carried out to assess the patient's general health followed by a detailed examination of the genital system. Details of feeding and management, including housing and work load, should be checked. The buck's fertility record should be examined. The buck's feet should also be checked, as pain from overgrown and infected feet can make the buck reluctant to serve.

Restraint of the patient Examination of the genital system is normally performed with the buck in the standing position. Goats resent being turned onto their hindquarters in the way in which rams are examined.

Testes These are quite large and pendulous. They are sometimes firmer in consistency than those of the bull. The two testes should be of the same size and consistency.

Orchitis may involve one or, less commonly, both testes. The affected testis is hard, warm to the touch and painful. The buck may walk with a wide stance to avoid increasing the testicular discomfort. Inflammation and heat in one testis with orchitis may result in some degeneration in the other testis. A decrease in testicular size and softening may be associated with *testicular degeneration*. An animal born with small testes may be suffering from *testicular hypoplasia*.

Epididymes These can be readily palpated. Inflammation of one or both can occur, sometimes associated with orchitis in the adjacent testis. The affected epididymis is enlarged, hard and painful to the touch. Abscesses and sperm granuloma may occur either as a result of infection or injury. Further investigation by ultrasonography is useful in establishing a diagnosis.

Accessory sexual glands   Manual rectal examination is not possible in the buck but the accessory sexual glands may be palpated using a gloved and lubricated forefinger. The glands may be involved in cases of orchitis and epididymitis. Gross enlargement of the seminal vesicles can be detected in this way.

Penis   The penis cannot be extruded from the prepuce in the conscious buck or at all in animals less than 6 months old. The anterior part of the penis including the glans can be palpated within the prepuce. *Rupture of the tunica albuginea* can occur as a result of injury sustained during mating. The lesions can normally be palpated as a firm mass just anterior to the scrotum. The sigmoid flexure is readily palpable caudal to the scrotum and below the perineum. A congenitally *shortened penis* has been reported, affected animals being unable to serve effectively. The caprine penis has a urethral process which is a common site for urolithiasis.

Prepuce   The prepuce is susceptible to local infection. In *balanoposthitis* the prepuce is enlarged and inflamed. A purulent foul-smelling discharge may be seen coming from the preputial orifice. Very occasionally a *foreign body* such as a grass seed may enter the prepuce and become embedded in the mucosa. The clinician should bear this possibility in mind in cases of balanoposthitis that do not respond to conventional therapy. In cases of severe preputial inflammation the penis cannot be protruded (*phimosis*) or sometimes retracted (*paraphimosis*).

(2) Assessment of libido
This is carried out as in the bull (see Chapter 11).

(3) Observation of mating behaviour
This is carried out as in the bull (see Chapter 11).

(4) Semen collection and evaluation
Semen can be collected by using an artificial vagina in the presence of a doe in oestrus. Alternatively, semen can be collected using an electroejaculator.

This should be used under heavy sedation or general anaesthesia with the buck in lateral recumbency. *Semen parameters* in the buck are very similar to those of the bull (Chapter 11).

(5) Further diagnostic tests
These may be needed in a number of areas, including evaluation of an orthopaedic problem causing difficulties with service.

The *main causes of infertility in bucks* are those that are found in bulls. They may be summarised with comments as follows:

Deficient libido   Causes include poor condition, immaturity, overuse, fear and other psychological problems.

Inability to mount   This can result from: orthopaedic problems including arthritis, laminitis and other causes of foot lameness; neurological problems including ataxia resulting from a spinal abscess or other space-occupying lesions; back pain.

Inability to achieve intromission   Causes include phimosis, paraphimosis, balanoposthitis, persistent frenulum and rupture of the tunica albuginea. Impotence may be a consequence of circulatory defects within the penis.

Inability to fertilise   This results from the production of abnormal or deficient semen and is usually associated with genetic defect, infection or injury.

As in the bull, a written report on the buck's clinical examination, service behaviour and semen quality should be prepared.

Udder

The goat has two mammary glands, each with a large and quite pendulous teat. *Supernumerary teats* are particularly common in pygmy goats. A full clinical examination must always accompany an examination of the udder to determine whether the animal is pyrexic as she may be in acute mastitis, or dull and toxaemic as she may be in peracute gangrenous mastitis.

The *udder* should be examined initially from behind the doe so that the two sides can be compared. Mammary tissue in the doe is quite firm to the touch, but also has a degree of elasticity. Shortly after kidding, the udder may be oedematous and the condition of *hard udder* is seen at this time. The animal is non-pyrexic but there is scant milk production. In many animals the abnormality is associated with caprine arthritis encephalitis virus (CAEV) infection. Serum antibody tests will confirm virus involvement. In cases of *peracute mastitis* the udder is warm and inflamed, but there may also be areas where the circulation is compromised and the affected areas are cold to the touch. There may also be areas of subcutaneous oedema extending forward from the udder into the muscles of the abdominal floor. In cases of *acute mastitis* the affected parts of the udder may be hard and painful when palpated. Some cases of *chronic mastitis* have areas of fibrosis within the affected half of the udder which may be smaller than the normal half (Fig. 17.7). *Pustular dermatitis* caused by *Staphylococcus aureus* on the skin of the udder produces dry crusty lesions from which the causal organism may be cultured.

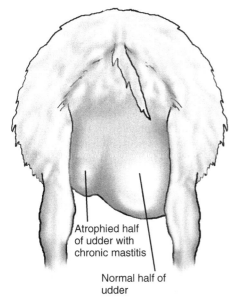

Atrophied half
of udder with
chronic mastitis

Normal half of
udder

Figure 17.7 Rear view of doe goat with chronic mastitis. Note atrophy of affected half of udder.

The *teats* should be examined and in lactating animals their patency checked. The presence of a '*pea*' or small round structure within the teat may result in obstruction of milk flow. Caused by small portions of granulation tissue adherent to the teat canal lining or mineral concretions, their identity can be investigated by radiography, including contrast studies. The skin of the teats is slightly roughened. Small skin lesions caused by fly bites or other injury may be seen. *Contagious pustular dermatitis* (orf) virus may produce dry crusty lesions covering inflamed moist skin.

Milk

Milk from both halves of the udder should be collected into a strip cup. In cases of mastitis there may be clots and sometimes blood in the milk. Blood is also seen in the milk of some young does for the first few days after kidding. Whenever clots or blood are seen, the milk should be cultured. Most cases of caprine mastitis are caused by coagulase positive *Staphylococcus aureus*. Other organisms associated with mastitis include *Mannheimia haemolytica* (*Pasteurella haemolytica*) and a number of streptococci.

Somatic cell count (SCC) tests and the Californian milk test (CMT) on goats' milk are often slightly raised in the absence of mastitis. Normal goats' milk contains a quantity of cellular debris from the breakdown of epithelial cells in the udder during milk production. These cells are responsible for the abnormal test results mentioned above.

Locomotor system

Lameness is quite a common problem in goats and mostly involves individual animals. Many cases of lameness involve the feet, but the clinician must examine the whole animal and all its limbs to make sure that other problems are not overlooked. All parts and all tissues of the limb can be involved in cases of lameness. If lameness involves one limb, the opposite limb must be examined and compared to ensure that suspected abnormalities really are a departure from the normal.

History

The history of the *animal and its herd of origin* must be investigated. Lameness may follow an accidental injury to an individual goat. A dietary deficiency or an imbalance of minerals may result in orthopaedic problems developing in groups of animals.

Signalment

The signalment of the patient is also important. Kids are very active and athletic animals, but they are prone to injury and may suffer from congenital problems. Septic arthritis (joint ill) caused by bacterial infection is much more common in kids than in adult goats. Degenerative joint problems such as osteoarthritis and infections of the feet are more common in older goats.

Observation of the patient

The patient should first be observed at rest and then when moving slowly. A painful leg may be non-weight bearing at rest and used reluctantly when the animal walks. If frightened or made to move quickly, the patient may carry the leg. On other occasions the goat may appear to use the leg normally when moving quickly, but become lame again when walking and less stressed. Lameness rapidly results in muscle atrophy in an affected leg. Animals with foreleg lameness may walk on their knees to avoid weight bearing on the lower limb. However, some normal goats habitually graze in this way.

Abnormal swellings anywhere in the limb and signs of obvious overgrowth of the feet should be noted for further investigation. *Reluctance to move* at all may indicate pain in both front feet or all four feet – signs that may be seen in cases of *laminitis*.

The *conformation of the limbs* should be observed from all angles. Lateral deviation of the lower forelimb is seen in cases of *valgus* involving either the carpal ('knock knees') or fetlock joints. One or both limbs are affected and the condition is seen chiefly in kids and goatlings. Bending of the hind limb in the region of the stifle is caused by deviation of the distal femur or proximal tibia (*varus*). Bending of the long bones is also seen in *rickets* and affected kids may show local enlargement of their costochondral junctions – the 'rickety rosary'. In older animals softening of the bones caused by severe imbalance of calcium and phosphorus in the diet may lead to *osteomalacia* or *osteodystrophia fibrosa* in which fracture or bending of the long bones is seen. Epiphyseal and growth plate abnormalities may be seen radiographically and identify the orthopaedic changes involved. Kids are occasionally born with severe *angular limb deformity* and a reduction or absence of normal joint movement.

Fractures of the metacarpus or metatarsus are not uncommon in adventurous kids. Affected limbs are mostly non-weight bearing, the bones are abnormally bent and crepitus is detected on gentle palpation. Fractures of the upper limbs also occur and are mostly the result of trauma. Radiography may be required to determine the exact injury sustained by the bone.

Some kids are born with *contracted flexor tendons* in their forelimbs and are unable to extend their legs. Tendon injury may produce a deformity in leg shape. Animals with a *ruptured gastrocnemius tendon* are unable to extend the hock or take weight on the affected limb. In this condition, obvious swelling may be seen on the caudal aspect of the leg just below the stifle.

Examination of the limbs

This should begin with the feet. Footcare in some herds is poor or non-existent. *Overgrowth of horn* may cause lameness, but also predisposes to infectious diseases such as foot-rot. The whole foot should be examined for signs of horn overgrowth, cracks or deficits in the hoof wall or sole, and inflammation in the coronary band region. Overgrowth of the toes may be associated with *pastern weakness* in which the goat takes more and more weight on its heels and the toes are not worn.

The hooves are normally slightly warm to the touch. An increase in horn temperature in one lame foot may indicate infection. If two or all of the feet show evidence of increased heat, the animal may be suffering from *acute laminitis*.

Gentle compression of each claw normally only causes discomfort if pathological damage is present. In addition to the claws, the interdigital area is also inspected. Red inflamed areas near the coronary band are seen in *strawberry foot-rot*. *Infection of the interdigital gland* with white purulent matter between the claws may cause lameness in young kids. Vesicle formation followed by ulceration may be seen on the coronary band and the interdigital area in goats suffering from *foot-and-mouth disease*.

Overgrown horn curling over the sole of the foot is carefully pared away using hoof clippers. The hoof should be scraped or washed and inspected for signs of penetration and other damage. In goats with *chronic laminitis* some pared horn has pink areas, and in some cases the animal has very hard feet with thickened soles.

The common condition of *foot-rot* may affect many members of the herd. Affected animals are lame in one or more limbs and have often had prolonged exposure to wet conditions. Areas of hoof wall and sole may be missing, and the deeper structures of the hoof may be exposed. Affected hooves have an unpleasant necrotic smell.

If the cause of painful foot lameness cannot be determined, the clinician should take radiographs of the affected foot. *Fractures of the third phalanx* (P3) can occur as can deep-seated infection of bone such as *osteitis* in P3 and *osteomyelitis* and joint lesions in the second or third phalanges.

After examining the foot, the clinician should methodically examine the rest of the limb. The tendons are examined for signs of strain. Each joint should be examined carefully. Radiography is useful to identify and indicate the degree of damage sustained by the articular surfaces of the joint. Distension of the joints may indicate *septic arthritis ('joint ill') in kids*. One or more joints may be infected and there may be evidence of infection in the umbilical region too. Affected joints are warm and painful to the touch. Joint fluid aspiration may reveal an increased quantity of watery, purulent fluid with a high neutrophil count. Older goats showing joint swelling with reduced movement and reduced synovial fluid may be suffering from *osteoarthritis*.

Joint enlargement in goats, especially those over 1 year of age, can also be a feature of *CAEV infection*. Often one joint (in many cases the carpus), but occasionally a number of joints, may be affected (Fig. 17.8). The affected joint is distended and joint movement is reduced. The degree of lameness is variable but may be severe. Joint fluid is red-brown in colour and contains large numbers of mononuclear cells. Serological tests can be used to confirm the presence of CAEV antibodies, but a negative result does not confirm that the virus has not been present. A subcutaneous swelling over the carpal joint not normally accompanied by lameness may be caused by a *carpal*

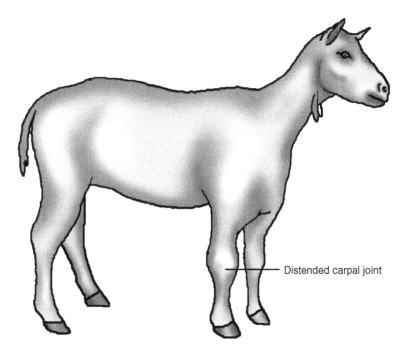

Distended carpal joint

Figure 17.8 Goat with chronic arthritis of the right carpal joint caused by caprine arthritis encephalitis virus (CAEV).

hygroma. This may develop in animals who habitually graze on their knees and who may have another form of lameness causing them to do so. In the stifle joint, instability and discomfort may be caused by *rupture of the cruciate ligament*. Lateral or medial *patella luxation* is seen occasionally in kids.

Lameness can also be caused by *muscle damage*. The hock and stifle joints normally flex and extend reciprocally. In goats with a *rupture of the peroneus tertius muscle* it is possible to extend the hock whilst the stifle is flexed. *Vitamin E and/or selenium deficiency* may lead to lameness in kids and goatlings. Affected animals may show sudden onset of lameness with painful distended muscle groups in the upper limb. In this condition (*white muscle disease*) high levels of creatine phosphokinase are found in the plasma of affected animals and methaemoglobin may be found in the urine. If the cardiac muscle is affected sudden death or signs of cardiac insufficiency may be seen.

Damage to nerves can give rise to signs of lameness. The cause of the damage is often traumatic, but can also be iatrogenic. Goats are rather poorly muscled and intramuscular injections can damage underlying nerves. An injection given into the gluteal muscles can damage the sciatic nerve causing *sciatic paralysis*. In this condition the leg cannot be flexed and the hock on the affected side is lower than the opposite joint. There may also be reduced cutaneous sensation over the tibial region on the lateral and on the lower parts of the leg. Electromyelography can be used to demonstrate areas of muscular denervation.

Neurological diseases

This important group of conditions requires careful consideration of the history, management (including feeding) and possible access to toxic materials, signalment and clinical signs of the patient. Neurological diseases in cattle have been considered in Chapter 14. The reader is advised to consult these sections for further general information. The comments here relate specifically to the goat.

Neurological clinical signs are caused by infection of, or some sort of damage sustained by the nervous system. Many other factors outwith the confines of the nervous system itself may be involved. The cardiovascular system in particular plays an important role in keeping the nervous system well supplied with oxygen. In terminal heart disease, signs of neurological problems may be seen. The clinician must consider all appropriate possibilities, use the information provided by the history of the case and the results of a detailed clinical examination – general and neurological – before reaching a diagnosis. Some examples of diseases with induced neurological signs affecting different age groups of goats are given below.

A group of goats of varying ages who have gained access to a food store may all be affected with varying signs of *ruminal acidosis*. Features of this condition include ruminal stasis, diarrhoea, ataxia and occasionally coma. Some conditions, such as *swayback*, are seen chiefly in young animals. Other conditions, such as *hypocalcaemia*, are seen most frequently (but not exclusively) a few days before and after kidding. *Pregnancy toxaemia* is seen mainly in late pregnancy.

Specific signs of neurological diseases in goats include the following:

(1) *Abnormalities of mental state* – such abnormalities may be immediately obvious but in other cases observations by the goat's owner may indicate that subtle abnormal behaviour is being exhibited.
(2) *Involuntary movements* – including muscular tremors.
(3) *Abnormalities of posture and gait* – the clinician should check that no orthopaedic problems are present which might also affect posture and gait.
(4) *Paralysis* – either flaccid or spastic.
(5) *Disturbance in sensory perception*
(6) *Blindness*
(7) *Abnormalities of the autonomic nervous system*

Clinical examination

This should start with observation of the undisturbed patient. The animal is then examined to determine whether a neurological abnormality is present and if so where in the nervous system it is located. The presence of upper and lower motor neurone deficiencies are among specific signs that may be seen. Additional tests including serology for CAEV and analysis of cerebrospinal fluid (CSF) taken from the lumbosacral space are useful in some cases. Clinical signs of a number of important caprine neurological conditions are given below.

Floppy kid syndrome   This affects kids in the first 10 days of life. Affected kids are normal at birth, but suddenly show severe muscle weakness, marginal consciousness and reduced reflex response. One kid only in a litter may be affected. There is no evidence of septicaemia, diarrhoea, pneumonia or colostral deficiency. The condition is thought to be the result of a metabolic acidosis.

Caprine arthritis encephalitis virus   Encephalitis can occur in both young and adult goats. In kids, the neurological signs are those of an ascending infection of the spinal cord. The patient may be initially bright but pyrexic. Within a few days the kid may show signs of ataxia, hemiplegia or tetraplegia and blindness. Terminal recumbency and coma follow. In adult goats, CAEV encephalitis may follow other manifestations of the disease including arthritis, pneumonia or mastitis. The animal may show incoordination of the limbs followed by paralysis.

Swayback in kids   The congenital form of the disease is uncommon in kids. Delayed swayback is seen in older kids which are normal at birth. Progressive hind-limb ataxia caused by copper deficiency induced demyelination is seen, although the kid appears bright and willing to eat. Blood copper levels are usually low in affected kids and in their dams. The latter may show other subtle signs of copper deficiency including anaemia, diarrhoea and hair discolouration.

Scrapie   This is seen chiefly in animals in the 3 to 4 year old age group. Initial signs may be subtle and non-specific. They include a slight change in temperament, weight loss and reduced milk yield. Later, more specific signs of pruritus and neurological changes are seen. Affected goats may nibble or scratch any accessible part of the skin, often causing quite severe damage. Stimulation of the skin caudal to the sacrum may cause the animal to make nibbling movements with its jaws and sometimes salivate. Neurological signs include incoordination and a high stepping gait. Muscular tremors are also seen. The animal may be dull or hyperaesthetic and temperament changes become more pronounced.

CLINICIAN'S CHECKLIST – CLINICAL EXAMINATION OF THE GOAT

Owner's complaint
History of the patient – long and short term
Signalment – breed, age, sex of the goat or goats
The goat environment – observation and inspection
Observation of the goat or group of goats
Clinical examination of the patient
Temperature, pulse and respiration
Mucous membranes, capillary refill time
Palpation of the carcase lymph nodes
Head and neck
Cardiovascular system
Respiratory system
Gastrointestinal system
Udder and perineum
External genital system of the female
External genital system of the male
Locomotor system
Neurological examination
Clinical pathology
Post-mortem examination if required

Bibliography

Andrews, A.H. (2000) *The Health of Dairy Cattle*. Blackwell Science, Oxford.

Arthur, G.H., Noakes, D.E., Pearson, H. & Parkinson, T.J. (1996) *Veterinary Reproduction and Obstetrics*, 7th edn. W.B. Saunders, London.

Baker, J.C. (1987) *Bovine Neurologic Diseases*, Veterinary Clinics of North America, Food Animal Practice, Vol. 3.1. W.B. Saunders, Philadelphia.

Brightling, P. (1995) *The Examination of a Sick Cow*. Proceedings No. 78, Postgraduate Committee in Veterinary Science, University of Sydney.

Clarkson, M.J. & Winter, A.C. (1997) *A Handbook for the Sheep Clinician*, 2nd edn. Liverpool University Press.

Greenough, P.R. & Weaver, A.D. (1997) *Lameness in Cattle*, 3rd edn. W.B. Saunders, Philadelphia.

Jackson, P.G.G. (1995) *Handbook of Veterinary Obstetrics*. W.B. Saunders, London.

Martin, W.B. & Aitken, I.D. (2000) *Diseases of Sheep*, 3rd edn. Blackwell Science, Oxford.

Matthews, J. (1999) *Diseases of the Goat*, 2nd edn. Blackwell Science, Oxford.

Meredith, M.J. (1995) *Animal Breeding and Infertility*. Blackwell Science, Oxford.

Radostits, O.M., Gay, C.C., Blood D.C. & Hinchcliff, K.W. (2000) *Veterinary Medicine*, 9th edn. W.B. Saunders, London.

Radostits, O.M., Mayhew, I.G.J. & Houston, D.M. (2000) *Veterinary Clinical Examination and Diagnosis*. W.B. Saunders, London.

Rosenberger, G. (1979) *Clinical Examination of Cattle*. Verlag Paul Parey, Berlin.

Searman, D.M. & Robinson, R.A. (1983) *Clinical Examination of Sheep and Goats*, Veterinary Clinics of North America, Large Animal Practice. Vol. 5.3. W.B. Saunders, Philadelphia.

Taylor, D.J. (1999) *Pig Diseases*, 7th edn. Glasgow (published by the author).

Wilson, J.H. (1992) *Physical Examination*, Veterinary Clinics of North America, Food Animal Practice, Vol. 8.2. W.B. Saunders, Philadelphia.

Appendix 1
Normal Physiological Values

	Cattle	Sheep	Goats	Pigs
Temperature (°C)				
Normal range	38.0–39.0	38.5–40.0	39.0–40.5	38.5–40.0
Average	38.5	39.0	39.5	39.0
Resting pulse rate (beats/min)				
Normal range	60–80	70–90	70–100	90–110
Average	70	75	90	100
Resting respiration rate (breaths/min)	15–30	20–30	15–30	10–20
Average	20	25	30	15
Oestrus cycle (days)				
Range	18–24	14–19	18–21	18–24
Average	21	17	20	21
Gestation (days)				
Range	279–291	140–160	145–155	110–116
Average	283	150	150	114

	Calves	Lambs	Kids	Piglets
Temperature (°C)				
Range	38.5–39.5	39.0–40.0	38.8–40.2	39.0–39.5
Average	39.0	39.5	39.5	39.5
Resting pulse rate (beats/min)				
Range	80–120	80–100	100–120	200–220
Average	100	85	105	210
Resting respiration rate (breaths/min)				
Range	24–36	36–48	20–40	24–36
Average	30	40	30	30

Appendix 2
Laboratory Reference Values: Haematology

The haematological values for cattle, sheep, goats and pigs are reproduced with permission from Radostits, O.M., Gay, C.C., Blood, D.C. and Hinchcliff, K.W. (2000) *Veterinary Medicine*, 9th edn, W.B. Saunders, London, pp. 1819–1822. Reference ranges supplied by individual laboratories should be consulted when interpreting results from these laboratories.

Table A2.1 Haematology – Conventional units

	Cattle	Sheep	Goats	Pigs
Haemoglobin (g/dL)	8.0–15.0	9.0–15.0	8.0–12.0	10.0–16.0
Haematocrit (packed cell volume) (%)	24.0–46.0	27.0–45.0	22.0–38.0	32.0–50.0
RBC ($\times10^6$/µL)	5.0–10.0	9.0–15.0	8.0–18.0	5.0–8.0
MCV (fL)	40.0–60.0	28.0–40.0	16.0–25.0	50.0–68.0
MCH (pg)	11.0–17.0	8.0–12.0	5.2–8.0	17.0–21.0
MCHC (g/dL)	30.0–36.0	31.0–34.0	30.0–36.0	30.0–34.0
Thrombocytes ($\times10^3$/µL)	100–800	250–750	300–600	320–520
WBC (per/µL)	4000–12 000	4000–12 000	4000–13 000	11 000–22 000
Neutrophils (mature) (per/µL)	600–4000	700–6000	1200–7200	3 080–10 450
Neutrophils (band cells) (per/µL)	0–120	Rare	Rare	0–880
Lymphocytes (per/µL)	2500–7500	2000–9000	2000–9000	4 290–13 640
Monocytes (per/µL)	25–840	0–750	0–550	200–2200
Eosinophils (per/µL)	0–2400	0–1000	0–650	55–2420
Fibrinogen (mg/dL)	200–700	200–500	200–300	

Table A2.2 Haematology – International System of Units (SI)

	Cattle	Sheep	Goats	Pigs
Haemoglobin (g/L)	80–150	90–150	80–120	100–160
Haematocrit (packed cell volume) (L/L)	0.24–0.46	0.27–0.45	0.22–0.38	0.32–0.50
RBC ($\times10^{12}$/L)	5.0–10.00	8.0–18.0	5.0–8.0	6.8–12.9
MCV (fL)	40–60	28–40	16–25	50–68
MCH (pg)	11.0–17.0	8.0–12.0	5.2–8.0	17.0–21.0
MCHC (g/L)	300–360	310–340	300–360	303–340
Thrombocytes ($\times10^9$/L)	100–800	250–750	300–600	320–520
WBC ($\times10^9$/L)	4.0–12.0	4.0–12.0	4.0–13.0	11.0–22.0
Neutrophils (mature) ($\times10^9$/L)	0.6–4.0	0.7–6.0	1.2–7.2	3.1–10.5
Neutrophils (band cells) ($\times10^9$/L)	0–0.1	Rare	Rare	0–0.1
Lymphocytes ($\times10^9$/L)	2.0–7.5	2.0–9.0	2.0–9.0	4.3–13.0
Monocytes ($\times10^9$/L)	0–0.8	0–0.8	0–0.6	0.2–2.2
Eosinophils ($\times10^9$/L)	0–2.4	0–1.0	0–0.7	0.05–2.4
Fibrinogen (g/L)	2–7	2–5	2–3	

Appendix 3
Laboratory Reference Values: Biochemistry

The biochemical values for cattle, sheep and pigs are reproduced with permission from Radostits, O.M., Gay, C.C., Blood, D.C. and Hinchcliff, K.W. (2000) *Veterinary Medicine*, 9th edn, W.B. Saunders, London, pp. 1819–1822. The biochemical values for goats are reproduced with permission from Matthews, J. (1999) *Diseases of the Goat*, Blackwell Science, Oxford, p. 332. Reference ranges supplied by individual laboratories should be consulted when interpreting results from these laboratories.

Table A3.1 Serum constituents (conventional units)

	Cattle	Sheep	Pigs	Goats
Electrolytes				
Sodium (mEq/L)	132–152	145–152	140–150	135–156
Potassium (mEq/L)	3.9–5.8	3.9–5.4	4.7–7.1	3.4–6.1
Chloride (mEq/L)	95–110	95–103	95–103	98–110
Osmolality (mOsmol/kg)	270–306			
Acid : base status				
pH (venous)	7.35–7.50	7.32–7.50		
PCO_2 (venous) (mmHg)	34–45	38–45		
Bicarbonate (mEq/L)	20–30	21–28	18–27	
Total carbon dioxide (mEq/L)	20–30	20–28	17–26	
Anion gap (mEq/L)	14–26	12–24	10–25	
Minerals				
Calcium, total (mg/dL)	9.7–12.4	11.5–13.0	7.1–11.6	9.2–11.6
Calcium, ionised (mg/dL)	4.8–6.2	5.7–6.5	3.5–5.8	
Phosphorus (mg/dL)	5.6–6.5	5.0–7.3	5.3–9.6	4.0–11.2
Magnesium (mg/dL)	1.8–2.3	2.2–2.8	1.1–1.5	3.5–5.2
Iron (µg/dL)	57–162	166–222	73–140	
Iron binding capacity (µg/dL)	110–350		270–557	
Renal function				
Urea nitrogen (mg/dL)	6–27	10–35	10–30	12–26
Creatinine (mg/dL)	1–2	1.2–1.9	1.0–2.7	0.6–1.6
Liver function				
Total bilirubin (mg/dL)	0.01–0.5	0.1–0.5	0–10	
Direct (conjugated) bilirubin (mg/dL)	0.04–0.44	0–0.27	0–0.3	
Bile acids (mg/mL)	<50	<9		
Metabolites				
Ammonia (µg/dL)				
Cholesterol (mg/dL)	65–220	43–103	28–48	
Free fatty acids (mg/L)	<30	30–100		
Glucose (mg/dL)	45–75	50–80	85–150	

(Continued on p. 304)

Table A3.1 Serum constituents (conventional units) *Continued*

	Cattle	Sheep	Pigs	Goats
Ketones				
Acetoacetate (mg/dL)	0–1.1	0.24–0.36		
Acetone (mg/dL)	0–10.0	0–10.0		
β-Hydroxybutyrate (mg/dL)	5.9–13.9	4.7–6.7		
Lactate (mg/dL)	5.0–20.0	9.0–12.0		
Triglyceride (mg/dL)	0–14.0			
Hormones				
Cortisol (μg/dL)	0.47–0.75	1.40–3.10	2.6–3.3	
Thyroxine (T4) (μg/dL)	4.2–8.6			3.3–7.0
Enzymes				
Alanine aminotransferase (ALT) (units/L)	11–40	22–38	31–58	
Alkaline phosphatase (units/L)	0–500	70.0–390	120–400	0–300
Amylase (units/L)				
Aspartate aminotransferase (AST) (units/L)	78–132	60–280	32–84	0–300
Creatine kinase (units/L)	35–280			0–100
GOT *see* AST				
GPT *see* ALT				
γ-Glutamyl transferase (GGT) (units/L)	6.1–17.4	20–52	10–52	0–30
Isocitrate dehydrogenase (units/L)	9.4–21.9	0.5–8		
Lactate dehydrogenase (units/L)	692–1445	240–440	380–630	0–400
Sorbitol dehydrogenase (units/L)	4.3–15.3	5.8–28	1–5.8	
Protein				
Total protein (g/dL)	5.7–8.1	6–7.9	3.5–6	6.2–7.9
Albumin (g/dL)	2.1–3.6	2.4–3	1.9–2.4	2.9–4.3

Table A3.2 Serum constituents (international units, SI)

	Cattle	Sheep	Pigs	Goats
Electrolytes				
Sodium (mmol/L)	132–152	145–152	140–150	135–156
Potassium (mmol/L)	3.9–5.8	3.9–5.4	4.7–7.1	3.4–6.1
Chloride (mmol/L)	95–110	95–103	94–103	98–110
Osmolality (mmol/kg)	270–306			
Acid : base status				
pH (venous)	7.35–7.50	7.32–7.50		
PCO$_2$ (venous) (mmHg)	34–45	38–45		
Bicarbonate (mmol/L)	20–30	21–28	18–27	
Total carbon dioxide (mmol/L)	20–30	20–28	17–26	
Minerals				
Calcium, total (mmol/L)	2.43–3.10	2.88–3.20	1.78–2.90	2.3–2.9
Calcium, ionised (mmol/L)	1.2–1.6	1.4–1.6	0.9–1.4	
Phosphorus (mmol/L)	1.08–2.76	1.62–2.36	1.30–3.55	1.0–2.4
Magnesium (mmol/L)	0.74–1.10	0.90–1.26	0.78–1.60	0.8–1.3
Iron (μmol/L)	10–29	30–40		
Iron binding capacity (μmol/L)	20–63		48–100	

(*Continued on p. 305*)

Table A3.2 Serum constituents (international units, SI) *Continued*

	Cattle	Sheep	Pigs	Goats
Renal function				
Urea nitrogen (mmol/L)	2.0–7.5	3–10	3–8.5	4.0–8.6
Creatinine (μmol/L)	67–175	70–105	90–240	54–123
Liver function				
Total bilirubin (μmol/L)	0.17–8.55	1.71–8.55	0–17.1	0–7
Direct (conjugated) bilirubin (μmol/L)	0.7–7.54	0–4.61	0–5.1	
Bile acids (μmol/L)	<120	<25		
Metabolites				
Ammonia (μmol/L)			7.6–63.4	
Cholesterol (mmol/L)	1–5.6	1.05–1.50	3.05–3.10	1.0–3.0
Glucose (mmol/L)	1.9–3.8	1.7–3.6	3.6–5.3	2.4–4.0
Ketones				
Acetoacetate (mmol/L)	0–0.11	0.026–0.034		
Acetone (mmol/L)	0–1.7	0–1.7		
β-Hydroxybutyrate (mmol/L)	0.35–0.47	0.47–0.63		0.0–1.2
Lactate (mmol/L)	0.6–2.2	1–1.3		
Triglyceride (mmol/L)	0–0.2			
Hormones				
Cortisol (nmol/L)	13–21	42–82	76–88	
Thyroxine (T4) (nmol/L)	54–110			43–90
Triiodothyronine (T3) (nmol/L)				
Enzymes				
Alanine aminotransferase (ALT) (units/L)	11–40	22–38	31–58	
Alkaline phosphatase (units/L)	0–500	70–390	120–400	0–300
Amylase (units/L)				
Aspartate aminotransferase (AST) (units/L)	78–132	60–280	32–84	0–300
Creatine kinase (units/L)	35–280			0–100
GOT *see* AST				
GPT *see* ALT				
γ-Glutamyl transferase (GGT) (units/L)	6.1–17.4	20–52	10–60	0–30
Isocitrate dehydrogenase (units/L)	9.4–21.9	0.5–8		
Lactate dehydrogenase (units/L)	692–1445	240–440	380–630	0–400
Sorbitol dehydrogenase (units/L)	4.3–15.3	5.8–28	1–5.8	
Protein				
Total protein (g/L)	21–36	24–30	19–24	62–79
Albumin (g/L)	21–36	24–30	19–24	29–43

Index